PUSH!

MCGILL-QUEEN'S/ASSOCIATED MEDICAL SERVICES STUDIES IN THE HISTORY OF MEDICINE, HEALTH, AND SOCIETY

Series Editors: S.O. Freedman and J.T.H. Connor

Volumes in this series have financial support from Associated Medical Services, Inc. (AMS). Associated Medical Services Inc. was established in 1936 by Dr Jason Hannah as a pioneer prepaid not-for-profit health care organization in Ontario. With the advent of medicare, AMS became a charitable organization supporting innovations in academic medicine and health services, specifically the history of medicine and health care, as well as innovations in health professional education and bioethics.

Push!

The Struggle for Midwifery in Ontario

IVY LYNN BOURGEAULT

McGill-Queen's University Press

Montreal & Kingston · London · Ithaca

© McGill-Queen's University Press 2006

ISBN 13 978-0-7735-2977-9   ISBN 10 0-7735-2977-2 (cloth)
ISBN 13 978-0-7735-3025-6   ISBN 10 0-7735-3025-8 (paper)

Legal deposit first quarter 2006
Bibliothèque nationale du Québec

Printed in Canada on acid-free paper that is 100% ancient forest
free (100% post-consumer recycled), processed chlorine free.

McGill-Queen's University Press acknowledges the support of the
Canada Council for the Arts for our publishing program. We also
acknowledge the financial support of the Government of Canada
through the Book Publishing Industry Development Program
(BPIDP) for our publishing activities.

Library and Archives Canada Cataloguing in Publication

Bourgeault, Ivy Lynn, 1967–
    Push!: the struggle for midwifery in Ontario / Ivy Lynn Bourgeault

    (McGill-Queen's/Associated Medical Services (Hannah Institute)
    studies in the history of medicine, health, and society; 25)
    Includes bibliographical references and index.
    ISBN 13 978-0-7735-2977-9   ISBN 10 0-7735-2977-2 (bnd)
    ISBN 13 978-0-7735-3025-6   ISBN 10 0-7735-3025-8 (pbk)

    1. Midwives – Ontario. 2. Midwifery – Ontario – History.
    3. Midwifery – Political aspects – Ontario. 4. Midwifery – Government
    policy – Ontario.
    I. Title. II. Series.
    RG950.B683 2005   618.2'0233'09713   C2005–904495-0

Typeset in Palatino 10/13
by Infoscan Collette Québec, Quebec City

To Ian and Rachelle Bourgeault
Jeff, Lauren, Tyra, and Adam Jutai

Contents

Contents

Foreword

Several factors influenced my decision to study the integration of midwifery in Ontario. As I embarked on my graduate career, my research interests were crystallizing around the issues of alternative health care, health professions, and women's health. Exploring midwifery in Canada seemed a natural topic as it touched upon each of these areas.[1] My fascination with midwifery became fully embodied (in the complete sense of that word) in the summer of 1990 when I became pregnant with my first child while an MA student. Already being theoretically curious about midwifery, I inquired into the more practical issue of the availability of midwifery services in Toronto. Naively looking up "midwives" in the Toronto telephone directory, I found the Midwives' Collective of Toronto. I subsequently became a client of midwives Arlene Vandersloot and Meryn Tate, and one of their "midwifery-friendly" family physicians, Howard Krieger. The birth of my daughter was a wonderfully positive experience due in large part to the support and education I received from these care providers. This experience cemented my interest and commitment to learning more about this unique form of maternity care.

Shortly after the birth of my daughter in 1991, I became a member of the Midwifery Task Force of Ontario, a midwifery consumer support organization. Being a young mother and graduate student, I was initially more a member in name. Nevertheless, I was kept apprised of significant social and political events. I became more politically involved in the broader alternative birthing movement in the fall of 1992 when I joined the Board of Directors of the Toronto Birth Centre, a committee which endeavoured to establish a free-standing birth centre in Toronto.

Although this involvement in the midwifery community was undertaken in large part for political reasons, it was instrumental in the development of the orientation of my research. Being a midwifery consumer meant that I was identified as an "interested" observer within the midwifery community from the outset. Through this involvement as a sort of observer-participant, I not only became immersed in the social and political context of the midwifery movement in Ontario, I developed important research contacts and became grounded in the internal dynamics of the movement. As I began to more clearly define my research focus, however, my position within the midwifery community became more complex.

I decided to examine the issue of the professionalization of midwifery; that is, how midwifery changed through the integration process from being a counterculture social movement to being more like a mainstream profession. Many researchers had examined Canadian midwifery from a historical perspective (Biggs 1983, Connor 1991, Laforce 1990, Mason 1987, 1988, Rushing 1991) and some had studied the remnants of an earlier form of midwifery that remained throughout the second half of the twentieth century (Benoit, 1991, Kaufert and O'Neill, 1995, 1996), but few social scientific scholars had focused on the rebirth of midwifery in Canada. Notable exceptions were Burtch (1994) and Rushing (1993). Burtch examined the re-emergence of midwifery in Canada from a law and society perspective, whereas Rushing described the ideological underpinnings of the legitimacy of the position of midwifery in the Canadian health care system. Critiques of the "new" midwifery in Canada were particularly rare (Benoit 1987, Mason 1990). A publication by Barrington (1985), regarding the new midwifery in Canada, although aimed at a lay audience, was an excellent source of background information. In addition, a fellow colleague, Fynes (1994), had begun to document the development of midwifery in Ontario but stopped short of official integration. My work was to take an analytical perspective informed by the literature on the professions and bring the analysis of midwifery integration up to date. In undertaking an examination of the midwifery professionalization project in Ontario, I asked the following questions:

1 How and why did midwifery become integrated into the Ontario health care system;
2 What factors and forces influenced the unique shape that midwifery took throughout the integration process; and
3 What impact has this integration process had on the structure and organization of midwifery care in the province and on the way midwifery is practised.

To help answer these questions, I employed a social historical research design. I collected data using two interconnected methodologies. The first form of data collection involved gathering primary and secondary source documents relating to the integration of midwifery in Ontario that spanned 20 years. The search for documentary material began in the libraries/collections of midwifery, nursing, and medical organizations. This included entire newsletters, articles in newsletters and journals, and policy documents. From there, I identified key committees influencing midwifery policy and later contacted them for publicly available correspondence, minutes from meetings, and official reports.

Second, to obtain information not available in these documents, I conducted in-person and telephone interviews with key informants who were identified through my involvement in the midwifery community and in the documents collected as knowledgeable and influential in the Ontario midwifery integration process. I took care to include a cross-section of key consumers, midwives, nurses, physicians, hospital administrators, midwifery policy makers, and state officials. Of 43 informants contacted, interviews were secured with 39.[2]

My participation in the Ontario midwifery movement proved to be very helpful in both the conceptualization and conduct of my research. Through my participatory work, I developed important research contacts that proved essential in securing interviews with the overwhelming majority of key informants I contacted for my study. In addition, because of my involvement with the birth centre committee, I had relatively easy access to documents and archival material which were key sources of data.

At the same time, however, my choice of research topic altered my role as a participant in the midwifery community. I quickly came to realize that having the issue of "professionalization" as the focus of my research recast my relationship with the midwifery movement. Now, I was not just doing research *for* the midwifery movement as other feminist social scientists had done in the past, but *about* it, as well (see Bourgeault 2002). My focus on professionalization meant exploring the controversies surrounding the pursuit of midwifery integration. These included dissent within the midwifery community regarding the content and process of key decisions involving organizational objectives, regulation and practice standards, and educational qualifications. Such dissent is typical of most professionalization projects (Witz 1992). Professionalization was a particularly sensitive issue for midwifery, given its anti-authoritarian roots. The more involved I became in my research, therefore, the more removed I felt from the midwifery community itself. My observer role came to supersede my role as a participant in the community.

This "academic outsider" status was cemented with the initial dissemination of my findings which were read by some members of the broader midwifery community as being much too critical, particularly some of my more sweeping conclusions. To a certain extent these criticisms were true. In the interim, I have gained much insight with time, two more midwifery-attended births, subsequent research on midwifery, involvement in comparative research on maternity care across Canada and in the United States and the UK, and further exploration of the theoretical literature on women's relationship with the state (much of which has been published since I originally conducted this research). Although these new sources of information have not significantly altered the description of the process of midwifery integration in Ontario I compiled, they have given me a more reflective viewpoint from which to analyse and frame critical events in the late '80s and early '90s. It is from this broader, more informed viewpoint that this book has taken shape.

Acknowledgments

Although I am listed as the sole author of this book, my ability to complete it is due to the involvement of many others whose inspiration, support, and encouragement I would like to acknowledge.

I would first like to express my appreciation to *all* of my key informants, especially the midwives and their politically astute supporters (both consumers and those within other professions, the government, and various ministries) for providing me with an incredible narrative to recount. I hope this book is something of a testimony to their efforts, enthusiasm, and vision. I would like to extend special thanks to my midwives, Chris Sternberg and Arlene Vandersloot, with whom I experienced a small part of this story through the birth of my children, Lauren, Tyra, and Adam. I would also like to thank the many midwives, most notably Holiday Tyson and Vicki Van Wagner, who have taken the time to provide me with feedback on my thesis. I hope these discussions are accurately reflected in the revisions herein.

I would like to thank my doctoral thesis supervisor David Coburn for helping me throughout the development of my dissertation from its inception as a problem statement to its completion. I would especially like to thank David for his swift (i.e., over the weekend) and insightful reading of my drafts which regretably ate into his sabbatical year. David should also be acknowledged for his insightful comments on how the confluence of female actors both within and impinging upon the state should be explored more fully. I cannot thank him enough.

Thanks are also owed to my committee members, Bonnie Fox and Linda Muzzin, thesis examiners, Ellen Hodnett and Dorothy Pawluch, for their helpful feedback. Bonnie's support in particularly helped me remain sane throughout my thesis writing/deadline meeting phase. Special thanks should also be extended to Joan Eakin and Merrijoy Kelner, both of whom have always been so supportive of my scholarly endeavours. I would also like to extend my gratitude to Greta Theobalds for her excellent transcription of my interviews.

To my friends and colleagues formerly of the Graduate Program in Behavioural Science at the University of Toronto, Jan Angus, Peri Ballantyne, Mary Fynes, Corinne Hart, and Ann Pederson, thank you for the many sympathetic and supportive discussions about studenthood, marriage, motherhood, and life. These women made my journey through graduate school significantly more enjoyable. I would also like to express my gratitude to the staff and faculty in the former Department of Behavioural Science and Graduate Department of Community Health, in particular to Karen Domnick for her support in helping me meet University deadlines; and to Danny Lopez for helping me scrape together some much-needed funding for the last few months of writing my thesis (including a University of Toronto School of Graduate Studies Bursary, Hastings Award, and Merrijoy Kelner Award).

Other sources of financial support for this research came from the Social Sciences and Humanities Research Council of Canada and the National Health Research and Development Program of Health Canada through both doctoral and postdoctoral fellowships. The teaching release time I have negotiated as part of my New Investigator Award from the Canadian Institutes for Health Research – first from the University of Western Ontario and then from McMaster University – has also proved to be instrumental in helping me see this project to completion.

I would also like to acknowledge the support I have received for the completion of this book from my social science colleagues who study midwifery: Lesley Biggs, Cecilia Benoit, Robbie David-Floyd, Ray DeVries, Pat Kaufert, Jacquelyne Luce, Maggie MacDonald, Sheryl Nestel, Anne Rochon Ford, Jane Sandall, Edwin van Teijlinden, and Sirpa Wrede; and students and staff who provided much-needed administrative assistance: Judi Winkup, Michelle Homer, and Terri Tomchick. Inspiration for the revisions of this manuscript came from several students in the various classes I have taught in medical sociology and on the health occupations, but most notably Kristine Hirschkorn.

Finally, I would like to acknowledge those persons to whom this thesis is dedicated. Though separated by a thousand miles, my parents, Rachelle and Ian Bourgeault, have always been there for me, supporting my endeavours with undying encouragement, reassurance, and support. To my husband, Jeff Jutai, thank you for your confidence and assurance that I would get things done, and again, to my children for their patience, understanding, and excitement.

Thank you all.

Ivy Lynn Bourgeault
2005

Acronyms

AOM	Association of Ontario Midwives
ACNM	American College of Nurse-Midwives
ACOG	American College of Obstetricians and Gynecologists
ARM	Association of Radical Midwives (UK)
BNA	British Nurses Association
CDC	Curriculum Design Committee
CMO	College of Midwives of Ontario
CNM	Certified Nurse Midwife (US)
CNO	College of Nurses of Ontario
CPSO	College of Physicians and Surgeons of Ontario
FIGO	International Federation of Obstetricians and Gynecologists
FNS	Frontier Nursing Service (US)
HPLR	Health Professions Legislation Review (Ontario)
ICM	International Congress of Midwives
IRCM	Interim Regulatory Council for Midwives (Ontario)
LMCO	Lebel Midwifery Care Organization (Ontario)
MCA	Maternity Centre Association (US)
MANA	Midwifery Alliance of North America
MIPP	Midwifery Implementation Planning Project
MOPP	Model of Practice and Payment
MRG	Medical Reform Group
MTFO	Midwifery Task Force of Ontario
NCW	National Council of Women (Canada)
NHS	National Health Service (UK)
OAM	Ontario Association of Midwives
OCFP	Ontario College of Family Physicians
OCHA	Ontario Committee on the Healing Arts

OHA	Ontario Hospital Association
OMA	Ontario Medical Association
OMCN	Ontario Midwifery Consumer's Network
OMP	Ontario Midwifery Programme
ONA	Ontario Nurses Association
ONMA	Ontario Nurse Midwives Association
RHPA	Regulated Health Professions Act
RNAO	Registered Nurses Association of Ontario
SOGC	Society of Obstetricians and Gynecologists of Canada
TCCMO	Transitional Council of the College of Midwives of Ontario
TFIMO	Task Force on the Implementation of Midwifery in Ontario
TPA	Transfer Payment Agency
VBAC	Vaginal Birth After Caesarean
VOHH	Victorian Order of Home Helpers (Canada)
VON	Victorian Order of Nurses (Canada)
WHO	World Health Organization

Introduction

Why *Push*? In addition to it being a catchy title drawing upon birth metaphors that are typical in the literature on midwifery (e.g., Barbara Katz Rothman's *In Labor*, Rose Weitz and Deborah Sullivan's *Labor Pains*, Cecilia Benoit's *Midwives in Passage*, and Brian Burtch's *Trials of Labour*), I chose it because it accurately captures the focus of this book: the active push by a group of lay and professional women (and some men) to achieve state recognition of the profession of midwifery in Ontario, where it previously existed only in obscurity. These women and men mustered key resources, sought strategic alliances, and pushed hard to deliver a new form of midwifery care that has garnered international attention and recognition.

Prior to the 1990s, there were few midwives in Canada and unlike every other developed nation in the world, their practice was neither legal nor officially recognized. Throughout the 1980s, a deliberate project was undertaken by midwives and their consumer supporters to fully integrate midwifery into various provincial health care systems. By 1993, midwives in one Canadian province – Ontario – had managed to achieve this previously elusive goal. This is a remarkably short time in which to advance from obscurity to official recognition. What is even more interesting, however, is how midwives were integrated in the province of Ontario.

In brief, midwives in Ontario have been integrated as independent practitioners, with government funding for a self-regulatory college; a direct-entry, university-based education program; and the provision of midwifery care for pregnant women and their newborn infants in both home and hospital settings. This is a model of midwifery that is truly unique in the world. Such a remarkable achievement raises a critical question *How was it accomplished*? I will answer this question by peeling back the various layers of this story in the pages that follow.

But this book is not simply about the struggle for midwifery in one Canadian province. The story about the integration of midwifery into the Ontario health care system can also be viewed as a case study of a successful, organized, largely female, and professional-based effort directed at the state. As such, it demands a broader consideration of the contemporary dynamics of the relationships between women (as consumers and as providers of care), the professions, and the state. This broader thread will be woven through the layers of the story of midwifery integration.

There is a substantial literature devoted to the professionalization and legitimation of various health occupations ranging from nursing and radiation therapy to chiropractic and naturopathy (Biggs 1989; Boon 1998; Cant and Sharma 1996; Coburn 1988; Coburn and Biggs 1986; Gort and Coburn 1988; Heap and Stuart 1995; Larkin 1983; Wardwell 1981; Willis 1989; Witz 1990, 1992). Limitation, subordination, and in some cases exclusion have been the primary outcomes of these *professional projects*. As a largely female-based professional project, midwifery in Ontario has managed to evade many of these negative outcomes. Examining how this was possible helps to more fully conceptualize the roles of the state and consumer supporters in female professional projects.

In the first section of the book, I lay out a map of the various contextual influences on this account of midwifery integration. I begin by briefly reviewing the two theoretical lenses through which the social history of the push to integrate midwifery can be viewed: 1) the literature on professional projects with a particular focus on gender, consumers, and the state and 2) the literature on the relations between women, women's groups, and the state. Following this theoretical background, I contextualize the integration of the midwifery profession comparatively and historically. I first outline the process and outcome of other midwifery professional projects in the UK, Australia, the US and the Netherlands (chapter 2). In the following chapter, I turn to the historic fall of midwifery in Canada, the factors leading to its decline and later to its rise as a new kind of midwifery movement. Together these contextual chapters help to make clear the unique features of the case of midwifery integration in Ontario.

In the next section of the book I provide a detailed description of the midwifery integration process in order to fully explicate the relationship between midwives, women, and the state. I begin by outlining the evolution of midwifery from a social movement into a professional project (chapter 4). In the following two chapters I detail both the factors leading up to the decision to integrate and regulate midwifery (chapter 5) and the decisions made about how midwifery would be integrated (chapter 6).

I then describe the evolution of and challenges to the midwifery model of practice experienced throughout the integration process – with specific reference to the integration of midwifery in hospitals (chapter 7) and the organization of funding for midwifery services (chapter 8). This is followed by a discussion of the development of the unique direct-entry midwifery education program in chapter 9 and how the midwives themselves were in fact integrated (chapter 10).

These chapters reveal that the unique configuration and context of the Ontario midwifery case enables an interesting discussion of the gendered nature of the relationship between the professions, its clientele and supporters, and the state. Specifically, I argue that midwifery became integrated due to a combination of factors each of which has an important gender dimension. This includes the astute lobbying on the part of the midwives, consumers, and other supporters – most of whom were largely female. There was also a conducive structural environment whereby the nursing and medical professions were preoccupied with other concerns and where some state representatives (increasingly female) regarded midwifery as a feminist cause and potentially cost-effective form of care. These factors played an important part in midwives' ability to achieve self-regulation and independence from the professions of nursing and medicine.

In the conclusion I revisit the model influenced by the conceptualizations of female professional projects and state-directed feminist initiatives described in chapter 1. In so doing, I attempt to reinvigorate some long-abandoned theories which help address this new strategic relationship between the midwifery profession, women, and the state. I also reflect upon over ten years of the integration of midwifery in Ontario, its integration (or lack thereof) in other Canadian provinces, and some of the implications of key decisions made during the 1980s and early 1990s for the future of maternity care in Canada.

PART ONE

Situating Midwifery

Theoretical, International, and Historical Contexts

CHAPTER ONE

Analytical Lenses:
Professions, Women, and the State

The struggle to integrate midwifery into the mainstream maternity care system in Ontario did not evolve in a vacuum. There were a variety of influences on its development including international examples of midwifery integration and the historical context it emerged from in Canada. But what are the most important factors of these contextual influences to draw upon? This is a critical question to ask because volumes of work have been devoted to each of these topics and there is limited space to fully capture them here. Moreover, how is one to fully tease apart the multiplicity of issues faced and factors involved in the struggle for midwifery in Ontario throughout the 1980s and 1990s? An analytical or conceptual lens is crucial in this regard. In this chapter, I briefly review the two analytical lenses that inform and are informed by this case study of midwifery integration.[1] I begin with a discussion of professional projects, highlighting the role of consumers and the state, drawing in large part on the work of Anne Witz (1992). Some of the gaps in this literature led me to turn to the more recent literature on the relations between women and the state. Together these two bodies of thought help to inform the conceptual framework that I present at the end of this chapter and more fully flesh out through this case study of midwifery integration.

"PROFESSIONAL PROJECTS"

Larson (1977, 1979) was the first to introduce the concept of a *professional project* in her treatise on the professionalization of medicine in Britain and the United States. She described it as involving 1) controlling a market of expertise; and 2) embarking on a collective process of upward social mobility. An upwardly mobile occupation must create a need for its services and at the same time create a scarcity of resources – its own members. This is accomplished by controlling the number of members through a standardized, mandatory system of professional training and through professional licensing and certification. Market conditions, however, are insufficient to guarantee professional power. Larson argues that as a profession attempts to rise upward, it "must form 'organic' ties with significant fractions of the ruling class (or of a rising class); persuasion and justification depend on ideological resources, the import and legitimacy of which are ultimately defined by the context of hegemonic power in a class society" (1977: xv). In the case of medicine, for example, she asserts that its collective rise was facilitated by the fit between its emerging doctrines and the ideology that was being used to justify the increasing power of the corporate capitalist class (see also Coburn, Torrance and Kaufert 1983).[2]

Larson's approach represented a profound reconceptualization of the process of professionalization, and one that has been followed by countless analyses of health occupations in a variety of system contexts (Biggs 1989; Boon 1998; Cant and Sharma 1996; Coburn 1994; Coburn and Biggs 1986; Gort and Coburn 1988; Heap and Stuart 1995; Larkin 1983; Wardwell 1981; Willis 1989). These "professional projects" often begin with some sort of organized effort, such as the development of a professional association, which comes to be controlled by a core group of members. These "elite" members not only lead the professionalization project, they also rally support for their endeavour, as well as seek out strategic alliances to help overcome the usual opposition to professionalization by those entrenched within the health care hierarchy, primarily medicine.

To overcome opposition, one of the strategic alliances sought by leaders of professional projects is often from within the "opposition" itself, that is, from key members of the medical profession. Larkin (1983), for example, notes how members of the medical profession were often "intimately associated with the foundation of para-medical associations" (notes 187) and how support from medicine is vital for such professional projects. In exchange for this sponsorship, the aspiring profession must often accommodate its sponsors' demands (Coburn and Biggs 1986; Larkin 1983). This usually results in the limitation of the aspiring professions' scope of practice or subordination of its practitioners. Indeed, Wardwell (1981) and Willis (1989) describe three main outcomes of professionalization in terms of the aspiring professions' relationship to the dominant medical profession: 1) *subordinate* professions, which function only under direct supervision of the medical profession; 2) *limited* professions, which practise independently of medical supervision but with a limited scope, either in terms of the part of the body dealt with or the range of treatment modalities; and 3) *excluded* professions, which practise outside of the mainstream medical system.

In addition to affecting the scope of practice and level of subordination of aspiring professions, professionalization may also impact on their ideology. Coburn and Biggs (1986), for example, note how chiropractic in Canada underwent a significant ideological shift during the professionalization process, away from its more traditional alternative roots to a more medicalized health specialty focused on musculoskeletal disorders of the spine. They highlight that this new scientific ideology is intricately connected with the perspective of the elite group that took over the organization and content of the occupation. Boon (1998) and Cant and Sharma (1996) describe similar processes within naturopathy and homeopathy respectively. This new professional ideology, as Davies (1983) argues, "is a leader ideology ... it is the "official" view as propounded by leaders ... [and] is not to be equated with the beliefs or sanctioned behaviours of all members of an occupational group" (49–50).

As Davies' quote suggests, efforts at organizing and seeking strategic alliances are more successful in some cases than others and can reveal substantial intraprofessional conflict, often between an elite group and the rank-and-file. But what is the impact of this intraprofessional tension? Wardwell (1981) argues that it has a positive effect, but Willis (1989) does not concur, pointing instead to how such divisions can severely diminish the chances of securing state legitimacy.

Just as the divisions within an aspiring profession are important, so too are the divisions between medical specialities. Willis (1989) and Larkin (1983), for example, both argue that various specialties can respond more successfully to competition from other health occupations in some cases than in others. This view concurs with Halpern's (1992) argument that "[medical] specialities best able to subordinate ancillary workers are those receiving support from established segments within medicine. Thus, relations between segments within a dominant profession powerfully affect its boundaries with other occupations" (994). It is important, therefore, not to regard medicine as an entirely homogenous profession; like any profession, it has many divisions, some of which are able to wield more power than others.

These points highlight the importance of drawing upon another complementary theory to that of professional projects, specifically Abbott's (1988) conceptualization of a *system of professions*. This "system," he describes, is a complex, dynamic, and interdependent structural network of a group of professions within a given domain of work, constantly struggling over areas of knowledge and skill expertise, called *jurisdictions*. Professions are said to develop from interrelations with other professions when a jurisdiction becomes vacant. Such vacancies occur in response to external system disturbances, such as technological or organizational change, or because an earlier tenant has abandoned. A profession's success in occupying a jurisdiction reflects on the situation of its competitors as much as it does the profession's own efforts. Subordination of one professional group by another occurs when a profession vacates a jurisdiction but maintains control over it through such strategies as supervising the new tenant. Audiences for jurisdictional disputes include the public, the legal system (i.e., the state), and the workplace. Both professions and their audiences influence the competitive process through reshaping the profession's knowledge base and/or changing the currency of legitimation.

As alluded to in this description of Abbott's *system* theory, seeking medical sponsorship is not the only method of enhancing professionalization. In many cases, sponsorship is sought directly from the state in its role as licensing agent. Such sponsorship is often bolstered by exhibitions of consumer support which if large enough can be interpreted as potential electoral support for state actors (Biggs 1989; Willis 1989). But the state is not simply a neutral arbiter of professional disputes. As the state comes to have increasing power within the health care division of labour, particularly in countries with systems of national health insurance or health services (Coburn 1993), seeking direct state support has proven to be a successful professionalization strategy (Coburn and Biggs 1986; Willis 1989). Indeed, Coburn (1993) argues that although state regulation of health occupations in Ontario was historically mediated through medicine's control over the health care division of labour, more recently the state's involvement has become less medically oriented as the profession has become increasingly seen as the major barrier to a more "rational" health care system. It has only been in the recent climate of health care rationalization, for example, that some professions have been able to gain legitimacy directly from the state.

This view of a supportive state is not a particularly new idea. Berlant (1975), for example, argues that the medical profession used state administrative structures to secure and further its collective interests. Portwood and Fielding (1981) also emphasize how negotiations with the state are a means by which professions enhance their privilege. But the state and the professions are not necessarily as separate as these statements suggest. Fielding and Portwood (1980), for example, argue that "a formal working relationship has in the case of almost all professions been established between them and the state ... for most professions the interdependent processes of bureaucratization and professionalization have been to the benefit of both themselves and the state" (48–9). Johnson (1982) also details how the formation of the professions and the state in Britain were historically interrelated processes. He describes how the state became more powerful with the development of the professions and in turn how professions attained power through newly developed state apparata (Johnson 1995). Larson (1977) earlier emphasized the symbiotic relationship between professions and the state, observing that "organizational professions are generated ... by the expansion of the bureaucratic apparatus of the state" (179).

These theoretical conceptualizations of the state's role in the professionalization process, however, focus almost entirely on the medical profession and its historic development. What of the relations between a more securely established state and other occupations seeking professional status? How is it that aspiring professions come to capture state interest? Is it that the state comes to see another possible extension of the domain it can "govern"? What impact do pre-existing relations with often competitive institutionalized areas of medical expertise have on these new state-profession relations?

To begin to answer these questions, one must take certain factors into consideration. First, it is important to acknowledge the role of a liberal democratic state in capitalist society in helping to ensure an environment conducive to the accumulation of capital as well as maintaining its own legitimacy vis-à-vis its citizenry or the electorate (Knutilla 1992; Simmons and Keohane 1992). Willis (1989), for example, notes that despite opposition, exclusion, and internal divisions, chiropractic flourished in Australia, mainly due to the support and lobbying efforts of chiropractic clientele. He also argues that there was a "compatibility of chiropractic knowledge with dominant class interests" (197) given that back injuries are a major source of productivity loss in capitalist society. Other than these insights, the mediating role of the public on the state has largely been overlooked as an element of professionalization.

Johnson's early work (1972) on the relations between professions and clients touches upon the role of the state. Specifically, he situates professionalism within a typology of practitioner-client relations. These relations include: *collegiate control*, where the practitioner defines the needs of the client and the manner in which these needs are catered to; *patronage*, where the client defines his or her own needs and the manner in which they are to be met; and *mediation*, where a third party, usually the state, mediates the relationship between practitioner and client, defining both needs and the manner in which the needs are met. Professionalism, he argues, is a subtype of collegiate control associated with a homogenous occupational community and a heterogenous client population. As is true of much of the literature on professional-client relations (see for example the thesis of medical consumerism by Haug 1973 and Haug and Lavin 1983), the relations between professions and the public are often cast in oppositional terms. While it may be true as Freidson (1970a) argues that "the relation of any service occupation to its clientele is inherently problematic" (105), this is but one view of profession-client relations. As we see from Willis' example and from the work by Biggs (1989) and Coburn (with Biggs 1986), consumers can be quite supportive of an occupation's efforts to gain professional status. We do not yet have a theory that adequately addresses the relations between consumers and professions that are not established,[3] let alone one that explains the mediating role of the public on the state as an element of professionalization.

In addition to taking into consideration the relations between the public, professions, and the state when examining professional projects, one must also look to broader social and cultural factors to help explain the outcome of such projects. For example, Willis (1989) argues that gender is an important determining factor in an occupation's legitimacy process. He states that subordination, or what Etzioni (1969) earlier called, "semi-professional" status, is the main outcome of efforts to integrate female health professions but he fails to explain why. In Larkin's analysis of the professionalization of paramedical professions, he briefly mentions the gender composition of the various groups but its impact is not fully considered in his analysis of occupational imperialism. Thus, in addition to professional, client, and state relations, the full impact of gender on the process of professionalization was in need of greater consideration.

GENDER AND PROFESSIONAL PROJECTS

Early theorizing about the influence of gender on professional status tends to take either an uncritical or a sexist view of professions dominated by female members.[4] Etzioni (1969), for example, argued that "the cultural value of professions, organization and female employment are not compatible" (vi). Simpson and Simpson (1969) asserted that women are less likely to maintain a high level of specialized knowledge and less able to attain societal support for professional autonomy. They added further that professions dominated numerically by women tend to be more bureaucratized than full professions dominated by men; in this sense they are only "semi-professions." According to this circular logic, female-dominated professions are not full professions *because* they are female (see also Hearn 1982). There is, however, no effort made to explain why this is so.

More recent examinations of the influence of gender on professionalization by feminist scholars offer a more critical analysis. Although they do not dispute that the lower-status professions are disproportionately staffed by women, they argue that this is not because of a difference in career commitment, years of education (Armstrong and Armstrong 1992b), or submissiveness by female professionals (Grandjean and Bernal 1979). They argue rather that women's lower status is due to the fact that they have been actively excluded from the established professions (Crompton 1987; Crompton and Sanderson 1990; Riska and Wegar 1993; Witz 1990, 1992), and experience different conditions as professionals (Armstrong and Armstrong 1992a; Butter et al. 1985, 1987; Kazanjian 1993; Lorber 1993). Indeed, some also argue that the very meaning of *professions* and *professionalism* has been shaped by gender (Adams 2000; Davies and Rosser 1986; Witz 1992). Specifically, professionalism came to be defined in terms of prevailing conceptions of middle-class masculinity, so that the traits valued by professionals – independence, rationality, education, authority – were precisely those that were most likely held by middle-class white men (Adams 2000). Thus, the term *profession* is assumed to denote maleness and dominance over both clients and other occupations (Benoit 2000). How this has influenced the professional projects undertaken by female health professions has been most explicitly conceptualized by Witz (1992) in *Professions and Patriarchy*.

In an attempt to advance the conceptualization of the influence of gender on the integration process of aspiring health professions, Witz (1990, 1992) expands upon the concept of *professional projects* originally introduced by Larson (1977, 1979) by gendering the agents of these projects, locating them within the structural and historical parameters of patriarchal capitalism. She argues that the professional projects women engage in employ different strategies and have different outcomes than the projects of male-based professions.

In an attempt to advance the conceptualization of how gender influences the professionalization process, Witz (1992) specifically elaborates upon two key elements of occupational closure that pertain to the relations between professions – *demarcation* and *dual closure* – to identify their gendered dimension. Briefly, demarcationary closure strategies are adopted by the dominant occupational group and involve the "encirclement of women within a related but distinct sphere of competence" (1992: 47) and are usually subordinated within the division of labour. The corresponding response of the subordinate occupational group to demarcation is *usurpation*, but *exclusion* against other subordinates is also enacted, which Witz labels *dual closure*. Both usurpation and this form of exclusion involve the *legalistic* tactic of seeking state-sponsored systems of registration, and the *credentialist* tactic of restricting ranks into professional training programs and institutional employment.

Witz further elaborates upon the efficacy of the legalistic and credentialist strategies employed by female professional groups through an examination of the historical projects undertaken by female health professions in Britain at the turn of the century, primarily nursing and midwifery. Based on these case studies, she argues that credentialist exclusionary strategies employed through institutions in civil society proved to be less effective at advancing female professional projects than legalistic strategies directed toward the state. Indeed, she argues that "it is in the sphere of civil society within which male power is organised and institutionalised where gendered exclusionary strategies operate to sustain patriarchal modes of occupational closure" (Witz 1990: 680). The institutions involved included hospitals, professional associations, colleges, all of which at the time were under strict medical control. How and why the state is less effective at maintaining patriarchal closure than institutions in civil society is not fully considered in her analysis.

Examining Witz' conclusions from an opposite perspective, one could argue that historically female professional projects such as nursing and midwifery were more successful in achieving legitimacy through legalistic means vis-à-vis the state than through credentialist means in civil society. This may be surprising in light of the fact that at the time of the initiatives Witz describes, women did not yet have the vote in Britain. Thus, the state may not only be a weaker sponsor of gender-based exclusion, it may also be a more viable source of support for female professional projects. This has already been noted to be the case for other aspiring professions discussed above (Coburn and Biggs 1986; Willis 1989) but without the additional analysis of the influence of gender. The idea that the state is increasingly becoming the site for "conflicts over jurisdiction" (Abbott 1988) is not new, but what has yet to be examined more fully is the complex dynamic of how gender intersects the relations between professions and the state. In particular, we need a more thorough analysis of the role of a liberal democratic state in female professional projects in the contemporary era when women have the vote and when, according to some, there has been a movement towards the feminization of the state.

Kazanjian (1993) begins to address this gap in our knowledge through her analysis of the recent regulatory environment in British Columbia. To contrast with this potentially more supportive view of the state, she argues that state policies in that province serve to perpetuate medical and by extension gender-based dominance within the health care division of labour. But how many of these state policies are vestiges of an era where the medical profession was at its pinnacle of dominance? (Coburn, Torrance, and Kaufert 1983). Does this necessarily negate the potential for change as indeed there has been evidence that the state has been more recently attempting to achieve change (Coburn 1993)? It does mean that the relations between female health professions and the state may be more complicated than initially thought and indeed, may be reflective of the gendered relationship between women and the state more broadly.

WOMEN AND THE STATE

From the first wave of feminism (1870–1930) with its initiatives on women's political and property rights to the second wave of feminism (from 1960) which concentrated on the control over women's sexuality, fertility, and experience of violence (Charles 2000), the state has been a focus of feminist efforts. Indeed, women's issues have moved from being a radical demand of feminists to a legitimate policy issue for various levels of government (Heitlinger 1993). Like the legalistic tactics Witz (1992) described in relation to female professional projects in Britain, other state-directed feminist initiatives have been relatively successful in advancing women's health and social justice issues. These include such issues as pay equity, access to abortion, anti-pornography legislation, and efforts to combat violence against women (Fox Piven 1990; Fudge 1996; Gotell 1996; McDermott 1996; Smart 1989). In the case of women's health initiatives in Canada, for example, Feldberg and Carlsson (1999) argue that "governmental institutions at a variety of levels have seemed to respond to women's organizing around health" (353).

While feminist activists have recognized the emancipatory potential of the state, feminist analyses have also revealed the oppressive nature of the state. Feminist authors of fiction, such as Margaret Atwood (1985),

depict the state as having hierarchical, centralized, and militarized political might (Brownley 2000). Many of the initial forays of feminist state
scholars follow the Marxist school of thought, which argue that the capitalist state acts primarily in the interest of capital (Charles 2000). Marxist
feminists, such as McIntosh (1978), argue similarly that the state, at least
historically, supports gender relations which are oppressive to women.
This support came to be known as "state patriarchy" (Eisenstein 1984)
and early radical feminists argued that on the whole, the state should
either be avoided (Waylen 1998) or acted against (Randall 1998). In the
case of Canada, for example, it has been argued that the welfare state is
shaped by policies that maintain the traditional sexual division of labour
which works both in the interests of capital and patriarchy (Bergqvist and
Findlay 1999).

The recognition, however, that engagement with a liberal democratic
state[5] can have positive outcomes for women has resulted in a modifica-
tion of this more one-sided view of the state by some feminists (Charles
2000, 18). That is, rather than reject the state, feminists need to rethink
their conceptions of it (Randall 1998). This shift in perspective of Marxist-
feminists has mirrored the acknowledgment of Marxist scholars of the
state that it is not monolithic; the state sometimes responds to political
pressure from the working class (Coburn, 1993). For example, Marxists
have argued that universal provision of welfare by the state also legiti-
mates its power by giving "the impression that the state 'cares' about its
citizens and give them a reason to support the existing system" (Charles
2000: 8). Similarly, Connell (1990) links the recent successes of feminist
initiatives to the need of the state to maintain its legitimacy. She argues
that a liberal democratic state is "obliged to respond to demands which
are phrased in the discourse of liberalism," for if it does not, "such
demands have the potential to call into question its legitimacy" (see
Charles 2000: 26). Thus, as noted earlier, the state must not only respond
to the interests of capital, it must also maintain its *legitimacy* vis-à-vis its
electorate, which now includes women who are increasingly constituting
an electoral force, voting in favour of their own interests as women
(Conway, Ahern, and Sterernagel 1999).

The impact of women on the state, however, is not limited to the state's
need to maintain legitimacy. One must also consider the internal workings of the state. In contrast to Marxist external representations of the
state, Weberian theorists focus on the exercise of power and domination
thereby fostering "a renewed interest in the internal organization of the
state ... its contradictions [becoming] apparent instead of appearing as a

monolithic entity" (Charles 2000: 13). That is, "viewed externally the state can be seen as a set of institutions which together constitute the state apparatus which has power over civil society ... viewed internally the state appears as a set of social relations which are in continual flux, it is seen as a process rather than a thing" (Charles 2000: 13).

Feminist theorists who follow a Weberian tradition argue that the internal organization of the state should be seen in terms of "institution-alized masculinity" (Connell 1990: 24), that is that it is controlled by men and policies are biased towards the interests of men. This often means women are left to attempt to penetrate the state indirectly from the out-side through interest groups. In the case of Canada, "women who took up the issue of women's equality were 'outsiders' in the male-dominated political system of representation, sidelined as lobbyists and forced to rely on the mechanism of a royal commission to influence the 'insiders.'" (Bergqvist and Findlay 1999: 126–7). As a consequence, Canadian women's organizations have tended to fall outside the domain of established pol-itics and remain isolated from standard sources of political power (Feldberg and Carlsson 1999). Organizations that have more power vis-à-vis the state, such as the medical profession, tend to be under-represented by women in the upper echelons of its organizational hierarchy (Conway, Ahern, and Steuernagel 1999). In Heitlinger's (1993) comparative analysis of the success of women's initiatives as state "outsiders" in Canada, Australia, and the UK, she argues that such initiatives work best where there are flexible political structures that are open to a variety of interest groups, and where innovative liberal feminist groups are willing and able to engage in "pragmatic reformist politics" (4). She further argues that "the ways in which feminist demands are formulated and translated into demands made on the state depends on the *ideological* predisposition of the women's movement and the political opportunities for feminist influ-ence on government" (20, emphasis mine). This idea is similar to Larson's arguments regarding the ideological compatibility of professional projects with the logic of capitalism, and likely refers to an argument based on the ideology of liberalism (to resonate best with the legitimacy of a liberal democratic state).

A more influential mode of interacting with the state could be described as the move from "outsider" to "insider" status (Conway, Ahern, and Steuernagel 1999). This mode of interaction may be accomplished by an increase in the number of elected female politicians, who may act as cen-tral agents for taking up the concerns of women. According to Arscott and Trimble (1996), the gender of legislators can influence "the expansion of the range of issues considered to be political, the bringing of a gender-specific perspective to bear on already established issues, ... and a symbolic presence that helps in the continuing task of eliminating sex-based discrimination" (16). This is particularly salient in those countries known for "state feminism," such as Sweden and other Nordic countries (Eduards 1991). There it offers an important strategic tool with which to challenge the existing legitimacy of male power within the state (Heitlinger 1993). An alternate strategy that was adopted in Australia was to create a group of *femocrats* (Eisenstein 1996), that is, community-based feminist "outsiders" who were integrated within state bureaucracies as representatives to help develop and implement policies to promote women's equality.

Together, these two strategies have been effective in creating a critical mass of women (Maillé and Wängnerud 1999) who have increased the feminization of the state, creating what Hernes (1987) has coined a "women-friendly" state. This has arguably resulted in states being more responsive to women's issues (Conway, Ahern, and Steuernagel 1999). Indeed, it has led to the creation of "opportunity spaces" (Waylen 1998) or "political opportunity structures" (Jenkins and Klandermans 1995) whereby existing patterns of gender relations are altered. These help to provide women or women's groups with opportunities to collaborate with influential state actors even if their intervention may be constrained and even shaped by such opportunities (Randall 1998). That is, as Briskin (1999) argues, "state responsiveness is not without contradiction: issues raised by women are often taken over by the state and solutions reshaped and managed in ways that might not have been foreseen and are not always in women's best interests" (12).

At the same time, however, if one teases apart the levels of the state, one uncovers a gendered order within it, where different branches of the state are more or less masculinized. For example, "the coercive sectors of the state are male dominated in comparison with those concerned with human service work such as health and education" (Charles 2000, 25). Indeed, the evolution of the welfare state into traditional feminine domains of health and child care may lead to the consequent increase in the proportion of women within the state both as elected representatives and as bureaucrats. Thus, the gender order of the family to a certain extent is reproduced in the various levels of the welfare state with the more powerful sectors still dominated by men. As a consequence, the strength of the resistance to the integration of women's interests remains embedded in the structures of representation and the practices of men who still dominate them (Bergqvist and Findlay 1999). Hence, to effect substantial change, women, both as insiders and as outsiders, still need to have allies in the upper echelons of government.

Thus, there exists a chameleon-like quality to the state when examined from a gendered perspective where it is "both enabling and constraining ... oppressive and responsive to pressure for change" by women and women's groups (Charles 2000: 28). That is, "although the state may be patriarchal and represent male power at a certain historical conjuncture, it is not essentially patriarchal and can therefore be changed" (Charles 2000: 5). The change, however, may be more incremental than radical (Conway, Ahern, and Steuernagel 1999). Thus, the state is not static with respect to gender relations but evolving, dialectic, and dynamic, making it important to examine the state at different conjunctures and periods of time. We must also recognize the dialectical relationship between the structure of and agency within the state as it is impossible to understand actions without analysing the structures that constrain those actions. The state also cannot be solely conceptualized as a unitary structure; rather it should be seen also as an arena where interests are actively constructed (Waylen 1998). Moreover, one needs to exercise caution not to assume that the interests of the state, capital, men, and women are homogeneous within the various sites of struggle.

SUMMARY

These two bodies of literature – on professional projects and on women and the state – are highly complementary and taken together help to inform the mapping out of the context of influences on the integration of midwifery into the Ontario health care system (undertaken in the next two chapters) as well as of the actual process itself (addressed in the second part). From this review, we see that there is a growing body of work delving into the specific role of the state in the professionalization process but little of this fully takes gender into consideration. To a lesser extent, we also find some literature highlighting the role that the public/ clients play in the professionalization process and the role this in turn plays on the state primarily as it pertains to class (Willis 1989). Again, however, there is little analysis of the influence of gender on either the profession or the public/clients. Indeed, most of the work on gender and the professions draws, not unexpectedly, upon the broader literature on women's work (Adams 2000; Benoit 2000; Crompton 1987; Witz 1992). Thus, these analyses have more to say about the internal dynamics of the "system of professions" than about external relations with either the

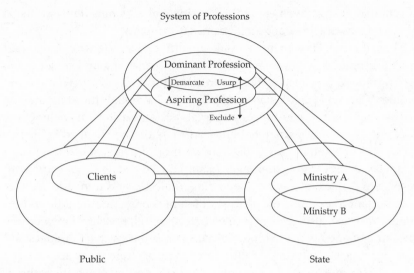

System of Professions

Figure 1
Preliminary model of interrelations between professions, public, and the state

public/clients or the state. What the literature on the relations between women and the state offers is a thorough analysis of women's role as consumers or clients of state services and policies. Unfortunately, it leaves the relations between women as providers and professionals inadequately addressed as it does their relations with consumers. In light of such gaps, what is required is a theoretical model that builds upon pre-existing theories, in order to simultaneously address the interrelations between professions, public/clients and the state, from a gender perspective. A preliminary model of this kind is presented in Figure 1.

This model situates Witz' (1992) model of female professional projects, specifically demarcation by the dominant profession and usurpation/ exclusion by the aspiring profession, within the system of professions as described by Abbott (1988) – which could be alternately referred to in this case as the health care division of labour. The jurisdiction under conflict is represented by the overlapping area of the "dominant" and "aspiring" professions. Consistent with Abbott, this model includes interaction between the public and the state – depicted here largely as the government and bureaucracy. These relations are presently conceived as being bidirectional, therefore expanding upon Abbott's depiction of the state and the public as merely audiences, and entailing either or both positive and negative feedback. Additional dimensions to the model include the relations between the public/clients and the state in order to capture the direct relationship that exists between these two bodies; these may in turn have an impact on the dynamics within the system of professions. Relations both between the bodies broadly (public, system of professions, state) and within them enables the deconstructing or unpacking of the state as much as the system of professions has been deconstructed in existing theory. Finally, the model is situated within a broader societal structure (not visually depicted) of capitalist relations of production and patriarchal relations of inequality.

Linking feminist theories of the state with the literature on the professions and relations with public/clients may help to advance a gendered perspective on both the sociology of the professions and the sociology of the state. Indeed, it allows us to pose the following critical questions:

1 What role does the state play in contemporary female professional projects?
2 How do internal female state actors in particular influence the professionalization process of female occupations?
3 How can one, theoretically, explain the affinity of state actors and agencies to particular professional projects, when gender is taken into consideration?
4 What role do consumers play in female professional projects and how does this intersect with the role of the state?
5 How can representatives from female professions become insider groups to the state influencing policy affecting its status? and
6 What is the impact of these varied and complex inter-relations on the occupation as it professionalizes.

It is in attempting to answer these theoretical questions that the illustrative nature of this case study is revealed. That is, in the detailed presentation of the contemporary midwifery professionalization project in Ontario, an attempt to uncover the interrelations between consumers, profession, and state is made possible.

But first, it is important to situate this contemporary professional project within international and historic context. We shall see that all three of these factors – professions, the public, and the state – both individually and collectively help explain the process and outcome of earlier and more recent attempts of midwives to professionalize and become integrated into the health care system in Canada and abroad. Reviewing this literature will also enable greater precision in the theoretical model presented herein.

CHAPTER TWO

International Inspirations
and Cautionary Tales

As noted at the beginning of Chapter 1, to fully understand the recent midwifery professionalization project in Canada, it is important to first situate it in historical and international context. What has come before and what exists in other settings has shaped this new initiative in some subtle and some not so subtle ways. I begin first with the international context in this chapter. I compare the efforts to professionalize midwifery in Britain, Australia, and the United States. The outcomes of these midwifery professional projects – old and new – provide a yardstick against which the efforts of Canadian midwives can be measured. The dynamics of these projects serve in part as "cautionary tales" (Davis-Floyd 1999) for Canadian midwifery. I then turn to a discussion of midwifery in the Netherlands. Canadian midwives turned to the Netherlands for inspiration because it offers an interesting contrast with the Anglo-American models that have dominated the professionalization literature on midwifery. Together these cases help highlight what is unique about the Ontario midwifery project and why it was so successful.

CAUTIONARY TALES:
MIDWIFERY IN THE UK, AUSTRALIA, AND THE US

The Professional Projects of Midwives in Britain

Efforts to obtain legislation regulating midwifery in England date back to 1865 with the work of the Ladies' Medical College, but it was not until the turn of the century, through the efforts of an elite group of midwives who formed the Midwives' Institute, that legislation was secured (Donnison 1977; Heagerty 1990). At that time, midwifery was practised primarily by informally trained, working class "handywomen" whose reputations had been *tarnished*. The subsequent *tarnishing* of the image of midwifery was due largely to the efforts of some vocal physicians. The Midwives' Institute, like the Ladies Medical College, sought to reform midwifery into a respectable occupation for upper and middle class women. To achieve this, the Institute recruited women considered to be of the highest moral character and competence to its organization; once selected, they were required to follow a strict code of conduct. The Institute also attempted to reform the handywomen who made up the majority of midwives, making them into more "lady-like" and respectable practitioners.

In concert with these reformist efforts within the profession, the Institute sought state legislation to regulate the practice of midwifery. Given that women did not yet have the vote, it was necessary for the Institute to mobilize proxy male power to represent their interests to the state (Witz 1992). To this end, the Institute enlisted the aid of women of position and through them attempted to gain the support of their male relatives and friends in Parliament. The Institute also realized that if it were to obtain legislation, it must seek the support of leading obstetricians. Obstetrical support, however, would only be forthcoming if the Institute pursued legislation to regulate midwives as competent to deal with *normal* labour only, precluding the use of instruments, and requiring midwives to seek assistance of a medical practitioner in difficult cases. Some elite physicians became more supportive of midwifery legislation once it was clear that midwives' efforts were not to create a group of rival maternity care providers, but to be watchers of the drudgeries of childbirth and competent assistants when difficult cases arose. Moreover, as Dingwall et al. (1988) note, physicians mainly envisioned midwives as women of working-class origin providing care for women of their own class, whereas doctors would provide care for wealthier women. To appease the medical elite, the Institute further stated that it was to seek legislation for trained midwives only (i.e., those making up the Institute) and not for the more numerous "untrained" handywoman.

In proposing such legislation, the Institute was to encounter resistance from their rank-and-file as well as from activists from the women's movement. Many working midwives and women's activists desired legislation for an autonomous rather than a dependent form of midwifery. Both groups opposed efforts to limit the sphere of midwifery competence and to subordinate midwifery to the medical profession (Witz 1992). They argued that male/medical imperialism was maintained by the Institute's proposed legislation and would result in the suffering of women, both as providers and as recipients of care. They also felt that the legislation proposed by the Institute would restrict women's ability to become licensed midwives and in turn restrict women's job prospects and women's choice of birth attendant.

General practitioners also expressed concern about the Institute's legislative proposal. They felt that licensed midwives would take over attendance at childbirth which was an important entree for GPs toward providing care for the entire family. Despite support for the proposed legislation by established obstetricians, opposition from rank-and-file general practitioners was fierce.[1] Allied with the general practitioners was the British Nurses Association (BNA). The BNA was also seeking legislation for the regulation of the nursing profession. After unsuccessfully attempting to entice midwives to join forces with the BNA to seek dual legislation, the BNA president sought to have midwifery subsumed under nursing legislation for the regulation of nurses and nurse-midwives.

In the end, the Midwives' Institute and its supporters were successful in persuading the British government to propose and pass the Midwives' Act in 1902 making midwifery the first health profession after medicine to be regulated in Britain. The Act, however, had several regressive elements in it which put midwives in a uniquely disadvantaged position (Donnison 1977). Most importantly, midwives were not in charge of their own regulation. They were denied official representation on the Central Midwives Board, the governing body of the profession. Instead, the Act specified that the majority of members on the Board were to be medical practitioners (Robinson 1990).[2] It is for this reason that Witz (1992) describes the Act as comparable to a "spider legislating for the fly" (109).

Legislation, therefore, severely limited midwifery and situated its practitioners in a subordinate position to physicians. That is, the price paid for state legislation and legitimacy for midwives was a loss of professional autonomy and a substantial degree of medical control (Donnison 1977). The Midwives' Act took this form mainly because of the need to obtain support for midwives' legislative efforts from more influential, often conservative, men. The overwhelming majority of midwives were poor, untrained, uneducated, and irregular workers. This did not make for a successful lobby, especially when women did not yet have the vote. The few elite midwives needed to solicit support from those with influence in state politics and in medicine. It was gaining this support that provided enough influence to table midwifery legislation.

The Act also did nothing to modify the two-tier system of midwifery that existed prior to regulation. The upper-middle class, educated midwife and the lower class, untrained handywoman were both licensed as mid-wives under the 1902 Act, mainly because there were too few trained midwives to serve all women, especially in rural areas (Robinson 1990). The inclusion of handywomen in legislation was regarded with dismay by the elite within the Midwives' Institute who felt this would hinder efforts to raise the status of midwifery. Following the 1902 Act, the Institute continually upgraded licensing requirements in the name of advancing midwifery, finally making nursing training a prerequisite for midwifery licensure. Although the "untrained" midwives resisted these exclusionary reform efforts, reform was achieved some 30 years later with the passage of the 1936 Midwives' Act (Heagerty 1990). Within that period of time, the proportion of trained midwives registered under the Midwives' Act increased dramatically from 44 per cent in 1902 to 96 per cent in 1933 (Dingwall et al 1988). Midwifery was essentially being cast as a profession most suitable to mainly single, middle-class recruits.

The 1936 Act also stipulated the development of a nation-wide, salaried, domiciliary service which was proposed as a means of improving the pay and working conditions of midwives during the Depression of the 1930s (Robinson 1990). The years between the 1936 Act and the introduction of the National Health Service (NHS) in 1948 have been described as the heyday of the domiciliary midwife (Barnett 1979). Rising institutional confinement rates increasingly drew midwives into hospitals as employees often under the direction of a physician, a trend which crystalized with the formation of the NHS.[3] Midwives' roles in maternity care was increasingly being eroded while the physicians' role enhanced. Changes in the organization of British maternity care during the 1960s and 1970s, including increasing hospitalization, medical intervention, and specialization of hospital midwives led to a further fragmentation of midwifery care and decline in midwives' independence (Oakley 1984; Robinson 1990). Midwifery practice became even more rigidly limited and specialized with fewer providing continuity of care. It was also increasingly being regarded as an obstetric specialty of nursing, a trend one could argue was linked directly to the exclusionary tactics used by the Midwives Institute decades earlier, and cemented with the replacement of the Central Midwives Board by the United Kingdom Central Council for Nursing, Midwifery and Health Visiting in 1979 (Sandall 1996). Not coincidently, rates of obstetrical interventions were on the rise.

In 1976, a pressure group formed to respond to the diminishing status of the midwife and to the increasing number of women who wanted more control over their birth experience: the Association of Radical Midwives

(ARM) (Weitz 1987). The rising feminist movement and maternity rights movement set the stage for ARM's support of a reduction in medical intervention into childbirth, the enhancement of natural and home birth, the development of more direct-entry training programs, and the promotion of systems of midwifery staffing that enhanced midwives' independence and responsiveness to clients (Flint 1986; Flint, Poulengeris, and Grant 1989; Weitz 1987). As Sandall (1996) notes, feminist writing validated midwifery as a career for women ... and several feminists entered midwifery because of their feminism" (219).

Thus, the British midwifery legislation experience suggests that midwifery has been limited by licensure schemes implemented there during the last century. This case also reveals that legislation results in the increased legitimacy of elite midwives and the ultimate exclusion of others seen as hindering the legitimation process. Midwives' role in maternity care slowly began to erode subsequent to these legislative efforts. Indeed, some could argue that legitimacy has lead British midwifery to become increasingly mainstream and medically oriented. This may be a direct result of the alliances made between the female midwifery elite and their male physician sponsors. A faction within the profession continues to strive to preserve midwifery independence and responsiveness to women's choices forging a new professional project from within the system of which they are acknowledged to be a part. The case of midwifery legislative efforts in Australia, as we shall see, shows striking similarities to the British example, but it also entails some interesting and unique features.

Midwifery Professionalization in Australia

Before examining the efforts to legislate midwifery in Australia, it is important to note that unlike Britain but similar to Canada (as we shall see), there was an indigenous form of midwifery care that existed in Australia before colonization. The development of non-aboriginal midwifery had a "frontier" aspect like early Canadian midwifery in that most of these 'midwives' were self-taught, independent practitioners who provided care to the majority of Australian women" (Robinson 1996/7). Another difference from the British context is that midwifery legislative initiatives came not from an elite group of midwives interested in professionalizing, but from state and public health officials during a time of concern over infant and maternal mortality and "race suicide" (Willis 1989). Following the significant losses of life in World War I, the Australian government established a national program of financial assistance for maternity care for both parents and practitioners.

As in Britain, these legislative efforts were largely accepted by elite, specialist physicians. Opposition was expressed by general practitioners, who for fear of competition did not want midwifery legislation at all; and nurses, who wanted midwifery to be legislated under the auspices of nursing. In its first draft legislation in 1920, midwifery in Australia was licensed as an independent profession separate from nursing, due primarily to the urgent need for midwives in rural areas. This legislation served to place several restrictions on the practice of midwives and bring them under considerable medical control. The "success" at preventing integration into nursing was short-lived when some ten years later, legislation was enacted that subsumed midwifery within the regulatory structure of nursing. This was due to the efforts by organized nurses who wanted to define midwifery within their scope of practice. This served to make midwifery a specialized branch of nursing and not an independent profession. The state, through the "maternity allowance" also encouraged pregnant women to use the services of a doctor rather than that of independent midwives (Reiger 2001). As a result of these initiatives, midwives not only suffered a significant loss of professional autonomy, they were also losing their place within Australian maternity care.

Australian midwives, therefore, experienced significant incursions into their jurisdiction by both physicians and nurses. By 1936, 80 per cent of births in urban areas were either attended or directly supervised by physicians with midwives assisting largely as obstetrical nurses (Robinson 1996/7). Midwives remained in rural and remote areas either as independent practitioners or autonomously within small cottage hospitals, but most of these closed down during the depression leaving few opportunities for this kind of autonomous practice (Reiger 2001). Thus, as Willis (1989) describes, midwifery was originally "limited" and then finally "subordinated" by medicine. He argues that the ultimate subordination of midwifery was achieved by its integration into nursing, an occupation which was itself in a position of subordination to medicine.

More recently, midwives in Australia have attempted to dissociate midwifery from nursing, and similar efforts to those proposed by the ARM in Britain, such as team midwifery, have been proposed (Rowley 1993). In 1983, a more independent professional association, the Australian College of Midwives, emerged out of the Royal Australian Nursing Federation to undertake a variety of initiatives to raise the professional profile of midwives (Robinson 1996/7). These efforts have been undertaken at professional, state, and international levels, and have included hosting the 1984 meeting of the International Congress of Midwives, which helped this new independent midwifery movement gain momentum (Reiger 2001). Reviews of maternity care like those undertaken in Britain have also been initiated by governments in Australia, also calling for a return to a wider role for midwives in the system. Continuity of care, which Sandall (1996) describes as being so integral to the new midwifery professional project in Britain, is also central to midwifery care reforms in Australia. And here in Canada too, we find resistance from many midwives to the newly emerging models of practice, in part because they fear that their roots in nursing may mean that they do not have the necessary skills to practice autonomously (Robinson 1996/7).

The Australian case illustrates that midwifery legislation can have a negative impact on midwifery independence and practice, but that midwives in turn can respond to these limits on their autonomy (and have done so) through organized lobby efforts. These efforts have been fostered both by women's desire to demedicalize birth and their emerging political power in Australia to achieve this (Robinson 1996/7). It is interesting to note how soon in its history midwifery came to be subsumed under the auspices of nursing and perhaps consequently how the fate of midwives' autonomy in Australia suffered more quickly and more dramatically. In the United States, where we now turn, an interesting hybrid form of midwifery was developed early on directly following the professionalizing efforts of the leaders of the Midwives' Institute in Britain.[4]

Midwifery in the United States: Competing Professional Projects

NURSE-MIDWIFERY

Unlike in Britain and Australia, midwifery in the United States was almost completely eradicated in the nineteenth century. In some small pockets, however, nurse-midwifery arose to attend to the needs of the some of the country's most vulnerable women. The first nurse-midwifery practices were established around 1920, one in a poor, inner-city area of New York City – the Maternity Centre Association (MCA), and the other in the remote mountains of Kentucky – the Frontier Nursing Service (FNS) (Hogan 1975). British-trained nurse-midwives and American public health nurses sent to Britain for midwifery training were recruited to work in these practices as it was not until 1932 that the first school for nurse-midwives in the US was established. These early nurse-midwives were quite different from the rapidly disappearing lay midwives (akin to the "handywoman" in Britain). They were predominantly young, white, middle-class, educated professional women who were granted approval to practise among the urban and rural poor, often where (and primarily because) medical services were not readily available.

Nurse-midwifery in the US did not develop without significant disagreements; these stemmed from the ideological disagreement between the FNS and the MCA regarding the autonomy of the nurse-midwife. The FNS nurse-midwives regarded the midwife as an independent health care provider, given that they practised independently by default since few doctors were available geographically. The MCA, which had easier access to physician's services, being located in the city, regarded the midwife as more of an assistant to the physician (Langton 1991). These two groups in turn developed separate professional organizations – the American Association of Nurse-Midwives (AANM) established in Kentucky in 1941, and the American College of Nurse-Midwifery.[5] Langton (1991) has argued that this division explains in part the slow development of the profession.

It was not until 1969 that the American College of Nurse-Midwifery and the AANM joined to create the American College of Nurse-Midwives (ACNM). The main concerns of the newly amalgamated ACNM became achieving legal status for nurse-midwifery (Litoff 1978). Around this time, the demand for nurse-midwifery services from middle-class clients had increased, due in part to the development of the Natural Childbirth Movement and a perceived physician shortage. This created a more socially and economically powerful clientele than before given that nurse-midwives previously worked almost exclusively among the poor. During the 1960s nurse-midwives also became increasingly involved in state-sponsored maternal-infant programs. The excellent outcomes of these projects, in combination with data from the FNS and MCA, increased nurse-midwifery's legitimacy. Nurse-midwives came to be valued by state agencies for their safe obstetrical outcomes, potential cost-effectiveness, and patient satisfaction (Matthews and Zadak 1991). The number of nurse-midwives increased rapidly along with a consequent increase in clinical opportunities and training programs (Rooks and Fischman 1980). These were primarily occurring within the mainstream health care system (Devitt 1977; Teasley 1983).

Along with increased public and state support, nurse-midwives came to acquire more acceptance from some physicians. For many years the ACNM worked diligently to earn the support of physicians for backup services by emphasizing the necessity of physician cooperation, consultation, and backup in their policy statements (Sharp 1980; Tom 1982). One might say that the focus of the ACNM reflected a less independent role for midwives more similar to the philosophy of the MCA-dominant American College of Nurse-Midwifery. Because of this position, nurse-midwives were successful in attaining a vote of confidence from the medical profession when the American College of Obstetricians and Gynecologists (ACOG) issued a joint statement in 1971 with the ACNM officially recognizing nurse-midwives as members of the obstetrical care "team." Nurse-midwives as "team" members were allowed to manage "normal" labour and delivery under the direction and supervision of an obstetrician-gynecologist (Langton 1991). The criteria of "normal" was central to nurse-midwifery's scope of practice, and given that obstetricians were defining normalcy it gave them significant power to control the potential market for nurse-midwifery services (Teasley 1983).

Not all physicians supported the development of nurse-midwifery. The American College of Family Physicians, for example, strongly opposed nurse-midwifery out of fear of being displaced from normal maternity care (Crawford 1968). Physician resistance, expressed by some physicians, medical societies, departments of obstetrics and gynecology, and physician-controlled malpractice insurance companies includes refusals of practice privileges, unreasonable restrictions on practice, unreasonable demands for liability insurance, misrepresentations of nurse-midwifery practice to the public, and professional ostracism of physicians who collaborate with nurse-midwives (Tom 1982; McCormick 1983). Some CNMs have responded with law suits, such as antitrust cases, claiming restraint of trade (Teasley 1983).

Despite this opposition, state legislation regulating and legalizing the practice of nurse-midwives has occurred. Whereas in 1968 only two states had licensure laws for nurse-midwives (Crawford 1968), currently all states have legislation recognizing the practice of nurse-midwifery. Fifteen states have legislation expressly for nurse-midwives and the others have special legislation under the practice of nursing (Evenson 1982; Barickman, Bidgood–Wilson and Ackley 1992; Bidgood–Wilson, Barickman and Ackley 1992). Nurse-midwives were also successful in attaining third-party reimbursement from government medical programs (e.g., Medicaid) and from some medical insurance companies in the late 1970s, due to the argument that nurse-midwifery is a cost-effective form of care (Tom 1982).With this increased recognition, the number of nurse-midwives in the US doubled between 1968 and 1976 from approximately 800 to 1700 (Evenson 1982).

Thus, organized nurse-midwifery in the US has been able to gain a fair degree of acceptance and partial integration into the American health care system. This move into the mainstream health care system increased the legitimacy of nurse-midwifery and the accessibility of nurse-midwives, but it represented a significant departure from the nurse-midwife being "in charge" (Sharp 1980). Nurse-midwives were not independent practitioners but part of a "team." Their practice patterns also changed within the hospital environment in that they began to do procedures that were part of normal obstetric practice as medically delegated acts, and many were forced to abandon traditional patterns of comprehensive care in favour of a more episodic mode in which the midwife attends only part of the woman's labour (Flanagan 1986; Sharp 1980). Many had to struggle to maintain their unique approach to care while at the same time easing the heavy workloads of obstetricians and maintaining cost-effectiveness in response to institutional imperatives (Flanagan 1986).

The subsequent form of state legislation for nurse-midwifery often followed the manner in which it was integrated into the health care system. Thus, state legislation also had a negative impact. In most states nurse-midwifery is not self-governing but is subsumed under the board either of medicine or of nursing, in some cases with a significant lack of midwife representation (Evenson 1982; McCormick 1983). Evenson (1982) asserted that "State legislation and regulations governing midwifery largely reflect medical establishment attitudes which perpetuate the dominant role of physicians ... The almost universal requirement that a nurse-midwife function under the supervision of a physician denies her the opportunity to practice as an independent health care provider" (319 and 321). Evenson argues further that legitimation carries with it a subordinate status within the health care system and limitations on the kind of work nurse-midwives do and on the women they are allowed to care for.

Thus, as was the case in Britain and Australia, integration and state legitimation of this uniquely US form of nurse-midwifery led to remarkably similar negative consequences in terms of the scope of practice and independence of midwives with legislation and integration into the mainstream maternity care system. But unlike the previous two cases, this professional project was to be challenged not from within, but from a lay group that developed outside the profession.

THE NEW LAY MIDWIFERY

The late 1960s and early 1970s not only marked a rise in nurse-midwifery, it also saw a resurgence of interest in the idea of lay midwifery.[6] This interest stemmed from the consumer backlash against medicalized childbirth promoted by the counterculture Home Birth Movement. Home Birth proponents argued that birth is a normal life process that should take place naturally within the supportive, familiar environment of one's home, and not in a hospital where it had become a medicalized, mechanized, and technologized event under the direction of a physician (Hosford 1976; Reid 1989). Within this counterculture birth environment, some women who had had a home birth or who had attended a home birth were invited to attend others, sometimes acting as assistants. These birth assistants were like traditional lay midwives in that they were usually friends or neighbours who had experience with birth, had observed some births, and had begun to help out at births; their training was derived from experience and participation in the home birth culture (Mason 1988; McCool and McCool 1989). But unlike the old lay midwives, these new lay midwives were more likely to be young, white, educated, and from middle-class backgrounds, and have a clientele with similar racial and class backgrounds.

Originally, these birth helpers did not regard what they were doing as a career or a profession, but the demands on their expertise and time from clients and apprentices rapidly grew beyond those originally required by close group of friends. In response to this increased demand, these birth helpers' practices became more formalized. They began to organize into small groups to share information, expand their educational repertoire, and get social support from others doing this kind of work (Reid 1989).

Lay midwifery practices expanded rapidly across North America despite being illegal or quasi-legal in many jurisdictions. This rapid expansion was regarded by many physicians with increasing concern. Physicians in the US generally dislike the idea of lay midwifery even more than they dislike nurse-midwifery because their concerns about competition are compounded with concerns about the safety of home births and the lack of formal training of lay midwives. Because their practice was officially illegal in most states, several physicians concerned with the encroachment of lay midwifery laid charges against these midwives for practising medicine without a licence and other violations. This resulted in a flurry of trials against midwives in the 1970s and 1980s (Sullivan and Weitz 1988).

Concurrent with this legal harassment of lay midwives, women's health activists became increasingly concerned with the fate of midwives. Although the women's movement originally engaged in "freeing women from the shackles of childbirth and mothering" (Barrington 1985: 151) by lobbying for access to contraception and abortion for women (Ruzek 1978), some activists within the women's health movement later began to focus on the oppression of women through maternity care practices (Arms 1975; Corea 1977; O'Brien 1981; Rothman 1981). One of lay midwifery's key philosophical principles – greater personal control and responsibility for birth – which arose from its roots in the Home Birth Movement, also prompted support from some women's health advocates. This was because it paralleled one of the central tenets of the rising women's health movement – women taking responsibility for and control over their health (Rushing 1993; Ruzek 1978). Lay midwifery soon came to be seen by some as a symbol of women controlling the reproduction process as it enabled women to be active and in control of the childbirth process (Rothman 1989). This midwifery was referred to as "subtle feminism" (Rushing 1993) and "feminist praxis" (Rothman 1989). The fate of midwives also came to typify the struggle of the women's movement (Ehrenreich and English 1973) with trials against lay midwives becoming a "feminist cause celebre" (Ruzek 1978).

In response to these trials, lay midwifery organizations, which had originally formed for self-education and social support, formalized around the issue of legalization and third-party reimbursement (Sullivan and Weitz 1988). The first effort to legitimate lay midwifery in the United States began in California after the arrests of three lay midwives in Santa Cruz in 1974 and their trial in 1976 (DeVries 1982). In 1977 a bill was introduced to the California state legislature proposing to establish a training and certification program for lay midwives. This bill was motivated by a concern for public health and was justified on the basis of reduced costs for state-supplied maternity care, given that midwives would charge less than physicians. Midwives generally supported the attempt at legal recognition, although a few were concerned about the possibility of excessive medical control. Physicians opposed the recognition of midwives and the California Medical Association lobbied strongly against the bill. The California Nurses Association also opposed the bill due to their fear of a loss of jurisdiction because the bill proposed that midwives be controlled by a medical rather than nursing licensing board. In the end, the bill failed to pass even after undergoing several revisions, each of which significantly increased medical control. The legal status of the California lay midwife remained uncertain for some time but they now have licensure as midwives in Arizona do (Midwifery Alliance of North America website 2004).

Integration efforts in Arizona proved to be more successful, as it became the first state to reintroduce legislation for the practice of lay midwifery. The process of legalization began when the Arizona Attorney

General prosecuted a lay midwife in 1977 after pressure from local physicians (Weitz and Sullivan 1986). The midwife's lawyer was able to locate
an old statute of licensure for lay midwives that was still active, the
requirements of which his client fully met. Soon after, thirteen other practising lay midwives applied for the licence. Neither the medical community in Arizona nor the medically dominated State Department of Health
Services approved of the reactivation of this outdated licensure program
and they responded by adopting more stringent rules and regulations the
following year. These new rules gave the state and the medical profession
greater control over the practice of midwifery, including the types of services midwives could offer and requirements for medical screening and
backup, and greater control over entrance to the occupation, including
training requirements and performance on the qualifying exam. Nevertheless, many licensed Arizona midwives feel that licensure has increased
their status and recognition (Sullivan and Weitz 1988).

Other attempts at state regulation, such as in Colorado (Tjaden 1987)
have also been documented. Bills proposing the regulation of the practice
of midwifery as separate from the practice of medicine and regulated by
an advisory board under the State Department of Health were submitted
to the state legislature in 1983, 1984, and 1985. The proposed advisory
board was to consist of two physicians, one nurse-midwife, three licensed
midwives, and one home birth client. Lay midwives and home birth
advocates, who had formed the Colorado Midwives Association, lobbied
strongly for the bills after facing dissent within the group over whether
or not legislation would undermine lay midwifery ideology and practice.
Opposition to the bill came from physicians, nurses, and certified nurse-
midwives, on the grounds that the proposal gave lay midwives too much
autonomy and freedom from supervision by physicians. Certified nurse-
midwives, who had been granted legal recognition as maternity care providers in Colorado in 1977, but not as independent practitioners, did not
wish to see another licensed practitioner achieve more autonomy with
less training. Compromises reached in subsequent drafts of the proposal
still did not meet with the approval of opponents and hearings on the
bill were postponed indefinitely.

Some efforts to legalize lay midwifery have clearly been more successful
than others. Lay midwives have also been successful in securing insurance reimbursement from a few small companies, based in part on the
argument that people are entitled to "alternative" health care.[7] General
trends in all of these three efforts to legislate lay midwifery in the US
point to the importance of liaisons between midwives, consumers, and

some feminist groups who strongly support legislation; and physicians, nurses, and nurse-midwives both individually and through their associations who oppose it. The opposition from nurse-midwives is particularly interesting and reveals a unique challenge to these two professional projects: *intraprofessional competition*.

THE "REAL" MIDWIVES?

One of the most salient issues in an examination of midwifery integration in the United States from a comparative perspective is the significant rift that exists between nurse-midwives and lay midwives. These two groups of midwives differ mainly in terms of the content and context of their educational background and in their relative recognition and legitimacy.[8] New lay midwives are educated through community-based apprenticeships alongside practising lay midwives attending home births. For the most part, they do not have any previous nursing education. More recently, lay midwives created a North American Registry of Midwives (NARM) and began to work on creating a new direct-entry credential, the Certified Professional Midwife (CPM) in the early 1990s and had it up and running by 1994 (Davis-Floyd 1999). Nurse-midwives, on the other hand, are educated first as nurses and later specialize in midwifery, usually within a formal program in an institutional setting. Furthermore, whereas nurse-midwifery is legalized in all fifty states, lay midwifery is currently legal in only thirty-five states, regulated by the state government in nineteen, and prohibited in ten (Barickman et al. 1992; Bidgood-Wilson et al. 1992; MCAP 1994, Midwifery Alliance of North America website).[9] Stemming in part from these differences in their education and legitimacy, there are important differences in their views regarding relations with the medical profession and the requirement of nursing education for the practice of midwifery.

Nurse-midwives tend to work in collaboration with physicians (Haas and Rooks 1986). This collaborative relationship was secured by the ACOG/ACNM Joint Statement in 1971, and has been strengthened by subsequent agreements in 1975 and 1982 (Langton 1991). Many nurse-midwives are unwilling to jeopardize the provisional acceptance they have recently garnered from some members of the medical profession by aligning themselves with the more radical home-birth/lay midwifery movement. It is noteworthy that soon after the ACNM made its Joint Statement with the ACOG in 1971, it made an official statement favouring hospital over home births (ACNM 1973).

Lay midwives tend to be less formally associated with members of the medical profession than nurse-midwives largely because of their differing opinions on the safety of home birth. Because of the close association with physicians, nurse-midwives have been depicted by some lay midwifery supporters as an extension of the oppressive medical establishment (Arms 1975; Rothman 1981). These concerns concur with those of others who argue that while the move by nurse-midwives into the mainstream health care system increased the accessibility, professional status, and work opportunities for nurse-midwives, the greater acceptance nurse-midwives garnered from physicians had a price – less autonomy. Their scope of practice and access to clients were controlled by physicians. Moreover, in most states nurse-midwifery is not self-governing, but is either subsumed under the board of medicine or nursing, and there has been a significant lack of nurse-midwife representation on these boards (Evenson 1982; Flanagan 1986).

Lay midwives and their supporters also point to problems with a reliance on nursing training in that it links nurse-midwives to nursing's history of subordination by physicians (DeVries 1986) and it thereby turns off many would-be midwives and substantially reduces the pool of potential applicants to nurse-midwifery educational programs. Some nurse-midwives argue that their nursing training is an important and essential element in the wider scope of practice necessary in many settings (Rooks 1983). This has been a significant factor in the continuing division between these two groups.

The division between lay and nurse-midwives is not completely clear-cut. For example, some nurse-midwives have come to wonder whether they were becoming too mainstream (Lubic 1976) and a few began to question interdependence with physicians (Flanagan 1986; Sharp 1980). Some nurse-midwives even became involved in the home birth movement and together with lay midwives developed a national organization representing all midwives in 1982, the Midwifery Alliance of North America (MANA) (Schlinger 1992; Ventre and Leonard 1982).[10] MANA's efforts to unify the profession of midwifery were initially met with opposition from the ACNM, who were concerned that an alliance with non-nurse-midwives would tarnish the CNM's professional image and jeopardize recent gains made by the profession (Shah 1982). The animosity between the ACNM and MANA was played out on the international scene when MANA's bid to become a recognized member organization of the International Confederation of Midwives (ICM) in 1984 was opposed by the ACNM. This opposition, although unsuccessful, caused many midwives, both lay and nurse, to regard the ACNM as an elitist organization that discriminated against lay midwives (Ventre and Leonard 1982; Walsh and Jaspan 1990).

Subsequent efforts have been made to unify these two groups; these included the Carnegie meetings held throughout the late 1980s and early 1990s and in the creation of the "Bridge Club" in 1997 (Davis-Floyd 1999). These efforts have reflected the convergence in the position of lay and nurse-midwives regarding the importance of nursing to midwifery education amongst nurse-midwives and the importance of standardization amongst lay midwives (Davis-Floyd 1999). Similar to perspectives in the UK and Australia, a large portion of American nurse-midwives now acknowledge that nursing need not be a mandatory part of midwifery education. Other nurse-midwives express acceptance of a direct-entry form of midwifery and advocate for multiple routes of entry and sites of midwifery practice with similar standards (Burst 1977, 1981; Lubic 1976). In light of this, the ACNM has begun to develop its own direct-entry educational programs and certification.

There has also been a move toward greater acceptance of standardization and credentialization amongst lay midwives with the creation of the Midwifery Education and Accreditation Council (MEAC) by MANA representatives in 1991 and the North American Registry of Midwives (NARM) created in 1987 (Davis-Floyd 1999; Garland Spindel 1995). One of the main reasons behind the development of this exam and registry was to enhance the recognition of the "direct-entry" midwifery.[11] Like nurse-midwives, "direct-entry" midwives now have a credential – the Certified Professional Midwife. The ACNM exhibited a more tolerant stance toward the development of direct-entry midwifery when it made an official statement in 1990 recognizing that direct-entry midwifery educational programs can augment nurse-midwifery programs (Muzio 1990). Despite this formal statement of mutual respect, the political reality is that organizations representing nurse-midwives and lay-midwives remain somewhat at odds.

Thus, midwifery in the US is still a profession divided, with lay midwifery being practised predominantly in home settings and nurse-midwifery being practised predominantly in institutional settings, and with lay midwives having less recognition than nurse-midwives. This is reflected in the numbers of midwives practising, which according to 1994/95 estimates is between 1500 and 1800 lay or direct-entry midwives (Garland Spindel 1995), and 4000 nurse-midwives (ACNM 1995). It is also reflected in the number of midwife-attended births, which has remained at less than 1 per cent of all births for lay/direct entry midwives, whereas the number of nurse-midwifery attended births has grown steadily from 0.6 per cent in 1975 to 3.2 per cent in 1989 and 7.5 per cent in 2001 (Declerq 1992, 2004; Martin et al. 2002).[12] Despite these differences, we nevertheless see similarities in the impact of integration on lay and nurse-midwives.

REFLECTING ON INTEGRATION IN THE UNITED STATES
As one of the first sociologists to critically analyze the impact of the legalization of lay midwifery, DeVries (1982, 1985, 1986, 1996), argues that the effect of licensure on lay midwives strongly resembles the effect of legitimation on certified nurse-midwives. First, licensed midwives and nurse-midwives both have a more interventionist stance regarding birth than do unlicensed lay midwives, due in part to their training within the mainstream health care system and to their more established working relations with physicians. Second, licensed and nurse-midwives both have a larger role-set with less emphasis being placed upon the practitioner-client relationship. Third, licensed midwives and nurse-midwives have strict boundaries of practice in terms of clientele, procedures, and the drugs and equipment they are able to use. Recruits into licensed midwifery and nurse-midwifery are also less likely to view midwifery as a calling than as a way to make a living. Finally, licensed and nurse-midwives are pressured into routinizing care and standardizing the birth experience.

DeVries makes a distinction between "friendly" licensing, which places the control of the practice in the hands of those to be regulated, and "hostile" licensing, which places control in the hands of others. In a comparison of lay midwifery regulation in three states – California, Texas, and Arizona – he argues that all of the laws proposed or enacted in these states are examples of "hostile" licensure. He asserts that legal recognition for midwives implies restriction and a decrease in autonomy, as it often requires supervision by physicians. Legalization serves to formalize medical control over the practice of midwifery. DeVries also claims that licensure subverts midwifery by: 1) restricting access to the profession to those who can afford lengthy training that socializes students into a more mainstream view of childbirth and childbirth practices; 2) restricting midwives' access to clients to those defined as low-risk by physicians; and 3) restricting midwives' use of techniques to those considered safe by medical superiors. DeVries (1986) concludes that licensure "frees midwives from the fear of criminal prosecution, but it sharply reduces their independence … [and as a result] is certain to diminish the alternative character of the profession in time" (1148–49). He concludes that licensure will destroy lay midwifery and that only "those who stay outside the law … have the benefit of remaining true to their own ideals of practice" (1986, 1147).

Sullivan and Weitz (1988) have questioned DeVries' conclusions about the effect of licensure on lay midwifery, criticizing his comparison of lay midwifery with the fate of certified nurse-midwives, a group with very different origins. They assert that discussing the medicalizing effects of nurse-midwifery tells us little about the true effects of licensure on lay midwives. DeVries' arguments, however, have been echoed by others (Annandale 1988, 1989; Butter and Kay 1988; Gaskin 1988; Kay et al. 1988; Ventre 1976). In a national survey assessing the current status and characteristics of state legislation regulating the practice of lay midwives, Butter and Kay (1988) found that in the twenty-one states with no legislation there were better opportunities for midwifery practice than in states with licensure. DeVries argues in a revisitation of his 1985 book that "where there are no clear regulations governing the practice of midwifery, an 'uneasy truce' between midwives and the medical community continues: midwives are free to practise until they attract the attention of medical professionals. If a client of a midwife comes to the attention of a physician and the physician believes something improper was done, then the law is invoked as a regulatory mechanism and courts become the arena of regulation. Over the past ten years, stories of this sort of regulation, many of them dramatic, have accumulated" (DeVries 1996, 175). Further, in those cases where obstetricians are unable to halt the integration of midwifery into the mainstream maternity care system, Annandale (1989) argues that they are still able to control the terms and content of the everyday practice of midwives. This means that midwives are not always able to maintain the naturalness of birth because of the need to standardize birth in conformity with obstetrical expectations (Annandale 1988).

Sullivan and Weitz (1984) also concur with DeVries, in part. In response to the rules that midwives had to operate under as dictated by legislation in Arizona, midwives consciously attempted to make their appearance, behaviour, and clients more acceptable to physicians. Midwives also modified their belief and practices towards a more medicalized model of care (Weitz and Sullivan 1985). Crucial aspects of this change have been midwives' increasing medicalization of three things: 1) the definition of childbirth, seeing the potential for medical problems to arise; 2) the management of childbirth, becoming more accepting of interventionist procedures; and 3) the practitioner-client relationship, moving towards a more hierarchical style of practice.

Although Weitz and Sullivan (1985) believe that licensing has been a major factor in these changes, they argue that it is not the only factor. Other factors eroding the alternative nature of lay midwifery include: "1) midwives' cumulative experience with handling obstetrical problems, augmented by their knowledge of problems faced by other midwives; and 2) the growing social acceptance of midwifery, which has led to changes in their clientele, the need for bureaucratic practice settings, and the desire to earn a living at midwifery" (Weitz and Sullivan 1985: 51). They (1988) argue, for example, that self-imposed training and voluntary self-certification programs, which several state lay midwifery organization have initiated (see Butter and Kay 1990 for example), are remarkably similar to those instituted by midwives working under a licensing system. One could argue that these self-imposed programs are a response to or otherwise reflect a desire for legitimacy or licensure. Regarding client relations, with the growing societal acceptance of midwifery, many clients now choose midwives because they are cheaper than physicians, and not because they share their midwives' "counterculture" values. This serves to create a larger social distance between the two and to open up the possibility of a more hierarchical relationship. Thus, Sullivan and Weitz (1988) conclude that "While licensure has contributed to midwifery's visibility, accessibility, and acceptability, similar developments have occurred in states without licensure laws, although not to the same extent. It is this natural growth – facilitated by but not dependent on licensure – that has changed the nature of midwifery's clientele and encouraged midwives to enlarge their practices, thus reducing to a *small degree* their ability to provide holistic, individualized, nonhierarchical care" (111, emphasis added).

Reid (1989) has also pointed to a combination of factors, other than licensure, that have led to the evolution of midwife relationships away from a model of friends and sisters to one of professionals. These include midwives' desire to progress and improve their working conditions, and the desire to grant more women the opportunity to experience a midwife-attended home birth. With an expanding clientele, midwives' relations with their clients and other midwives changed and became more formal and their practice more business-like. In addition, the national organization of lay midwives, although crucial for the legitimation process, also served to distance the midwife from her immediate friendship circle – she was now part of a larger entity called lay midwifery. The setting up of standards of practice within these groups added to the conflict and dissension, as it signified to some a departure from the individualistic approach to birth that lay midwives originally promoted. Reid (1989) states that many of these changes pre-empted any form of legislation. Specifically, she argues that the "radical nature of original lay midwifery had already been modified ... Legislation spelled out the parameters even more clearly" (236).

It is clear from this example of legislation of lay midwifery in the US that although licensure creates significant changes in the practice of midwifery, other factors that have accompanied the evolution of midwifery have also had their effect. Taken together, these legislative examples suggest that lay midwifery also suffers serious consequences upon receiving state legitimacy, as has nurse-midwifery and British and Australian midwifery. Midwives' practices come increasingly under medical control and in turn their philosophy regarding natural birth becomes more medicalized and their relations with clients and other midwives more hierarchical. One could argue that the more integrated midwifery becomes the more limited it is. But this is not always the case. Indeed, midwives everywhere have looked to the situation of midwives in the Netherlands in particular for inspiration. Here we see some striking differences in the role and recognition of midwives within the health care system.

INSPIRATION: MIDWIFERY IN THE NETHERLANDS

The Netherlands is noted worldwide for its unique system of maternity care in which midwives and home birth remain a critical element (DeVries 1996; van Teijlinden and van der Hulst 1995). For example, in 1992 midwives attended 45.8 per cent of the births and 31.5 per cent took place in women's homes, with excellent perinatal and maternal mortality outcomes (DeVries 1996). The Netherlands also has the lowest Caesarean section rate among several European and North American countries. These numbers tell only part of the story.

Dutch midwives are known for their high degree of professional autonomy (DeVries et al. 2001, DeVries 2004); they are considered to be medical practitioners regulated under the same college as physicians, dentists, and pharmacists (Eberts et al. 1987). Training has always been direct-entry and since 1912 takes three years to complete (Smulders and Limburg 1988; van Teijlinden and van der Hulst 1995). Midwives are expected to work independently and not under hospital or medical authority. This helps ensure that midwifery training remains separate from nursing. The majority of midwives (approximately 70 per cent) work in independent practice and their primary mode of reimbursement is based on a fee-for-service model (Benoit 1991). In these situations, the midwives are on call twenty-four hours a day, particularly in cases where they do not share care (i.e., most midwives are in solo practice, though group practices are increasing) (Benoit 1991; Smulders and Limburg 1988). Some midwives work as salaried employees in clinics and in the obstetrical units of hospitals (Smulders and Limburg 1988).

Thus, as Benoit (1991) describes, "in the Netherlands crucial aspects of the traditional maternity care system based on independent midwifery practice have been retained, with institutionalized practice complementing rather than replacing homebirth attendance" (28). In comparison to mid-wifery in other jurisdictions, van Teijlinden and van der Hulst (1995) argue that it is more than a semi-profession as it has more power and autonomy vis-à-vis the medical profession than exists elsewhere: "Dutch midwives have their own jurisdiction over normal childbirth reflecting a psychosocial model" (184).

When one questions why this situation exists, DeVries (1996) points out that "[t]he most common explanation of this phenomenon focuses on the structure of Dutch medical care: historians and sociologists point to early legislation that favoured midwives, to an insurance system that gives midwives an advantage over their competitors, and to a well-developed program of postpartum care in the home" (Hingstman 1994). The legis-lation officially recognizing Dutch midwives as independent practitioners in 1865 was early by comparative standards (van Teijlinden and van der Hulst 1995) even when midwives were confined to "normal" deliveries (Smulders and Limburg 1988). This early legislation was probably enabled by the fact that the modern state in the Netherlands developed prior to the development of the medical profession (which lagged behind in the Netherlands in comparison to other countries) (van Teijlinden and van der Hulst 1995). As we have already seen, the medical profession in the UK (by way of comparison) was more organized and, as a result, the legislation in Britain – which happened later – was more restrictive of midwives' professional development. We will see that in Canada, where legislative attempts came much later, the result was so restrictive as to cause the near eradication of midwifery. So, timing is important.

It is also important to note that the medical profession was never against midwifery recognition in the Netherlands. Smulders and Limburg (1988), for example, highlight the importance of the sponsorship by prom-inent physicians midwifery has had. They state, "In Holland, the midwife has assumed this unique position in public health because throughout history she has always been able to rely on the support of influential doctors and obstetric surgeons" (238). Similarly, van Teijlinden and van der Hulst (1995) say, "rather than lobbying against midwives in the late nineteenth and well into the twentieth century, prominent obstetricians advocated the cause of the Dutch midwife." Dutch midwives also enjoyed more assistance from the academic medical establishment in the form of training (Smulders and Limburg 1988). In fact, there was much coopera-tion as opposed to confrontation between physicians and midwives early on; this continues with the professional custom (DeVries et al. 2001, DeVries 2004) that specialists do not attend normal deliveries.

State support was also important and, following its early recognition, continued to protect midwifery through subsequent legislative efforts. For example, in its attempt to reduce high infant mortality rates, rather than mandate hospital birth as was done in other jurisdictions, the government introduced regulation and training of maternity home care assistants through the National Institute for Maternity Aid (Smulders and Limburg 1988; van Teijlinden and van der Hulst 1995). Under this legislation, maternity home assistants would assist the midwife by providing care and support for new mothers and their babies in the postpartum period (van Teijlinden and van der Hulst 1995).[13] Home care assistants provide nursing care to the mother and baby, breast-feeding advice, and other health education, as well as domestic help in the form of cleaning, shopping, or looking after other children (van Teijlinden and van der Hulst 1995). Maternity care assistants help to relieve midwives of most of their post-delivery nursing activities (Smulders and Limburg 1988). In developing maternity home care assistance, van Teijlinden and van der Hulst (1995) argue that the state legitimizes an occupation whose role included being an assistant to the midwife and furthermore whose existence was fundamental in enabling birth to remain in the home, traditionally the domain of the midwife. They state, "the midwife's sense of professional autonomy is [also] strengthened by the existence of maternity home care assistants ... they have some degree of authority over another occupation in their field" (180).

DeVries also alluded to the protection of midwife-attended births in the Dutch health insurance system. In 1941 the government, through the Sick Fund Act, sought to protect midwives' central role in maternity which had started becoming more tenuous with increasing competition by GPs. The Act stated that women covered by national health insurance would not be reimbursed GPs' fees for providing maternity care when there was a midwife practising in the area (Vans, Smulders, and Limburg 1988). Moreover, both the state and private health insurance plans[14] do not cover birth attended by specialists unless it is warranted by risk factors (Benoit 1991; DeVries et al. 2001, DeVries 2004).

Thus, although the Netherlands is not completely immune to the trends toward the increasing medicalization of birth that exists in other developed nations (DeVries et al. 2001, DeVries 2004)[15], as van Tiejlinden and van der Hulst (1995) argue, "the elevated position of midwives is due in large part to the influence of the state on the provision of health care in general and the regulation of health occupations in particular" (178). Smulders and Limburg (1988) argue similarly that "the government has consistently protected the midwife by guaranteeing her an income, by institutionalizing home delivery and by fully subsidizing the maternity aid system" (238). In the face of declining home birth rates, the Dutch government has joined forces with midwifery professional associations in a public education campaign emphasizing the importance of home birth in Dutch society (DeVries 2001, 2004). The Dutch government has also defied some obstetricians who feel their system of maternity care is severely lacking in part because the structure of the Dutch state resists pressure by powerful medical lobbies (DeVries 2001, 2004). But what remains to be asked is why the state was so supportive in the Netherlands. Smulders and Limburg (1988) allude to the fact that "midwives have represented a more affordable delivery option for the poorer people in Holland" (238) but do not explicitly link this to state support.

Despite these analyses of the historical development of the unique situation that Dutch midwifery finds itself in, we are nevertheless left asking, as DeVries poses: "why did this structure emerge in the Netherlands and not elsewhere" (1996: xvii). DeVries is particularly interested in the issue of home birth and so delves into a thoughtful analysis of the unique culture of the Netherlands and its early emphasis on the "nuclearized" family, solidarity, and domesticity (DeVries 2001, 2004). As he describes, "in the seventeenth and eighteenth centuries the Dutch were renowned for their domesticity. Homes were small, tidy and the center of family life – a perfect setting for birth." The small, densely populated geography of the Netherlands where women are never far from hospitals and specialist care is offered by DeVries (2001, 2004) as another explanation for the persistence of midwifery-attended home birth.

SUMMARY OF MIDWIFERY PROFESSIONALIZATION LITERATURE

In sum, we find from this review of the midwifery professionalization literature that the integration of midwifery in various countries faces similar challenges and includes comparable dynamics as those of other health professions seeking integration discussed in the previous chapter. Specifically, attempts at integration by midwives in the UK, Australia, and the US, like other aspiring health professionals, are faced with varying degrees of opposition from physicians and in some cases also from nursing. That Dutch midwifery has less medical opposition makes it a truly unique case. In all cases, however, support elicited from a few significant medical elites was integral to midwifery, ability to survive or thrive.

Midwifery across these cases also exhibits varying degrees of conflict within its ranks, or between the elite and rank-and-file, throughout the process of integration, as do other health professions. This is particularly salient in the deep division between nurse and direct-entry midwifery in the US, which likely has an important impact on midwifery's status and professionalism. Conflict was also evident earlier in Britain when, relatively early on, midwifery became *nurse*-midwifery to reflect the desires of its professionalizing elite members.

By and large, the outcomes of integration efforts by midwives in the UK, Australia and the US are similar to those that have been described for other health professions. This includes the limitation of midwives' scope of practice, subordination of midwifery practitioners, bureaucratization of their occupational organizations, and medicalization of their ideology and practice. That is, the trend seems to be that the more integrated midwifery is in the various health care systems analysed – the more limited, subordinated, bureaucratized, and medicalized is their care. By way of contrast, this is not true of midwifery in the Netherlands. The unique set of circumstances for midwifery in that country make it less comparable to the Canadian context than its Anglo-American counterparts. Therefore, it seems likely that any effort to integrate midwives in Canada would likely result in similar negative circumstances to those witnessed in the US, the UK, and Australia.

Consumer support of midwifery integration or professionalization is most salient in the emergence of lay midwifery in the US but is also noted as being important for the revitalization of independent midwifery in both the UK and Australia. It is unclear from the literature on Dutch midwifery whether this is a critical feature in the maintenance of midwives' status in their system of maternity care; in fact it is only in the last few years – with Dutch midwifery under threat because of a decline in home births – that parents began to organize in support of midwives (DeVries 2004).

State support also arises as an important factor – particularly in the Dutch example – and this, coupled with less medical opposition and perhaps fewer internal divisions, has led to the maintenance of a significant role for midwives in their system of maternity care. State support in this context has helped quell any attempt by physicians intent on reforming a maternity care system which significantly favours midwives. State support for midwifery is emerging (or re-emerging) in the UK, but this is less clear in the Australian and American contexts.

Although many insights can be gained from this review of midwifery in other settings, one issue that remains overlooked is the specific gendered dynamics of state support and how this might be linked to consumer support. DeVries (2001, 2004) has chosen to credit the culture of Dutch society as the key to the support the state has so willingly provided to the midwifery profession. This offers us an important new perspective on this issue. A gender perspective on the nexus between state and consumer support for this female health profession offers us another. Thus, informed by the profession's literature and the literature on midwifery integration, I focus on precisely that issue in the case of "the re-emergence of midwifery" (Burtch 1994) in Canada.

Canadian midwifery, which I present in a historical perspective in the next chapter, offers us an interesting case in which to analyse the key factors influencing midwifery integration as a female professional project. That there was no legislation devoted to midwifery prior to the 1990s – making Canada unique among developed nations – meant that there was a sort of *tabula rasa* from which midwifery could be recreated. The examination of this case also helps to reveal the contemporary dynamics of the relations between women, professions, and the state.

CHAPTER THREE

The Fall and Rise of Midwifery in Canada

Before the turn of the twentieth century, midwives in Canada, as in many other countries, were the predominant attendants at childbirth. Prior to European contact, traditional Aboriginal midwives played a fundamental role in the childbirth process (Carroll and Benoit 2004). Native women often served as midwives to new Canadian settlers, and their birth practices were as effective as, and in some cases more effective than, European ones (Rushing 1991). Colonial governments also appointed midwives, an indication of the importance of midwifery to early colonial life and the respectability of this position (Rushing 1991). For example, in New France (what was later to become Quebec) midwifery was considered a profession in its own right and a distinctive branch of medicine (Laforce 1990). Physicians, surgeons, and midwives practised with little conflict and with mutual respect, reinforced by the fact that many came from similar socioeconomic backgrounds. Each of these three groups was governed by rights and obligations and structured according to a strict hierarchy. In the larger cities midwifery services were remunerated with a set fee, whereas in the villages it was part of a system of community support. Some women in New France even had the privilege of electing their midwife, a right that women elsewhere in Canada never enjoyed.

Caution should be taken in generalizing from the organization of midwifery in early Quebec to that in the rest of Canada. Indeed, the system of midwifery care in New France rapidly deteriorated with the British conquest. Midwifery in English Canada largely did not exist as an organized profession. Childbirth, particularly in rural areas, was considered a community affair often handled by female neighbours of the parturient woman (Mason 1987) and repaid with services rendered in kind (Connor 1994). These women's training was derived less from formal study and apprenticeship than from participation in a birth culture that expected neighbour women to help each other out (Mason 1987). Support included material aid, such as a layette for the newborn baby, as well as emotional support during labour and delivery, and afterward. In general, little physical interference in the birthing process occurred. Although women whose primary function was being a midwife was rare, some women in certain communities did act as midwives and were regarded and called upon for their special knowledge and skills in childbirth attendance (Biggs 2004).

THE FALL OF MIDWIFERY IN CANADA

This early, informal system of midwifery care in English Canada and the more formal system which existed in French Canada were soon eclipsed by various factors and forces. The first was a rise in medical interest in childbirth attendance toward the end of the eighteenth century. The medical profession in Canada was relatively late to develop and initially was not seriously interested in the practice of midwifery or the exclusion of midwives. It was only towards the end of the eighteenth century when their numbers grew and they began to organize as a profession that the first male medical practitioners entered the childbirth scene, primarily as an entrée into family practice (Barrington 1985; Rushing 1991).

The first act in Upper Canada established to limit the practice of midwifery to members of the medical profession dates back to 1795 (Biggs 1983; Connor 1989, 1994; Mason 1987). Given the scant population of Ontario at that time and the lack of physicians,[1] this exclusionary Act was considered ridiculous. It is notable that this law was never enforced and when it was revised in 1815, an exemption for midwives was made. A similar law was in effect in Nova Scotia exempting all midwives in the province except those practising in Halifax (Rushing 1991). Acts that followed in Ontario (Upper Canada) in 1818 and 1827 also exempted midwives. It was not until 1865 that the practice of midwifery in Ontario required a licence. It was not considered illegal to practise midwifery, however, what was illegal was to pretend to be licensed as a physician under the Act (Mason 1987). Midwifery outside medicine, therefore, was not illegal but it was also not legal nor recognized. Physicians and legislators did not attempt to make the practice of female midwifery illegal because it would have been unenforceable and moreover it would have resulted in public condemnation of the medical profession (Rushing 1991).

At this time, Ontario had the lowest population to physician ratio in the country (Naylor 1986). Connor (1994) argues that physicians were much more concerned with other medical practitioners than with midwives, as evidenced by one Ontario physician's comments regarding midwifery that "there were larger fish to catch" (Connor 1994, 1). That is, physicians were concerned about controlling the numbers of their competitors – the "irregular" practitioners, not the midwives. This in part explains the logic of the act's omission of stipulations about female midwifery.

In 1874, when this act came up for revision, there was a renewed attempt to include female midwifery and to grant licences to midwives practising within a specified district, regulated by territorial medical divisions. This amendment, however, never became law because it was felt by many within the medical profession that such provisions were unnecessary. This continuing "alegal" situation in Ontario apparently did not prevent women from seeking help from neighbour women, but this was likely due to necessity rather than to any form of organized protest on the part of midwives or the women they were attending. Moreover, although these laws were often not enforced, and in some cases exempted midwives from prosecution, they likely served to intimidate and discourage midwives from pursuing or continuing this line of work (Connor 1994).

Concurrent with these licensing efforts was the promotion of medicalized childbirth, in large part through the efforts of some medical practitioners. Increasing public distaste for midwifery-attended births ensued, reflective of the increasing societal desire for the progressive and modern world which medicalized childbirth came to exemplify (Barrington 1985; Biggs 1983; Mason 1987). Physicians, in contrast, were promoted as superior birth attendants trained in "scientific" technological childbirth practices (Connor 1994).[2] Canadian women's confidence in giving birth and in attending birth was slowly being eroded, a trend beginning with the upper class and moving to the middle class (Mason 1987).

The increase in physician attendance at childbirth, however, was not without its critics. Opposition came first from the more conservative members of society, including a few notable physicians, and involved a concern with the preservation of female modesty (Biggs 1983). Another source of opposition came from those who argued that a medical monopoly in maternity care both not warranted – due to the lack of scientific evidence of its efficacy – and not beneficial to the community. This concern about a medical monopoly is likely to have been connected with the ideas promulgated by the Popular Health Movement of the 1840s and 1850s in the United States (see Ehrenreich and English 1973). Mason (1987) argues, based on various mortality surveys, that medical birth in a hospital was statistically more dangerous than birth accomplished at home in the traditional manner. She adds that studies that were not supportive of doctor-attended births were never published nor investigated further.

Despite this opposition, the redefinition of childbirth spearheaded by the medical profession was having an effect. Assertions that childbirth was dangerous and required the assistance of a trained attendant spurred Lady Aberdeen, the wife of the Governor General and head of the newly formed National Council of Women (NCW), to propose the development of the Victorian Order of Home Helpers (VOHH) in February 1897. This idea was initially proposed by the Local Council of Women of Vancouver who were concerned with the scarcity of health care in rural areas (Rushing 1991). Lady Aberdeen recommended that experienced women already serving as midwives in rural communities should have their education upgraded in a six-month to one-year course including instruction in midwifery, first aid and simple nursing, household economy and sanitation, food preparation, and "ladylike" manners such as tact and self-control. The redefinition of childbirth originally intended to support medical attendance at childbirth was being used to challenge it through the NCW proposal.

Many physicians came out strongly against the proposal for the VOHH, asserting that it would lower standards of medical care by sending out inadequately trained nurses (Rushing 1991). Attendance at childbirth was regarded by physicians as a successful entrée into general practice and into providing care to the family as a whole. Birth offered a way for a young doctor to gain access to the family and exhibit his skills. Mason (1987) points out that general practitioners in Canada were in competition for this entrée with women who did not regard midwifery as a career and therefore often did not charge a fee. Physicians were concerned that midwives were taking their potential "business" away, and that the licensing laws enacted to discourage midwifery practice were not acting as a deterrent. Any proposal to license such competitors met with fierce opposition.

Some physicians began to emphasize the dangers of childbirth and the need for trained attendants (i.e., physicians) to manage childbirth (Mason 1987). Many physicians sent threatening letters to midwives. This behaviour was augmented by negative articles in the medical and lay press detailing the horrors of midwifery-attended births and claiming that midwives were ignorant, dirty, and potentially dangerous (Biggs 1983). Connor (1989) recounts some of the cases described by physicians of midwives who, out of ignorance, dismembered or severely bruised unborn children or incompetently left women to labour for prolonged periods of time (i.e., days). Mason (1987) accedes there were no doubt serious cases of incompetence on the part of some midwives, but that these accounts were successful in attempting to discredit *all* midwives. It should also be pointed out that there were numerous incidents of incompetence on the part of male physicians with similar disastrous outcomes which were hidden from the public gaze.

Connor (1994) is careful to note that not all physicians in Ontario were against midwives, but rather a small vocal group of doctors. Female midwifery, he argues, was tacitly approved of by many doctors including the president of the Ontario College of Physicians and Surgeons, who in 1879 ordered that midwives be exempt from College prosecution. He states further that, generally speaking, physicians were tolerant of midwives' practices, especially when they blundered, and in their published reports they often did not mention the midwife's name, a favour that he states was not extended to reports about their blundering medical colleagues. Many physicians acknowledged the wide range skill in midwives, from the highly competent to those who were ignorant. In fact some physicians felt that midwives could and should be trained and a few elite physicians supported the VOHH proposal (Rushing 1991). So physicians' opposition to midwifery was nuanced but most would agree that, as a group, they were hostile to midwives (Mitchinson 1991, 2002).

The NCW proposal also garnered opposition from the newly developing nursing profession (Buckley 1979). Nursing was just developing and was beginning to gain public recognition for its services (Mason 1987). Nurses were struggling to gain acceptance by physicians and they were also struggling for better working conditions, opportunities, and wages (Buckley 1979). Attempts to create a new health worker with shorter training, and in direct competition with these nurses, were regarded with dismay.

In response to this perceived attempt to usurp nursing turf, nurses made an uneasy and unequal alliance with physicians to promote medically attended, nurse-assisted births preferably in the hospital setting (Barrington 1985). In aligning with the physician, the nurse took a less direct role in the amount of care she gave. Her role became that of health educator, public campaigner, and propagandist of physician-assisted births (Mason 1987). Nurses educated physicians as to the benefit of having a nurse as an assistant and they also educated the public through home, school, and church group visits that health and pregnancy should be managed by a trained physician, with the assistance of a trained nurse.

In the face of such opposition, Lady Aberdeen's efforts to upgrade the existing system of childbirth attendance by neighbour women was derailed. "Behind-the-scenes" lobbying by organized nursing put pressure on the Council, who in turn yielded to these pressures and redefined the new Order as including only trained nurses (Mason 1987). In April 1897, The Victorian Order of Home Helpers was changed to the Victorian Order of Nurses (VON).

Lady Aberdeen still insisted that the VON's tasks included midwifery. Because of nursing's precarious alliance with the medical profession, they remained on the sidelines of this midwifery debate. In the end, however, the NCW proposal succumbed to the fierce opposition of the medical profession. The VON revised its proposal so as to devote its services only to the urban and rural poor. The charter of the VON expressly forbade nurses from doing anything but emergency midwifery. They were required to call in a physician for women in labour, or else face permanent dismissal from the Order. Rushing (1991) describes how the final outcome of the VON's proposals served the interests of nursing as well as medicine: "Nurses had their professional interests realized in that the VON became trained nurses rather than competitors to nurses. Physicians' interests were achieved in that nurses were more directly subordinate to the medical profession" (18). Renewed efforts at establishing midwifery came after World War I. In 1917, it was proposed that the VON launch an inquiry into the need for trained midwives in Canada, the attitude of professionals and laymen towards their introduction, and the workings of the system of midwifery in Britain. Influential nursing supporters argued against such efforts and further, that nursing would surely relinquish its support for the VON rather than be associated with such a backward organization. The inquiry was promptly cancelled.

In 1918, Charlotte Hannington, the new superintendent of the VON, again brought up the issue of upgrading women already helping out at childbirth. She secretly sent several nurses to the Bellevue Midwifery School in New York to investigate the system of training and regulation of midwives. She circulated the information gathered by these visiting nurses to women's groups and nurses' organizations in order to garner some interest in her aspirations. She found that there was little interest in attempts to upgrade neighbour women. Her efforts to import British nurses, who had training in midwifery, to serve in the remote areas also faced fierce opposition from organized nursing (Buckley 1979). In fact, her efforts served to put the VON in disfavour with the more "progressive" women's groups, such as the Red Cross.

Amid the attempts to renew midwifery, the Red Cross set up the first outpost hospitals staffed by nurses in remote areas of Ontario. Between 1922 and 1933, 3600 births took place in these outpost hospitals and another 500 births took place at home, many without the assistance of a physician (Mason 1987). The maternity work that Red Cross nurses did was never regarded as midwifery. They were, however, successful in meeting the needs of the women in their community without antagonizing physicians and their birth statistics were quite successful despite attending a relatively poor clientele.[3] The combined efforts of the Red Cross and the VON, however, never recruited enough nurses to make this lonely, tiring, and unacknowledged form of midwifery viable (Mason 1987). The outcome of these various unsuccessful attempts to recognize midwifery was that at the turn of the twentieth century physicians were beginning to attend the majority of births and more and more midwives were occupying only a minor role in childbirth attendance.

Analyses of the Fall of Midwifery in Canada

One of the first authors to comment on the history of midwifery in Canada, Biggs (1983), attributes their decline to the organized efforts on the part of the male medical profession to enact restrictive laws against midwives and to undermine the credibility of midwifery, increasing public skepticism about the safety of birth and of midwives as birth attendants, and the promoting of physicians as superior birth attendants trained in the more advanced scientific technological childbirth practices. Mason (1987) largely concurs with Biggs' argument and adds that this strategy on the part of physicians was used during a time when, for more than three decades, medical birth had been statistically more dangerous than births attended by traditional birth attendants.

By way of contrast, Connor (1994) and others (e.g., Mitchinson 1991, 2002) argue that the demise of midwifery in Ontario was not the result solely of physicians' efforts but instead was due to a confluence of factors. He asserts that the medical profession in nineteenth-century Ontario was far from an organized cohesive group, and that physicians displayed considerable tolerance towards midwives. He argues that the medical profession lobbied for protective licensing laws not solely to oust midwives but rather to deal with physicians' other competitors, such as irregulars and homeopaths. He does concede, however, that such laws likely served to intimidate and discourage midwives from pursuing this line of work. Rather than actively attempting to change societal attitudes regarding the safety of birth, Connor argues that physicians were conservative in their use of obstetrical instruments and medical technology and that these were not employed solely to oust midwives. He also points out the active involvement of parturient women in the increased use of instruments and technology in that they often implored physicians to do something and use anything to relieve their suffering. Physicians, it could be argued, were simply responding to patient demand. Connor argues that one must look at other important factors leading to the decline of midwives other than simply the actions of the medical profession.

Connor (1994) suggests that midwives' failure to organize was an important factor that led to their decline. Others, such as Michinson (2002) concur: "Midwives were in no position to protest their weakening position. They had little contact with one another and had few influential champions. There was little, then, for physicians to actively oppose" (97). Midwives tended to be new immigrants or of advancing age and were often isolated from one another, geographically and through language (see also Van Wagner 1988). Younger women did not take up midwifery, therefore there were few new recruits into the profession. They also did not establish any training programs to transmit their knowledge and skills. Mason would agree with this argument, but she reframes it by highlighting the informality of much of early Canadian midwifery and its location in the community. That is, she claims that midwifery was not conceived as a career around which women should organize. Lack of organization was also likely to be due to time pressures given that many midwives were faced with the numerous demands of being a midwife, mother, wife, and farm worker.

Connor (1994) also points to how changing societal attitudes toward childbirth and larger social forces such as urbanization also served to bring about the demise of the midwife. He also notes that midwives were closely associated with the practice of infanticide and this served to further erode midwives' practice as society became less willing to condone of such practices. Mason (1987) concurs, observing that there came a disdain for the traditional (which midwifery came to represent), and a desire for the progressive and modern (which obstetrics came to represent). It is also likely that local birth helpers were not unwilling to hand over their arduous duties to the physician. These arduous tasks often included travelling long distances in less than seasonable weather. The trend towards hospital births also had an additive effect, but it occurred much later in midwifery's decline process (Oppenheimer 1983).

Mason (1987), following Buckley's arguments (1979), also points to the negative influence of the nursing profession. Opposition from nursing served to divide support from the women's movement for a legitimate female health profession; some early feminists supported midwifery and others supported nursing. Rushing (1991) focuses attention on the market forces which affected the occupational strategies of medicine and nursing. She argues that it was when medicine and nursing were faced with an oversupply of practitioners that they turned their efforts to controlling competitors, and became anti-midwifery. If the market conditions of oversupply did not exist, she argues, midwifery may not have been so fiercely opposed.

It is important to recognize that there were a combination of factors that led to the decline and near eradication of the midwife in Canada. But to take a totally "pluralist" approach in accounting for the decline of midwifery is to obscure the connection between some of the key underlying causes. The consequence of the use of obstetrical instruments, whether intended or not, was to create a distinction between physicians and midwives, with medical attendance being more highly valued. The origin of women's demands for the use of obstetrical interventions can be traced back to medicine's claims to produce speedier and easier births. Changing societal attitudes can be linked to the promotional efforts made by some physicians. Nurses' opposition to midwifery can be linked to the subordination they experienced at the hands of physicians. So although there are a multitude of factors leading to midwifery's decline, there are nevertheless intricately interconnected.

Moreover, in a revisitation of the issue of midwifery decline some twenty years following her first study, Biggs (2004) notes that there are many gaps in the history of midwifery in Canada. "There is, for example, in my article no mention of aboriginal midwifery; it is as if the history of midwifery began with the arrival of the settlers. In addition, almost all of the sources cited are by commentators of English origin" (18). Further, she questions the universality of the "neighbour midwife" described by Mason (1987), an image which has dominated Canadian midwifery history. Instead, she argues that "rather than being a universal form of midwifery practice, the 'neighbour midwife' emerged within a particular historical context, namely the settlement of Upper Canada throughout the nineteenth century and the first wave of immigration on the prairies in the twentieth century" (18). Her subsequent research reveals a diversity of cultural understandings of the figure of the midwife, and shows that not all women who attended births were called midwives but that this distinction was more often reserved for those women who had acquired a specialized set of skills conferred by some sort of formal authority or by the community. Finally, she highlights that the "demise of midwifery" thesis has served to obscure the persistence of midwifery in several parts of Canada, most notably Newfoundland (Benoit 1990, 1991; McNaughton 1989), and the survival of Aboriginal midwifery particularly in Northern areas until the 1960s (Benoit and Carroll 1995; O'Neil and Kaufert 1995, 1996).

REMNANTS OF MIDWIFERY
IN THE CANADIAN LANDSCAPE

Although midwifery was nearly eradicated by these factors and forces, there remained pockets of midwifery practice in Canada (which were nonetheless) endangered by modernization and restrictive legislation (Mitchinson 2002).[4] These included remnants of midwifery in tightly knit ethnic communities, such as the Mennonites in Southern Ontario and in some native settlements. One of the largest pockets of midwifery that remained was in Newfoundland and Labrador, due in part to the isolated nature of many areas of the province, the greater influence there of Britain where midwifery was an accepted part of the health care system, and its late joining into the Canadian confederation. Benoit (1987, 1991, 1997) describes how midwifery evolved from traditional home birth practices to local cottage hospital practice, and ultimately into the larger district hospitals. Unlike other Canadian provinces, lay midwifery continued in isolated communities of Newfoundland well into the post-World War II period. These lay midwives focused primarily on attendance at childbirth in their client's homes and trained through apprenticeships and active participation in the birthing community (Mitchinson 2002).

Between the 1930s and 1960s, small cottage hospitals began to be set up in several communities and midwives began to work in these settings. In these small hospitals, midwives had access to other colleagues, undertook more formalized training, and practised with a great deal of professional autonomy. Like traditional midwives, they were responsible for pre- and post-natal care in addition to attendance at childbirth. This setting offered practising midwives an organized time schedule as well as a separate and uniform work site.

With increasing modernization, including the building of roads and the development of larger regional hospitals, many of the small cottage hospitals were closed. As a result, midwives who had practised relatively independently in the cottage hospitals were forced to take work as rank-

and-file maternity nurses assisting physicians rather than attending child-birth as autonomous practitioners. That is, in the larger hospitals they experienced a significant narrowing of their occupational role and were placed under direct supervision of the attending physician and nurse administrators. Thus, midwifery in Newfoundland and Labrador too eventually succumbed to external pressures toward the norm of physician-attended, nurse-assisted birth in hospitals.

In addition to these remnants of traditional midwifery, unofficial forms of "nurse-midwifery" in remote areas developed mainly during the 1960s but began with the efforts of the nurses in Red Cross outposts as noted above, and those of the United Farm Women and United Farm Men of Alberta following World War I (Mason 1987). Prompted by the scarcity of physicians, these Alberta organizations lobbied the government to supply midwives to remote areas of the province. This need was originally met by British-trained nurse midwives. These organizations also lobbied for a local institution to provide such training. In response, a nurse-midwifery training program entitled Advanced Practical Obstetrics Course for District Nurses was established in Edmonton in 1944, the first of its kind in Canada (Hurlbert 1981). The three-month program specifically recruited public health nurses and the word "midwife" was not to be used in connection with the program (Mason 1987). Other educational programs were developed much later in Halifax, Nova Scotia, in 1967 for nurse practitioners and in St. Johns, Newfoundland, in 1978, boldly titled Nurse-Midwifery. The establishment of these two programs reflected the development of nurse-midwifery practice opportunities in the Canadian north.

The development of federal health programs in the north during the 1950s and early 1960s also resulted in a growth in the number of nursing stations in the newly created Inuit settlements and an increase in nurse-midwife-attended births. Like the remote practices in Alberta and Ontario, British trained nurse-midwives were recruited to staff these stations, but some were graduates of Canadian nurse-midwifery programs in Edmonton, Halifax, and St. John's. Although these nurse-midwives came to replace traditional native midwives, they were nevertheless regarded as a positive contribution to the community (Kaufert and O'Neil 1993).

There was also little opposition to the development of nurse midwifery in the North from the medical profession because it was specifically directed toward native women. Federal health policy changes during the 1970s resulted in a policy of increased evacuation of pregnant women to physician-attended facilities in southern cities. This trend and the discontinuation of the hiring of foreign-trained midwives, in part because of tighter immigration policies, led to a decrease in the opportunities for these nurse-midwives to practise, an overall decline of nurse-midwifery in the north, and a convergence towards physician-attended birth in the north as in other areas of Canada (Mason 1988). Women in the north complained bitterly about the disappearance of the midwife, seeing her as the key to the returning of birth to the community setting (Kaufert and O'Neil 1993).

Analyses of the Remnants of Midwifery

In contrast to the sizable literature on the historical demise of midwifery in Canada, little research has focused on the remnants of midwifery that remained in the mid- to late part of the twentieth century. What is available helps inform our understanding of midwifery in the past and the implications of its demise. For example, unlike others who tend to glorify the independent practice of lay midwives of the past, Benoit's work on the vestiges of midwifery in Newfoundland reveals that although free of bureaucratic controls experienced in large hospital settings, traditional lay midwives lacked autonomy in many areas of their work lives. The traditional lay midwife had little control over her remuneration, choice of practice site, time schedule, and pace of work activities and lacked sufficient association with colleagues to keep her knowledge base sharp and up to date. Often they had to work under less than desirable conditions in many women's homes (see also Mitchinson 2002). Benoit argues that it was in the small cottage hospital that midwives achieved the most desirable occupational status. Unlike home birth midwives, they experienced less control over their work from the community of attending families and friends, and unlike the hospital midwives they experienced less control over their work from physicians and the hospital bureaucracy.

Kaufert and O'Neil's work reveals the important position that midwives played in Aboriginal communities in the North (see also Jasen 1997). Similarly Benoit's work with Carroll (1995, 2004) on the decline and rebirth of Aboriginal midwifery which paralleled the rebirth of midwifery among non-Aboriginal Canadians reveals the critical role midwifery plays in Aboriginal culture (see also Couchie and Nabigon 1997). While some attention has focused on these important remnants of midwifery, more attention has been paid to what has been referred to as the "new" midwifery, that is the re-emergence of a more counterculture form of midwifery in the 1970s and 1980s.

REBIRTH OF MIDWIFERY

Despite the decline in practice opportunities for midwives located in outlying areas of the country, interest in the concept of nurse-midwifery in non-remote areas of the country began to peak (Hurlbert 1981). For example, Hays (1971) argued in an article in *The Canadian Nurse* that nurse-midwives could function effectively in urban as well as rural and remote settings. Several regional nurse-midwifery associations began to discuss the idea of promoting the integration of nurse-midwives as a member of the obstetrical care team (Hurlbert 1981). The Registered Nurses Association of Ontario (RNAO), for example, made an official statement in 1972 supporting the development of nurse-midwifery in Ontario (Hurlbert 1981). These efforts were supported by the Canadian Nurses Association which recommended in 1974 that the nurse-midwife be recognized as "the health professional best equipped to meet the growing needs for counselling services and for greater continuity of care within this area of the health system" (as cited in Hurlbert 1981, 31). The RNAO then attempted to initiate negotiations with the College of Nurses of Ontario (CNO), the College of Physicians and Surgeons of Ontario (CPSO), the Ontario Medical Association (OMA), and the Ontario government regarding enabling legislation for nurse-midwifery (RNAO 1973). These efforts were buoyed by an earlier recommendation of the Ontario Committee on the Healing Arts, a government-appointed health committee, that nurse-midwifery be integrated into the existing health care system (OCHA Report 1970). The OCHA proposed nurse-midwives be clinical nurse specialists who would work in hospital settings and/or outpatient clinics, under the general direction of a physician (167). The negotiations between the nursing and medical associations regarding the implementation of the recommendation to integrate nurse-midwifery, however, never materialized. When the minister's advisory body, the Ontario Council on Health, reviewed the OCHA nurse-midwifery recommendation, it concluded that there was not sufficient need for nurse-midwives in the health care system in Ontario (Fynes 1994).

Concurrent with the efforts of the RNAO, several nurses in the province who had midwifery training from other jurisdictions (predominantly the UK) had organized around a similar agenda of integrating nurse-midwives into the health care system. These "nurse-midwives," many of whom were working as public health nurses or as labour and delivery room nurses, created the Ontario Nurse-Midwives Association (ONMA) in 1973, which later became a special interest group of the RNAO. Later that year, nurse-midwives in BC, Alberta, Saskatchewan, the Northwest Territories, and the Yukon organized into the Western Nurse Midwives Association adopting the Ontario statement, and a Canadian National Committee on Nurse Midwives was formed to nationally promote the nurse-midwifery concept. But similar to the efforts of the RNAO earlier, implementation would not be forthcoming.

In the midst of the stalled efforts to introduce nurse-midwifery in the south came a "rebirth" of a new form of lay midwifery in Canada. The development of this form of midwifery stemmed in part from the grass-roots and in part from the influx of ideas and proponents from emerging social movements in the United States, namely the Home Birth and Women's Health Movements (see discussion in previous chapter on lay midwifery in the US). It originated on the west coast in the early 1970s in large part because that was the counterculture centre of Canada.

One of the main US influences on west coast midwifery was a midwife from Santa Cruz, California, Raven Lang. In the same year that her *Birth Book* was published, 1972, Lang was invited to help establish a medical program providing care for residents in the BC interior (Edwards and Waldorf 1984). There she met Cheryl Anderson, a lay midwife-to-be. Anderson had worked at the Vancouver Free Childbirth Education Centre, which had opened one year earlier. Funded by the federal government to provide free prenatal education to transient youths on the west coast, the Centre marked the first organized attempt in Canada to meet the needs of a growing population who were opting out of the formal maternity care system by giving birth at home (Barrington 1985). When Lang returned home to California after this short placement in BC, Anderson returned with her to learn more about midwifery. The following year, Anderson, with the help of Lang and others, founded the Vancouver Birth Centre (Barrington 1985, Edwards and Waldorf 1984). Activities at the Birth Centre included workshops, conferences, and midwifery classes for their growing number of apprentices. Lang also helped foster lay midwifery on Vancouver Island when she moved there in 1974. Throughout the 1970s and 1980s, other communities of lay midwives became established.

As was the case in the US, the development of lay midwifery in Canada was not unproblematic. Expanding lay midwifery practices gar-nered increasing attention by physicians as "[h]er work, and her very existence, ran completely counter to obstetrical logic" (Mason 1990, 1). Two main reasons lay behind the concerns expressed by physicians: com-petition and safety, particularly of home birth attendance. As was the case historically, physicians saw midwives as unwelcome competitors. The president of the British Columbia Medical Association, for example, stated, "[midwifery] is only one tentacle of a thrust in the direction to take over general practice" (As cited in Barrington 1984, 6). Canadian estimates are that childbirth services made up approximately 5 per cent of general practitioners' billings in the late 1970s (Evans 1981).

These concerns over competition, however, should be countered with the reality that many physicians in Canada, both specialists and generalists, are abandoning the practice of obstetrics (Barrington 1985; Benoit 1987) and that in general Canadians are faced with an obstetrical care shortage (Cohen 1991; Rosser and Muggah 1989; Wysong 1998). Barrington (1985) states, "due to time pressure, complex obstetrical procedures, and escalating medical insurance premiums, it is no longer practical or possible for most family doctors to continue attending their patients' births" (155–6). General practitioners are also opting out of hospital privileges, especially in urban centres, due to the added effort of maintaining these privileges. Obstetrician/gynecologists are also practising obstetrics less and less due to increases in malpractice insurance and the comparatively smaller financial remuneration. As Barrington (1985) states, "[G]ynaecology is more profitable and less time-consuming than obstetrics. Some specialists basically take on maternity patients as loss leaders, hoping to serve their ongoing gynaecological needs" (156). Although the trend was for physicians to be quite opposed to midwives and the practice of midwifery, a number were (and continue to be) enthusiastic supporters who have developed professional relationships with midwives (Barrington 1985; see also Anderson 1986; Goldman 1988; Kinch 1986; Reid and Galbraith 1988). Many of these physicians helped spark the rebirth of lay midwifery. Some also attended home births or provided backup support for midwives, but the negative attitudes of their medical organization and the sanctions brought against them, such as by their provincial medical colleges, served to keep these numbers low (Barrington 1985).

As in the US, the strategies employed by physicians opposed to midwifery in Canada have included legal tactics, but initially included having the provincial medical colleges pass rulings against physician involvement in home births. This occurred in Alberta in 1981 and in Ontario in 1983 (Barrington 1985). These rulings served to put midwives in a legally vulnerable position, since they require medical consultations in emergencies, including backup for hospital transfers. Court cases and "quasi-judicial" inquests against midwives have also occurred in those cases that resulted in baby deaths. Any case of a baby death occurring outside an institutional setting must be inquired into by a provincial coroner, a medical practitioner. Two such inquests occurred in Ontario, in 1982 and 1985.

It was not until 1983 that Canadian lay midwives faced trials either for practising medicine without a license or for criminal negligence (Barrington 1985). The case against three Halifax midwives in 1983 became a national media event. The three midwives were charged with criminal negligence causing bodily harm when they transferred an infant born at home to hospital (Burtch 1988b). The baby died six months after her birth when removed from a respirator; she was said to have suffered massive brain damage from asphyxia. The physicians who laid the charges argued that the baby would not have died had she been born in the hospital. At the preliminary hearing of the case some ten months later, expert witnesses did not concur. The judge decided that the case would not be brought to trial due to insufficient evidence much to the dismay of some within the medical community.

Other trials have come against midwives in other provinces for practising medicine without a license or for criminal negligence causing harm or death. No prosecutions had been successful until 1986 when two Vancouver midwives were found guilty of criminal negligence causing death following assistance at a home birth (Burtch 1988b). The judge had concluded that the midwives failed to exercise reasonable knowledge, skill, and care in managing the birth.

Burtch (1986, 1988a, 1994) asserts that one should not assume that midwives are completely powerless against the official powers of the state and the medical profession. Indeed, in some cases, legal proceedings created a platform through which midwives could openly promote their practice and defend the legitimacy of their work, of home births, and of the right of women to choose the manner and place of birth of their children (see also Arms 1975; Barrington 1985; Burtch 1988b). In several cases where midwives have been brought to trial, courtrooms have filled with consumer and feminist supporters. Midwives have also been able to draw upon expert witnesses to argue the case for midwifery care.

One should also not exaggerate midwives' power in the courts, however, particularly in light of successful convictions. Despite some of the positive aspects of trials against midwives, there are some obvious negative effects. Midwives lack a substantial defence fund (such as that available to physicians through the Canadian Medical Protection Association) when legal charges are laid against them (Barrington 1985). Thus midwives suffer severe financial losses during trials from loss of income and through the retention of a defence lawyer. They also have to cope with the uncertainty of the verdict and in a few cases midwives have had to deal with the consequences of being convicted (Burtch 1986, 1988a, 1994). Faced with the threat of trials, midwives operate under the constant fear of arrest and in a state of paranoia (see Lyons 1981 for example).

Midwives have responded to their vulnerable position in two main ways. First, midwives began to formalize their practices by increasing their documentation of clients and by increasing conformity to evolving standards of practice (Mason 1988). The newly developed pattern of practising in pairs proved to be beneficial for the possibility it provided of back-up support against legal charges. Strict, formalized screening procedures began to be employed throughout prenatal care in order to screen out mothers who were more likely to have problems in a home birth setting. Women were also strongly encouraged to consult with a physician to assess risk.

Second, legal proceedings also provoked midwives and parents to adopt more sophisticated patterns of political action and organization. Barrington (1985), for example, describes court cases and college rulings as catalysts "the political activities of the midwifery community ... are a direct response to the legal non-status of midwifery in Canada ... Legal proceedings, and the rulings of medical authorities intended to curtail midwifery practice, have provoked increasingly sophisticated organization in the midwifery movement (142 and 144)." Organizations that included parents, midwives, and their supporters, which originally formed for self education and social support, formalized in pursuit of legalization and began to lobby for favourable legislation and regulatory policies. The first of these organizations in Canada was developed by midwives and their supporters in British Columbia making up the Interdisciplinary Midwifery Task Force of British Columbia (MTFBC) and the Midwives' Association of British Columbia (MABC). Although it was the groups in BC who first proposed the idea of securing legislation regulating midwifery and integrating it into the health care system, it was a group of lay midwives in Alberta forming the Alberta College and Register of Domiciliary Midwives Association (ACRDMA) who made the first formal attempt (Barrington 1985).

The ACRDMA made an argument for state endorsement of midwifery as a designated health occupation before the provincial Health Occupations Board (HOB) in the fall of 1983 (Barrington 1985). This proposal was in direct response to the ban on physicians providing backup for home births made by the College of Physicians and Surgeons of Alberta (CPSA) in 1981 and the resulting increase in demand for midwifery services. In response to the ACRDMA proposal, the CPSA declared to the HOB that any effort to legalize midwifery was unprogressive. Local consumer groups, the Calgary Association of Parents and Professionals for Safe Alternatives in Childbirth (CAPSAC), and the Edmonton Association for Safe Alternatives in Childbirth (ASAC), countered with a thoroughly researched and well documented brief to the HOB supporting midwifery legislation. In the end, the proposal was not accepted, but the HOB did respond favourably to the idea of integrating midwifery and it encouraged the ACRDMA to seek an alliance with nurse-midwives and resubmit a proposal for a unified midwifery (Barrington 1985). It would be the efforts of midwives in Ontario – discussed herein – that would prove to be the first successful integration project in the country.

Reflections on the Rise of the New Midwifery

Although the historical demise of midwifery in Canada has garnered a great deal of attention by social scientists, the more recent rise or rebirth of midwifery has begun to interest scholars as well. For example, similar to the work of DeVries (1982, 1985) and Sullivan and Weitz (1988), Canadian commentators describe how efforts to seek state legitimacy for midwifery in Canada are cause for concern. Mason (1990), for example, outlines how the struggle of the alternative childbirth movement was "carried out in a context of a passionate NO to institutional and professional management of our lives," (2, emphasis in original) and discusses how contemporary midwifery emerged from this struggle. She now has difficulty "recognizing the connection between the present-day midwifery movement and the alternative birth culture that came into being in the seventies" (2). In her view, there has been a change in focus towards the establishment of midwifery rather than on the mother and child, contrary to the origins of lay midwifery (Mason 1988). She argues that there has been a subtle shift in the language and assumptions of contemporary midwives away from their feminist roots, obscuring the issue of control with the less confrontational issue of choice. Midwives, she asserts, have also shifted from regarding childbearing women as their "friends" to regarding them as "pupils," and in so doing have repudiated their non-medical birth culture. She expresses concern that legislating midwifery will simply establish a new monopoly of state-employed midwives who will be forced "to exchange their independence for financial security, [and] to curb their ingenuity in favour of the grander goal of universal, quality-controlled midwifery care" (3).

Barrington (1985) counters some of the concerns about integration by focusing on the issues of equity and sustainability. Although she documents that some midwifery advocates fear that the midwife's role will be co-opted by the system and her philosophy of care corrupted, she asks, "how can one conscientiously enjoy the services of a midwife when the majority of the population, including those most in need are not even aware of her existence?" (159). She argues that only a minority of women, with the time, money, and information, have access to the few midwives that were available. She asserts that the status quo is not only difficult to justify, it is impossible to sustain. Indeed, it was becoming increasingly difficult for midwives to continue quietly practising, without fear of legal reprisal. Moreover, she argues that if midwives and their supporters did not take the initiative to advance their own ideas about legislation, someone else would define it for them or worse yet, seize the opportunity to eradicate midwifery altogether. At the same time she cautions that "the kind of midwifery most readily won in the political arena will not necessarily provide the quality of care we now know. Advocates must be careful not to make disastrous compromises in their efforts to hasten legislation. They need to carefully assess various models and options, identifying priorities and safeguards for the kind of midwifery they seek" (160). In other words, in order to safeguard the central tenets of midwifery philosophy and practice, including client control and midwifery autonomy, midwifery in Canada must become an independent self-governing profession with substantial consumer input.

Burtch (1994) comments on the multitude of paradoxes that exist between midwifery, the state, and the public in its recent re-emergence. For example, he argues that while the state endeavours to promote safe maternity and infant care and women's choices in reproduction – in essence promoting midwifery – it at the same time has prosecuted midwives through a crude system of regulation in the courts and coroner's inquests. He outlines how the prosecution of midwives makes clear the vulnerable legal position of practising midwives in Canada, particularly prior to state-endorsed self-regulation. Paralleling this, the media also tend to focus on the most dramatic aspects of midwifery and birth, often drawing much public attention to infant deaths associated with an attempted home birth. Simultaneously, however, the media have been an important forum for the alternative perspective on birth that midwifery has come to typify. Legalization, therefore, draws midwifery into this complex environment that will ultimately change its face in some expected and some unexpected ways.

Rushing (1993) also focuses on the agency of midwives in her description of how they draw on two key ideologies in their efforts to legitimate their position: science and feminism. The ideology of science (the medical professions' most frequently invoked source of power, according to Rushing) is used by midwives and their advocates to support the safety of home births and midwives' non-interventionist practice style (Buhler, Glick and Sheps 1988; Kaufman and McDonald 1988; Reid and Galbraith 1988; Schneider and Soderstrom 1987; Sides 1981; Sullivan and Beeman 1983; Tyson 1991; Weatherston 1985). Rushing argues that the ideology of science has been especially important for lay midwives whose independence from the mainstream health care system necessitates the use of an ideology with more widespread currency. Feminist ideology is used to support midwives' distinctive woman-centred practice style and emphasis on personal control and responsibility.

Taking an even more critical perspective informed by the sociology of professions literature, Benoit (1987) questions whether it is truly possible for the new Canadian midwife to become an autonomous professional and at the same time continue to be a true partner of pregnant women, given that women as "clients" and midwives as "professional workers" often have divergent interests (see also McCrea and Crute 1991; Richards 1982). She argues that professionalism and client partnership are inherently contradictory:

Professional status for midwives involves the opportunity to acquire experience attending abnormal as well as normal pregnancies, to work alongside like-minded colleagues, to gain easy access to the latest birth technology and to enjoy a degree of autonomy in organizing their working hours. However, such professionalization of working conditions is likely to result in the midwife's estrangement from the pregnant woman, who will now have to confront a new stranger in place of the doctor – the midwifery specialist – and not the hoped for partner sharing her reproductive passage. (276)

Benoit also argues that midwifery philosophy, regarding the sharing of information between midwives and their clients, is problematic given that many midwives and their clients often do not share the same cultural backgrounds. Moreover, she asserts, this philosophy assumes a great deal about midwife compliance with and client receptivity to the sharing of information.

Nestel's (1996/97, 2004) examination of the fate of immigrant midwives of colour in Ontario throughout the integration process begins to address some of the social cleavages that exist within midwifery itself. Similar to Witz's analysis of the exclusionary closure strategies employed by elite midwives in the UK, Nestel critically reveals the paradox represented by the absence of women of colour in Ontario midwifery, given the presence in the province of many who possess formal training. She argues that a combination of the pre-legislation social environment and various bureaucratic decisions made throughout the midwifery integration process together served to systematically exclude immigrant midwives of colour from the profession. Specifically, the precarious legal context for the practice of midwifery throughout the 1980s prevented many immigrant women with midwifery training from practising largely because of their concerns about their own equally precarious immigrant status. In turn, their lack of recent midwifery practice experience led them to be excluded from processes that could fast-track them into the profession. Although some might argue that Nestel's argument about systematic racism is overstated, reality clearly shows that there are few immigrant women of colour practising as midwives in the province of Ontario.[5]

What these analyses of the rise of midwifery highlight is that there exists a complex web of relations – between midwives and the state, the media, the public and between midwives themselves – that must be mediated in the process of integration (or re-integration as the case may be). Both Burtch (1994) and Nestel (1996/97, 2004) encourage us to look beyond midwifery as a largely homogenous, like-minded group to see its heterogenous nature as a group enacting its own internal systems of control. Specifically, Burtch (1994) draws out the differences between nurse and community midwives and within these groups, the varying degrees of willingness to conform to particular standards of practice. Benoit's (1987, 1991, 1997) work also challenges the basic tenets and assumptions underlying midwifery, such as independent practice and the midwifery model of care. These are important features of the rise of midwifery which inform the present study.

SUMMARY OF LITERATURE ON MIDWIFERY IN CANADA

In this chapter, I present the documented *fall* and *rise* of midwifery in Canada alongside the commentaries other scholars offer about the relevant factors and forces influencing this trajectory and the impact these events have had and continue to have. As noted in the introduction, the events preceding the integration in Ontario help to fully contextualize

Ontario Midwives' contemporary professional project. Indeed, midwives in Ontario and across Canada were emerging largely out of obscurity. Physicians came to almost exclusively dominate the system of maternity care in Canada and the state did not seem particularly interested in changing this situation. Midwives, therefore, faced a rather insurmountable task in attempting to permeate and change this system.

The social commentaries on the rise of midwifery are also important sources which help inform the present study. Scholars had begun to trace the rebirth of midwifery across Canada and to highlight the key factors that were beginning to emerge in that process. This helped to inform the framework upon which I built this case study. At the same time, outlining what has been done before reveals the gaps in the literature. In the next chapters, the description of the integration of midwifery in Ontario aims to address a few of the unanswered questions.

PART TWO

Integrating Midwifery
The Nexus between Midwives, Women, and the State

CHAPTER FOUR

From Social Movement to Professional Project

Throughout the late 1970s and early 1980s, what came to be known as the midwifery community evolved from an amorphous social movement of women and men who attended women at birth; women who had given birth, were giving birth, or planning on giving birth; and family members and other supporters of alternatives to mainstream childbirth into a professional project aimed at integrating midwifery into the system of maternity care in the province. One of the primary motivators behind this integration project was the establishment of a review of the legislation of all health professions in Ontario by the provincial government in 1982. There were other objectives to this project as well, not the least of which included the increasing recognition of this somewhat "underground," grassroots movement. Although the integration project caused some apprehension from members of this alternative childbirth community, it was ultimately undertaken. In this chapter, I outline the development of the social movement behind the professional project and its evolution throughout the negotiations with the government, other professions, and the public regarding the inclusion of midwifery in the Regulated Health Professions Act.

THE ORGANIZATION OF MIDWIVES AND CLIENTS PRIOR TO INTEGRATION

As midwifery re-emerged in Ontario in the late 1970s, midwives and the women they served existed as an amorphous group with few divisions and little hierarchical separation of caregiver and client. In fact the terms *caregiver* and *client* may not be entirely appropriate in describing the roles of each, as a more egalitarian, friendship-oriented relationship than these terms connote existed. Indeed, in some cases, a woman would help a friend at birth and that friend would in turn help her out at childbirth. Many of these "midwives" in fact were not really midwives yet, since many practised as birth educators and/or as birth helpers to the few physicians who were sympathetic to the practice of home birth.[1] These "midwives" and the women they cared for were not seen as having different interests from each other. Together, they made up a small, but politically active community striving for more choice and control in childbirth.

Some physicians who were sympathetic to the practice of home birth were also important members of this community. These physicians often had experience practising with midwives from other countries, or had been asked by women from countries where home birth was practised to attend their birth at home.[2] Some were also part of the larger counterculture movement. To a large extent, these home birth doctors helped spark the revival of midwifery. One of these physicians was Dr John McCoulagh. McCoulagh was a family physician who had attended home births throughout the 1960s and early 1970s in Toronto before it became fashionable among the counterculture crowd. His services were used largely by a conservative clientele who, for largely religious reasons, did not want birth in a hospital (Conservative Catholics, Orthodox Jews, etc.). McCoulagh had a profound impact on the young family practice physicians he supervised, many of whom then became the "second generation" home birth physicians. Together he and these young physicians helped create the conditions for birth attendants to become involved in home birth attendance.[3]

Clients would often approach a sympathetic physician about attending their birth at home. Many physicians encouraged clients to arrange with an additional attendant (ideally one with home birth experience) to be at the birth and to help throughout the labour as the physician would often arrive just for the birth. Frequently these physicians knew of potential birth attendants to whom they would refer women requesting a home birth. These birth attendants (who were almost exclusively women) were not necessarily trained in midwifery but rather were women interested in promoting childbirth alternatives through helping out at home births. For many, their own home birth experience sparked their interest.

One of the first instances of organization among this amorphous group of birth helpers, consumers, and home birth physicians was the Toronto-based Home Birth Task Force. In the latter part of the 1970s before there were many birth attendants from whom to draw support, home birth physicians on occasion sought the assistance of nurses in the Victorian Order of Nurses (VON) (Fynes 1994). Upon request, VON nurses provided assistance during labour and delivery, and followed up with home care to the mother and infant for a few days postpartum. In the spring of 1976 funding for this service was discontinued. In response, home birth supporters organized the Home Birth Task Force (HBTF) to lobby the government to reinstate the VON service. Although they were unsuccessful in their bid to reinstate the service, the HBTF continued as an information and support group for parents considering a home birth. As midwife Vicki Van Wagner recalled, "[the HBTF] carried on because it had a community function that was perhaps more important than its original political function" (personal communication 1995).

One of the community functions of the HBTF was to organize and sponsor an information seminar called Birth Day held in Toronto in May 1978 (Fynes 1994). Among the guest speakers at the conference was Shari Daniels, a lay midwife from El Paso, Texas, who had established her own maternity clinic serving largely migrant women from Mexico. Daniels agreed to make a presentation at the conference if she could also give a workshop on basic midwifery skills. Daniels had told the attending group of birth helpers, "from now on consider yourselves as midwives." For many midwives, this workshop was an important turning point in their view of themselves as midwives. Following the workshop, Daniels invited interested participants to El Paso to work in her birth clinic to expand their skills in midwifery. Several midwives subsequently took up Daniels offer and obtained training at her clinic.

Following this pivotal conference, home birth consumers, supporters, and assistants formed a Midwives' Support and Study Group as an offshoot of the HBTF. Meetings of this group were held informally in the homes of its members. These women came together to share information and resources about childbirth and it generally became an occasion to share birth stories and experiences. Birth attendants in areas where few physicians attended home births (i.e., outside Toronto), set up similar groups to draw on each other's expertise and experience.

Thus, the organization of midwives and their clients was originally an egalitarian grouping of like-minded individuals without clear separation of interests or even, in some cases, of knowledge. It is interesting to note that this amorphous group organized initially for political reasons through the HBTF to lobby the government to reinstate a previously funded service. It was from this organization around a political cause that a community support network formed. Many of the women involved did not lose sight of the inherently political nature of the social movement in which they were involved.

FROM SOCIAL SUPPORT GROUP
TO PROFESSIONAL ORGANIZATION

The Ontario Association of Midwives

One of the midwives who accepted Daniels' invitation to El Paso was Ava Vosu. While in El Paso, Vosu became aware of developments in the midwifery movement in the United States and of how the movement was beginning to develop organizations for social support (Fynes 1994). One of the groups with which Vosu became involved was a group of lay and nurse-midwives who later organized as the Midwives Alliance of North America (MANA) in 1982. MANA was envisaged as a means to unite lay midwives[4] and nurse-midwives in the United States. It was felt that these two groups together would have broader support and greater political strength in promoting midwifery than they would separately (Schlinger 1992).

Upon her return to Ontario, Vosu saw the potential advantages that a Canadian organization similar to MANA could provide to women practising as birth helpers/midwives and those who supported and drew upon their services (Fynes 1994). Vosu introduced her idea at a gathering of the Midwives' Support and Study Group. Given the obscure legal status of midwives in Ontario, compounded by the increasingly frequent prosecutions of lay midwives in other jurisdictions (primarily in the US), some midwives "felt nervous about doing anything official" (Vosu as quoted in Fynes 1994). Despite this initial reluctance, Vosu was successful in securing enough support from women practising as midwives and their supporters to create the Ontario Association of Midwives (OAM) in January 1981.[5] She described the informality of this newly established organization: "It wasn't really an official organization. It was just a support group to help each other ... We opened the membership to anyone who supported midwifery ... and we got all kinds of people who supported us ... people who had had midwives, and other who were interested in learning about them" (as quoted in Fynes 1994: 72–3). The membership, which included birth helpers/midwives, consumers, and other supporters, quickly rose to 200 members (Toronto Star, June 17 1982, E4). Within the OAM, membership was categorized as practising midwife, student midwife, associate midwife (midwives who were not practising), and supporting members (the category including both consumers and supporters); only practising midwives had voting privileges. Although membership did not exclude those who did not practise midwifery, the differentiation of membership categories, in addition to Daniels' assertion that birth helpers were midwives, marked the initial steps in the demarcation of midwives as a group distinct from the women they served.

The 1982 Inquest

The establishment of the OAM support structure was timely, as soon thereafter came one of the first of many significant challenges to the development of midwifery – the tragic death of a baby following a planned home birth attended by two midwives in the Kitchener-Waterloo area in February 1982. During the home birth, complications arose and the midwives transferred the woman to hospital. Hospital staff delivered the baby but it later died of pneumonia. The hospital staff blamed the midwives for the death. They argued that the woman should have been induced immediately after her membranes ruptured (four days earlier); this, they felt, would have prevented the baby's death. These accusations led to an inquest which was held in July 1982. Ironically, this inquest, which was focused on condemning the practice of midwifery, was actually to play a key role in bringing midwives in Southern Ontario together to work for a common cause.

The midwives involved in the death – Ava Vosu and Mary Molnar – initially considered keeping a low profile at the inquest. The serious possibility of legal consequences, however, spurred them and the midwifery community to take more decisive action: "The inquest really helped to motivate midwives to get more politically organized ... We knew that in California midwives were being charged with criminal charges ... but [the possibility of it] happening in Ontario made people feel very vulnerable" (Vicki Van Wagner, as quoted in Fynes 1994: 76). Midwives focused their political action in three directions. The first was a decision to hire one of the top criminal lawyers in the country, Clayton Ruby, to defend their case. In hiring Ruby, the midwives wanted to send a clear message that they "meant to challenge the system, rather than just [remain] sort of a quiet underground" (Van Wagner 1993, as cited in Fynes 1994). The second action was to set up a letter-writing campaign to help raise funds to pay for their legal expenses. In response to a letter the OAM sent out to former clients requesting a fifty-dollar donation to cover the legal costs of the inquest, they netted $10,000 in donations and several letters of personal support (Barrington 1985). The third action taken by the midwifery community was to elicit support from women's health advocates in the Toronto-based Women's Health Network to help organize a public demonstration to increase public awareness and support for midwifery and homebirth. All three actions proved to be highly successful.

At the inquest, Ruby argued that the midwives were not on trial; rather, his case challenged a health care system that did not include them as essential caregivers for birthing women. He called directly for the integration of midwifery into the health care system. With respect to the specific circumstances surrounding the baby's death, internationally prominent obstetrician and midwifery supporter, Murray Enkin, argued that the blame for the death lay not with the midwives, but with the attendants at the hospital who did not heed the information given to them by the midwives when the baby was transferred. He felt that the hospital staff waited an "unconscionably long time" to attend to the woman (personal communication 1995).

When the jury members made their recommendations on the case, they included a call for the regulation and official recognition of midwifery. The jury had specifically proposed that the College of Nurses (CNO) and the College of Physicians and Surgeons of Ontario (CPSO) set up standards and establish a program of study in midwifery leading to a licence to practise in the Province of Ontario. The jury also requested that available information on home and hospital births be made public.

Midwives and their supporters regarded these recommendations as the first official public endorsement of midwifery in the province. At the same time, the inquest highlighted the precarious legal situation in which midwives were practising. They realized that they needed to more clearly articulate their standards of practice and education to make their care more defensible (Eberts et al. 1987). Consequently, the OAM developed specific committees to address these very issues. Midwives and their supporters also realized that they would have to become more sophisticated in their dealings with the public and the media. The demonstration organized by the Toronto Women's Health Network was helpful but it made clear how much more needed to be done in this regard. For some members of the midwifery community, inspiration was drawn from the lobbying efforts of the pro-choice movement – in particular the connections it had established with the larger women's movement. Midwife Vicki Van Wagner describes the influence of the women's movement on midwifery organizers: "We made an effort to look to the women's movement for political influence about the challenge of what we could do with midwifery as a semi-legal profession. Definitely we made a very clear choice to seek out mentors in the women's movement, to look at how the pro-choice movement organized itself and learn whatever we could from it, to make alliances within the women's movement" (personal communication 1995). Although the midwifery community still viewed itself as a social movement looking to the pro-choice movement for insight, it was quickly becoming a professional movement, creating standards of practice and education for its practitioners. In mapping out their professional project, midwives were to face numerous other challenges.

The CPSO Statement on Home Births

The CPSO had known about physician attendance at home birth but for the most part considered it a fringe activity practised by only a few physicians. Some hospital-based physicians had made complaints to the College regarding what they considered an unacceptably high incidence of emergency obstetric cases arising from home birth situations. Often these emergencies were a result of the relative lack of experience of home birth physicians and the general reluctance of physicians, birth attendants/midwives, and clients to transfer to hospital because it was regarded as a hostile environment and inappropriate for birth. Decisions to transfer were frequently delayed until the woman and/or baby were clearly in crisis.

In response to the increasing awareness of home birth practices, the CPSO sent to its members the following notice in January 1982:

The current interest in home births has created an opportunity for certain individuals to offer their services as "Home Birth Attendants." Non-medical practitioners are not entitled to provide obstetrical services which are clearly within the practice of medicine. It is professional misconduct for a member to permit, counsel or assist any person not licensed as a physician to engage in the practice of medicine. Some physicians have been urged by their patients to attend them at home when they go into labour. The College would discourage this practice because it does not consider home births to be safe or in the patient's best interest. (College Notices, January 1982: 2)

Following this notice, the CPSO sent letters to the physicians they identified as attending home births or backing up midwives attending home births, threatening to bring them before the College on charges of professional misconduct.

The Kitchener inquest and another inquest in 1982 into a baby death in Toronto (the latter attended by a physician with the assistance of a midwife) brought the increasingly prevalent practice of home births to the forefront of the CPSO's attention. In response to the recommendations of the juries of both these inquests that the CPSO develop standards for home birth, the CPSO created an Ad Hoc Committee on Out-of-Hospital Births. The Committee, headed by obstetrician Roy Beckett, requested briefs from interested parties. The OAM was contacted directly by Beckett. He requested information regarding midwives' feelings about their place in this process. At that time, he stated that the Committee would likely accept home births given adequate safeguards.

In their response to Beckett's letter, the OAM argued that midwives were a necessary component of the health care system. Midwives provided a continuity of care that consumers were increasingly demanding. OAM members cited international precedents in which midwives conducted deliveries under their own responsibility. They asserted that the integration of midwifery into the health care system, as recommended by the inquests, would help maintain the quality and integrity of obstetric care (Fynes 1994).

The "acceptance" of home births that Dr Beckett alluded to in his letter to the OAM never came to be. When the CPSO issued an official position statement on out-of-hospital births in early 1983, it reiterated the main elements of its 1982 notice. Although it did not ban physician attendance at out-of-hospital births, the statement strongly discouraged it. This position was based on British research which the College interpreted as indicating that home birth posed an additional risk to mothers and babies.

In response to this formal statement, the OAM asserted that the College had come to untenable conclusions about the safety of planned home births. Midwives criticized the CPSO for grossly misinterpreting British statistics; they argued that these statistics in fact supported the safety of home births. The OAM also questioned the "motives of the College in not revealing the sources of information on which they based their conclusions to their members" (*Issue* 3, no. 2, Spring 1983, 6). The OAM strongly urged midwifery supporters to write to the College registrar protesting the statement. Angry consumers did more than write letters. They formed an ad hoc organization, Choices in Childbirth, and held a week-long picket of the CPSO offices to protest the limiting of women's options. This protest was successful in gaining considerable publicity for the home birth issue. Indeed, midwifery consumers were becoming increasingly media savvy.

Midwives "Go It Alone"

Following the strong recommendations of the CPSO, several physicians who attended home births discontinued this practice.[6] With fewer physicians left to attend home births, most would-be midwives decided that they would "go it alone" and practise without the assistance of a physician.[7] More and more, these women began to regard themselves as independent midwives rather than as birth educators and attendants. Thus, the CPSO Statement had the contradictory effect of not shutting down the practice of homebirth, but rather further politicizing midwives and increasing their self-confidence as independent practitioners (Eberts et al. 1987: 30).

The trend toward more independent practice, in concert with the implicit threats symbolized by the inquests, increased midwives' concerns regarding their legal status. Midwife Robin Kilpatrick recounted "lengthy discussions about ... the legal responsibility ... midwives would be shouldering" (personal communication 1995). As a result, several midwives began to consider pursuing legitimacy and integration into the Ontario health care system using the newly created OAM as the vehicle to steer these efforts.

The goal of integration became strongly influenced by the establishment of a Health Professions Legislation Review (HPLR) by the incumbent provincial Conservative government in 1983. Midwife Vicki Van Wagner described how the 1982 inquest and the HPLR together spurred midwives to seek integration: "In the debate about whether we should be overtly working for legislation ... pressure came from the outside. First, legal challenges to midwives being able to exist, the first being the 1982 inquest into the death of a baby after a birth attended by midwives in Kitchener ... The other was the Health Professions Legislation Review which started in 1982" (personal communication 1995).

REORGANIZING TO ENHANCE THE CASE FOR INTEGRATION

The Health Professions Legislation Review

In response to various pressures for change in the way health professions were regulated, the provincial Conservative government announced the establishment of the HPLR in November 1982. The mandate of the HPLR, which was more clearly defined on April 20, 1983, was to make recommendations to the Minister of Health in draft legislation with respect to: 1) which health professions should be regulated; 2) updating and reforming the existing Health Disciplines Act; 3) devising a new structure for all legislation governing the health professions; and 4) settling outstanding issues involving several health professions (HPLR 1989). The HPLR's primary objective was to design a new regulatory framework that would more effectively advance and protect the public interest.

The Review committee was kept at arms length from the Ministry of Health and was composed almost entirely of legal experts. It was coordinated by Alan Schwartz, also a lawyer. The committee set out on an exhaustive search of existing health care groups to respond to their first mandate. Throughout the spring and summer of 1983 more than 200 groups were contacted, including approximately seventy-five would-be and established health professional groups. The OAM, representing practising midwives, and an older organization representing nurse-midwifery in the province, the Ontario Nurse-Midwives Association, were two of the groups contacted. In this initial contact, the Review panel asked simply if midwifery was a profession that they should regulate under a health profession statute. As midwife Vicki Van Wagner recalled, "In 1983 they approached us and said, do you want to be regulated? So we had to say to each other, do we want to be regulated?" (personal communication 1995).

The Ontario Nurse-Midwives Association

As noted briefly in the previous chapter, the Ontario Nurse-Midwives Association (ONMA) was developed in late 1973 by a British-trained midwife, May Toth, in response to the desire of some foreign-trained nurse-midwives to practise midwifery in Canada. A catalyst for the establishment of this organization was Toth's attendance at the International Confederation of Midwives (ICM)[8] Conference in Washington DC in 1973. There she met with other Canadian-based nurse-midwives and discussed the idea of setting up an organization to promote nurse-midwifery. The nurse-midwives who joined the ONMA worked largely on labour and delivery wards but some also worked in departments of public health. For the most part, they were unclear about the role they would like to play in the health care system. Therefore, they consulted widely with various women's groups, such as the National Council of Women; sympathetic physicians; health policy makers; and nurse-midwives from the US, about various models of integration. As most members of the ONMA were

British-trained nurse-midwives, the preferred model was the British independent midwifery model. Options that May Toth proposed for consideration ranged from having nurse-midwives provide care for parturient women throughout their pregnancy to assisting women only in labour and delivery. In the end they felt that pursuing an American nurse-midwifery model, in which a more limited role for nurse-midwives was delineated, would be politically easier to implement in the Canadian context.

Soon after its development, this independent organization became a special interest group within the Registered Nurses Association of Ontario (RNAO). The negotiations that the RNAO had proposed with the College of Nurses of Ontario (CNO), representative organizations of the medical profession, and the Ontario government regarding enabling legislation never came to fruition and neither did the efforts of the ONMA.[9] Throughout the 1970s, the membership of the organization ranged from sixty to seventy-five though there were estimates that 5,000 to 7,000 nurses registered with the nursing college had prior midwifery training (TFIMO 1987). These nurse-midwives never practised the full range of care often associated with midwifery either within or outside the hospital setting. In hospitals, they were limited to practising as labour and delivery nurses. They also strictly avoided practising midwifery out of hospital due to concerns that they might lose either their nursing licence or their hospital jobs or both.[10] Given the opposition to the practice of home birth, these concerns were valid. Many nurse-midwives were recent immigrants to Canada who on occasion experienced discrimination on the job. Most did not feel confident in challenging the system. Because they did not practise, nurse-midwives were not able to amass consumer support for their services as the practising home birth midwives had. Although the members of the ONMA were initially enthusiastic about the possibility of practising midwifery in Canada, their interest and commitment to the pursuit of legislation soon waned.

In the early 1980s, some members of the ONMA became aware of the organization of lay midwives represented by the OAM. The ONMA extended an invitation to OAM members to attend their information session on midwifery at the annual RNAO Conference in 1981. This initial interaction was positive, as members of both groups agreed on the need for midwives in the maternity care system (Fynes 1994). ONMA Vice President Rena Porteous became "interested in this group [the OAM] because it seemed to be a really active group; they had a lot of energy; they were younger women doing what we were talking about what should be done" (personal communication 1995). The following March, the OAM extended an invitation to ONMA members to attend one of their meetings to discuss gaining acceptance for midwifery. They held subsequent meetings between members of the two groups. The initial contacts between the ONMA and the OAM would prove to have important repercussions for the advent of the HPLR.

The OAM's Decision to Integrate

Although the ONMA was organized with the sole purpose of integration, contact with the HPLR thrust the issue of integration to the forefront of the OAM agenda, causing a contentious debate within the ranks of the organization. Midwife Vicki Van Wagner described how differences in perspective within the midwifery community were likely present at first but crystallized as time went along: "Some people who began to work as birth assistants and evolved into midwives felt ... 'let's just be quiet, let's just keep this underground' and that perhaps an underground movement would be the best way to go. And there were other midwives ... who solicited American midwives to come and do workshops and had writers from the *Star* and the *Globe and Mail* coming to interview them and who were talking about women organizing to provide these services" (personal communication 1995). The debate between these two groups regarding the integration issue came to a head at a one-day conference held in Toronto in June 1983. With more than 300 midwives and supporters present, the two sides broke out into what midwifery supporter Jutta Mason described as a "big fight ... [which] became very emotional with people yelling at each other" (personal communication 1995).

Pushing the idea of becoming integrated into the mainstream maternity care system in a community that had developed out of a distrust of the professional management of childbirth would be difficult. As alluded to in the quote from Van Wagner above, opposition to integration came from those midwives and supporters who wanted to continue practising quietly. Opposition also came from those espousing a more radical feminist agenda who expressed concern over the primacy of the midwifery issue (i.e., a focus on the caregiver) over the broader issues of choices in childbirth alternatives (i.e., a focus on the woman and her choices).[11] For these women, midwifery was seen as a means to the end of women having more choice and control in childbirth, and not as an end in itself.

Concerns were also expressed that seeking legal recognition through integration into the mainstream maternity care system, which midwifery had arisen in reaction to, was fundamentally contradictory: "It was easier in a way to present the anti-legislation argument because it was more articulated at that point. And it seemed to have a gut level appeal with midwives ... because why were we there except that we didn't like bureaucracy. We were an alternative!" (Midwife Vicki Van Wagner, personal communication 1995). As Jutta Mason (1990) later documented, "these midwives were marginal by choice" (1).

The midwives promoting the integration project, however, felt it important to channel these "anarchist tendencies" into creating change within the system: "One of the interesting things that one often faces around building midwifery as an alternative movement, which is both its strength and its enormous weakness, is the anarchist tendency to have the individual courage to look at things and critique them and say, 'I don't want to do them that way' ... The challenge is to channel those energies into changing a system from within it as opposed to from outside of it" (Midwife Holliday Tyson, personal communication 1995).

Several of those opposing integration also pointed to the effects of integration in the United States, which suggested that integration led to serious negative consequences for midwives and their clients (see discussion of DeVries and others' work in chapter 2). The following points made by the Michigan Midwives' Association were reprinted in the OAM newsletter (*Issue* 3, no. 1, Winter 1983) for consideration:

We affirm the mother's right and responsibility to study the birth process and to make an informed choice regarding the type of birth attendant and environment that feel most suited to her needs ... Parents choose midwives for a variety of reasons and purposes, therefore no single standard of certification will meet all parents' needs ... Parents can be better "protected from incompetent practitioners" through education than through licensing, which does not encourage them to be responsible ... Certification tends to lead to a false sense of security, and the unquestioning acceptance of the midwife as an authority figure by her clients ... Certification will define our practice as midwives and therefore limit the complete use of our skills ... To certify ourselves ... we would run the risk of merely creating a new class of birth professionals. (10–11)

In addition, as noted by Anne Frye in an article from *Special Delivery* reprinted in *Issue* Winter 1981, 1, no. 4: "Certification tends to lead to a false sense of security and the unquestioning acceptance of the midwife as an authority figure by her clients. By creating this artificial separation we're in danger of dehumanizing our essential relationship with one another" (1). Several midwives agreed with these cautionary statements.

Many also opposed any rapid change and simply wanted to take things more slowly. Others expressed concern that midwifery was being thrust into the political arena prematurely when it was only in its early stages of development.

On the other side of the debate were the midwives who tended to be more politically active, not just in dealing with midwifery but also with the broader women's health and pro-choice movement. These midwives and supporters pushed for integration. They countered arguments made by those against integration by asserting that the only way to avoid potential legal repercussions was to seek protective legislation. Midwifery consumer and supporter Holly Nimmons described the precarious legal situation in which midwives found themselves: "There could be witch hunts. There could be one inquest after another. And without any legal structure to protect a practising midwife, it just seems like a horrible way, a sacrifice, a penalty for a woman to want to put herself out on the line to be constantly in that potential" (personal communication 1995). In seeking integration, these midwives also hoped to gain government funding for midwifery services to help increase the accessibility of midwifery care to all women (i.e., beyond those who could afford to pay for their services privately) (Van Wagner 2004). In attaining legislation, midwife Robin Kilpatrick argued that "it could strengthen the profession and provide more options for more women" (personal communication 1995). Midwife Vicki Van Wagner concurred, arguing that whatever kind of midwifery care was implemented would result in better care for women:

We looked at midwifery systems that were regulated all around the world, and we still thought that even the most oppressed, regulated, restricted midwifery would be better than nothing. We compared, for example, the average Canadian obstetrical birth, and the average birth in Britain in a very oppressed and fragmented midwifery system, and realized that women were less likely to have a caesarian in Britain ... less likely to have an episiotomy ... and even though as a woman in Britain I've never met my midwife before ... there is still some of what midwifery is left there. So the worst case scenario ... was we become oppressed and over-regulated ... [but] it's still better than nothing. And the other part of it was ... access. We realized that the literature very clearly showed that in the US even nurse-midwifery – another fragmented and oppressed midwifery system that we didn't want anything to do with creating – was doing so much good for teenagers, poor women, minority group women. In inner city New York – at the North Bronx hospital – it's like a miracle what they have done for prematurity, rates of intervention, for women who probably get abused most by the system. And an underground, sort of alternative practice of midwifery would never be able to be accessible to those poor women and teenagers. (personal communication 1995)

Indeed, the accessibility issue would become a critical point in the pursuit of integration. As midwifery supporter, Jutta Mason (1990) described: "In Ontario, the framing of midwife-attended birth as the privilege of a prosperous elite originated as a propaganda tool: to present the exclusion of the midwife from the government health care system as direct discrimination against the poor and helpless, and therefore to ring the moral alarm bells of the public conscience" (7). But to be sure, there was much more than propaganda to this issue.

The strongest argument made by advocates for integration was that "midwifery had come up [to the HPLR] in terms of the inquests ... and that there were going to be proposals from medicine and nursing about a kind of midwifery ... It became really clear to some of us that if we don't regulate ourselves, they will" (Vicki Van Wagner, personal communication 1995). ONMA President Rena Porteous believed that the nursing profession would make a submission regarding midwifery whether midwives did or not: "One of the reasons why we actually decided to do the submission even though we thought, Good Lord, we're not prepared ... [was that] we knew if we didn't, nursing would and they would probably get it ... by default" (personal communication 1995). Thus, it was primarily because of the HPLR that midwifery rather than other childbirth alternatives became the focus of the movement. Midwife Larry Lenske argued that "[t]his may be the only opportunity during the foreseeable future for midwifery to be legalized" (*The Ontario Midwife* 1, no. 3, 6). The sense of urgency in pursuing integration was considered real. It was argued that the HPLR, initially envisaged as a two-year process, was going to regulate midwifery with or without the input of midwives. The status quo was not considered to be a situation that would continue. Change was believed to be inevitable.

In the end those promoting integration prevailed and the OAM decided to focus its efforts on the HPLR. Nevertheless, the concerns regarding integration lingered. Attempts to unite behind the issue of integration were paralleled by attempts to unite midwives in Toronto into one practice group – the Midwives' Collective. These efforts failed, however, and two practice groups were set up: the Midwives' Collective, those midwives who supported integration; and the Midwives' Cooperative, those more hesitant of entering the whole HPLR process. Soon after, the Collective set up an office practice, whereas midwives in the Cooperative continued to practise largely out of their homes.

Not surprisingly, the midwives in the Collective became the political centre of midwifery in Ontario. This trend had begun during the 1982 inquest when some Toronto midwives took over the organizational tasks of the OAM from Ava Vosu (as she was the subject of the inquest). When the Collective set up office space, they shared it jointly with the OAM. Subsequently, the midwives in the Collective became the principal political contacts. The midwives operating out of the Collective had developed important political skills and connections within the women's health movement. Some argued they had more time to focus on political activity because they had fewer children than less politically active midwives. The Collective also created practice conditions which not only strongly supported political activity but also financially reimbursed midwives for the time they spent on political work at the same rate as midwifery care activities.

Creation of the Midwifery Task Force of Ontario

Once they decided to pursue integration, midwives began to employ various political strategies to promote their quest. The midwives advocating integration were strongly influenced by a visiting midwife from British Columbia, Patti Mayr. In that province, midwives tended to have a stronger sense of professionalism and had already begun to seek integration through an Interdisciplinary Midwifery Task Force. Mayr brought these ideas to Ontario and encouraged midwives there to do the same; that is, to create a midwifery consumer advocacy and support organization, the Midwifery Task Force of Ontario (MTFO), separate from the OAM.[12] Consumers had started to become more organized following the 1982 inquest and after the 1983 Out-of-Hospital Birth Statement made by the CPSO (the Choices in Childbirth group). Following Mayr's recommendation, an interdisciplinary group of consumers, professionals, and others supportive of the midwifery integration project came together in June 1983 to create the MTFO. They held the first general meeting in Toronto a few weeks later. The official mandate of the organization was to lobby for the legal recognition and integration of midwifery into the health care system. Midwife Betty-Anne Davis highlighted the importance of having established the MTFO for midwives' pursuit of integration: "It's better to have a consumer group rather than blowing your own trumpet to say the things that need to be said not just about the need for midwifery but about what is best for clients" (personal communication 1995).

The first item on the MTFO agenda was a major campaign to attract more consumer supporters. In the opening statement of *Issue*, now the MTFO newsletter, MTFO officials rallied support from consumers to take up the midwifery integration cause: "Many of us have already enjoyed the support and caring of our midwives, in those important times around childbirth. Your midwife has been your advocate. Now, it is time for consumers to come together to share the task of advocating for the legal recognition of midwifery as part of our health care system ... We are wrong to suppose that their services will always be available to us – unless we are willing to work for their recognition" (*Issue* 1983:1). Membership campaigns were successful. MTFO membership grew steadily, and by the spring of 1984 it had reached 400 (*Issue* 1984) and almost 1,000 soon after (Nimmons, personal communication 1995). Members came from all around the province as regional chapters of the MTFO were set up in London, Kingston, Ottawa, and Thunder Bay. Calls for members attracted support from a well-educated group of individuals (the majority with college/university education). This included many concerned professionals who had training, experience, and professional connections which could be drawn on to promote midwifery (Fynes 1994; *Issue*, Winter 1984:3). Concurrent with these membership drives, the MTFO became actively involved in a public education campaign to increase public awareness of the benefits of midwifery, the formulation of draft legislation proposals along with the OAM and ONMA, lobbying efforts to increase the awareness of the public demand for midwifery care among members of the Ontario provincial parliament (MPPs), and fund raising to help support the attempts to achieve legislation.

The establishment of the MTFO as a consumer support group would prove to be an effective political strategy facilitating the integration process. But reflected in this organizational separation of the interests of consumers and midwives was another step in the creation of midwives as professionals separate from the women for whom they provided care. The OAM was now a separate association representing midwives' professional interests. Membership in the OAM was largely limited to midwives (this was paralleled by the ONMA); consumers and supporters were channelled into becoming members of the MTFO. MTFO took over the newsletter *Issue* and the OAM newsletter became *The Ontario Midwife*, which they described as "a professional publication for midwives ... (a place to publish professional quality, research articles on midwifery) ... while *Issue* is designed to appeal to everyone, with a mix of articles" (*The Ontario Midwife* 1, no. 2, 1). Although there was significant cross membership on OAM and MTFO committees and much shared interest, the development of this separate consumer group nevertheless marked the first time that consumers were organized separately from midwives. This, in addition to the decision to pursue integration, marked a general change in the amorphous midwifery community from an egalitarian social movement striving for alternatives in childbirth, to the beginnings of the professional project.

The HPLR Process

CREATION OF THE MIDWIFERY COALITION

Having been contacted by the HPLR, the two midwifery groups, OAM and ONMA, discussed the idea of making a single submission to the Committee. Given that members of the OAM and ONMA had already met and established good rapport, both groups were open to the possibility of collaborating on the HPLR submission. They agreed that if the members of the two groups found that they held similar views, they would make one submission. A key player in the decision to make one submission was Rena Porteous, then ONMA president. She recalls that, "as we talked more and more we ... realized that – or at least I had certainly realized – that there was really no difference in philosophy between the OAM and the ONMA" (Porteous, personal communication 1995). This philosophical compatibility was in terms of both women-centred care and the independence of midwifery from nursing (following the British model with which many Ontario nurse-midwives were already comfortable). Porteous described how they "always came back to the bottom line that midwifery needed to serve women [and they] wanted what was best for women – that women have a choice over medicalization" (Porteous 1993, as quoted in Fynes 1994). Realizing that their goals and philosophies of care were compatible, and that the strengths of the one group complemented the weaknesses of the other, the groups agreed to make a single submission to the HPLR committee as the Midwifery Coalition.

THE FIRST SUBMISSION TO THE HPLR

In making a submission to the HPLR, the members representing the Midwifery Coalition had to respond to twenty-two points set out by the HPLR Committee. These areas focused on the regulation of the profession, education and entry to practice issues, and scope of practice. To elicit submissions from the broadest possible range of participants, the Review panel also met in person with many groups. The Midwifery Coalition, including representatives from the ONMA, the OAM, and the MTFO, first met with the HPLR panel in August 1983. At this meeting, members of the committee provided assistance to midwives, as it had to other groups interested in regulation, to make the review process easier as well as to obtain the best possible information from the groups to help them in making decisions about regulation.

Members of the MTFO worked closely with the midwives in the Coalition, and were consulted and given the opportunity to have input into the content of the HPLR submission. In *Issue*, frequent updates of the issues were presented, not only to keep members informed, but also to invite comments and critiques on materials relevant to the submissions (Fynes 1994). The MTFO also provided support for midwives' legislative efforts through its publicity campaigns. For example, to coincide with the Midwifery Coalition's first submission to the HPLR, MTFO representatives encouraged members to write to the Minister of Health, Keith Norton, and their respective MPPs (between mid-January and early February "for greatest impact" (*Issue* 1983:2) to indicate their support for the legalization of midwifery. Midwife Larry Lenske (1984) stated that "[t]hese endorsements, in essence, become part of the submission and indicate to the provincial review committee the level of support which exists for legalized midwifery" (6). This was to ensure the government recognized the level of public demand for the integration of midwifery.

KEY ELEMENTS OF MIDWIFERY COALITION'S
FIRST SUBMISSION TO HPLR, 1983

---

1 Recognition of Midwifery as an Independent, Autonomous Health Profession
2 Self Regulation
3 Licensing of Midwifery with Exclusive Right to Practice
4 Multiple Routes of Entry to Practice

In their first submission to the HPLR, the Midwifery Coalition made four major points. The first was the recognition of midwifery as an independent, autonomous health profession, distinct from nursing and medicine: "Midwifery is a separate entity distinct from nursing and medicine. Its specific focus on normal pregnancy and childbirth contrasts sharply with both the broad scope of nursing and general practice medicine, and the focus on the abnormal of the obstetrician ... Midwifery is the only profession whose primary responsibility is the continuous care of mother and child from conception through labour and delivery to six weeks post partum. No other profession is specially trained to monitor and assist throughout the normal childbearing cycle" (Lenske 1984: 9). The second argument was for the establishment of a College of Midwifery, a self-regulating body for midwives, with significant consumer representation to help maintain the quality of midwifery care. The third point was for the licensing of midwives with an exclusive right to practise. The final argument was for multiple routes of entry to practise, including training through formal programs and through empirical experience (Lenske 1984, *The Ontario Midwife* 1, no. 2: 6).[13]

These four proposals drew on the international definition of a midwife for support, and were bolstered with references to the "wide acceptance of midwifery in other countries" (Midwives Coalition, First Submission to HPLR, December 1983: 2). The proposals were also supported with references to consumer demand: "Recent trends, including consumer demand for more personalized family-centred maternity care, have emphasized the void in our health care team system" (10). The members of the Coalition regarded all of these elements essential in preventing midwifery from losing its unique approach to care of the childbearing family.

In making the submission to the HPLR committee, those heading the Coalition did what they deemed necessary to help achieve state recognition. In doing so, some argued that midwifery was moulding itself to the demands of the HPLR process by espousing such principles as standardization and compliance (Mason 1990). Midwife Jane Kilthei countered these assertions:

My general sense of [the HPLR submission process] was that ... a lot [of it] was a learning process for us as midwives and what do they really want to know about. So it wasn't that we were shaping answers to make some of the answers they want; it's more like oh, they want us to tell them about that area. Or they're concerned about safety of home births so we have to go and find all the research about home births and compile that and give them something rational to base it on. Because a lot of the first responses as I remember it were more reactive than ... based on knowledge and information ... They had a lot of misconceptions. (personal communication 1995)

Some midwives and midwifery supporters made criticisms not only of the content of the submission, but also about the process of making the submission. Lenske (1984) described some of the dissent in *Issue*:

Due to the pressure involved in meeting the submission deadline, there was only limited opportunity for midwives and consumers to voice their ideas and concerns ... I've heard both criticism from midwives who disagree with points of the submission and who are feeling excluded from the process; and pleas from the committee members who feel they are out on a limb as well as overworked. This is to be expected given how rushed the initial process was ... It is ... important for midwives, individuals, and consumer and health care groups to give their feedback, (whether supportive or critical), to the OAM/ONMA committee drafting revisions, and to the OAM and MTF boards as soon as possible. Bear in mind that the legalization procedure is a political process. The OAM/ONMA committee will not only be ... drafting and revising the submission, but forging alliances with non-midwifery groups. Some of these alliances may necessitate compromises on issues which may not be acceptable to you. (9)

Thus, the HPLR had begun to create an environment to which midwifery, as represented by its leaders in the Midwifery Coalition, had to a certain extent conform. In trying to fit within the parameters of this environment and gain acceptance by the Review, the divisions within the midwifery community arising from the decision to seek integration intensified.

SUMMARY

Although the midwifery community in Ontario developed as a grassroots movement of like-minded individuals intent on creating a place where a different form of maternity care could exist, the organization of this community from its inception with the Home Birth Task Force was political. This Task Force formed to respond to the discontinuing of government funding for home birth service by the Victorian Order of Nurses (VON). Given that these services were no longer available, this prompted a new group of birth helpers to develop. Later when the physicians these home-birth helpers assisted were being harassed by their College to discontinue providing care at homebirths – another external challenge – these birth helpers were faced with the decision to either take on a larger role in childbirth attendance or cease practising. But perhaps the two largest external influences on the development of midwifery and midwives' decision to seek integration were the Coroner's inquest and the HPLR. Midwives and their supporters viewed these fora as potential threats to the movement to challenge traditional forms of maternity care in the province. It was in response to these cumulative challenges (or opportunities) that this community was transformed from a social movement to a midwifery professional project. Thus, the decision was either seek inclusion or potentially be excluded. Concurrent with this transformation of the community, the challenges it faced were also reshaped into opportunities through which midwives and the practice of midwifery could seek public support and protection through integration.

In their decision to pursue integration into the Ontario health care system, midwives and their supporters made significant changes to the way they were socially and politically organized. The original broad focus of the alternative childbirth community narrowed over time to the professional project of integrating midwifery into the health care system.[14] Not only did the focus of the movement narrow, but groups representing the shared interests of a social movement evolved into separate, more bureaucratically organized structures representing the "different" interests of midwives and the women for whom they provided care. Although much of this could be viewed as strategic, increasingly midwives' interests were being seen and treated differently from those of their clients. Midwives had "professional" interests, such as liability and the legal context of their work; women were organized as consumers to indicate support for midwifery and also to help promote the midwifery integration project.

It is important to note that although accomplished within the confines of the midwifery community, these changes were made largely in response to these external forces either implicitly or explicitly. That is, leaders of the midwifery integration project were reconfiguring midwifery initially in response to external challenges and later to increase its likelihood of inclusion within the implicit agenda of the HPLR. This included exhibiting a more professional appearance through an association that was not an undifferentiated mixture of consumers, supporters, and practitioners (see figure 2). This reconfiguring process resulted in some apprehension from those within the midwifery community who expressed concern with the entire midwifery integration project and the establishment of a new professional expert in maternity care.

The strategic political importance of the separation of midwifery and consumer organizations, however, should not be devalued. When it was decided to pursue integration, the separation of organizations was envisaged as enhancing midwives' case for inclusion in the health care system. Through their association, midwives could exhibit their appearance as professionals worthy of inclusion in the system of health professions. Through a separate consumer group, the constituency support for midwifery could be made evident. This strategy was proving to be successful in increasing public and political support for the integration throughout the early 1980s. Several studies of professionalization highlight the importance

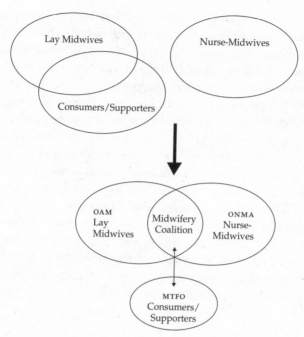

Figure 2
From social movement to professional project: the evolution of the organization of the midwifery community

of consumer support (Coburn and Biggs 1986; Willis 1989), which was particularly noteworthy of this midwifery project. As we shall see in the forthcoming chapters, this consumer support was especially important in garnering state support.

One also should not underestimate the importance of the coalition between nurse- and lay midwives in the Province. This would help prevent some of the divisiveness within midwifery along nurse- and non-nurse lines, which in the United States has resulted in significant negative consequences in the attempt to legitimize midwifery (Bourgeault and Fynes 1997; Davis-Floyd 1999), and hopefully quash any efforts to implement a limited nurse-midwifery model. Internal divisions are also something that many other professional projects had to overcome in order to succeed (Willis 1989). Together, these organizational moves would prove to be critical political decisions significantly bolstering midwives' overall chances of securing state legitimacy and professional status.

Despite the changes to the organization of the social movement, one could argue that midwives, childbearing women, and their supporters maintained their interconnectedness by having significant committee cross-membership and minimal barriers in general to communication and decision-making. That is, although the interests of midwives and clients were bureaucratically separated, at the level of everyday practice, a concerted effort was made to ensure involvement and coordinate activities. Indeed, the midwives' professional organizations and the consumers' support organization were both focused on the same project of gaining the integration of midwifery into the health care system. They both thought that having some form of legitimate midwifery was better than it remaining marginal at best or non-existent at worst. They hoped that through their continued, coordinated involvement, changes to midwifery throughout the integration process would help to ensure that the fundamental nature of midwifery as it had begun to evolve in the province would not be significantly altered. Representatives of both organizations were beginning to develop some expertise in strategies to publicize and politicize their project. These strategies would become well-honed as they faced even more significant challenges in their integration project.

CHAPTER FIVE

Deciding to Integrate Midwifery

During the early 1980s, the midwifery community had begun to poise itself for integration into the health care system largely in response to the initiation of a review of the legislation governing health professions, the HPLR. Leaders of the midwifery community realized that legitimacy and public support were necessary not only to convince the HPLR and the government to integrate midwifery, but to integrate it in a manner that preserved what they considered the essential and unique aspects of midwifery that had begun to evolve in the province. One of the essential elements desired by the leaders of the integration project was self-regulation and the HPLR was critically important in this pursuit. The HPLR not only sparked the political reorganization and reorientation of the midwifery community to focus on integration, it was also fundamentally important in altering the manner in which midwifery was regulated in Ontario.

THE REGULATION OF MIDWIFERY PRIOR TO INTEGRATION

As it emerged in the late 1970s, midwifery has been described as an "unregulated" profession. This assertion, however, is not completely accurate. Midwives, as one early observer described, were "regulated" in part by the women they served: "Midwifery ... is an earned position in the birthing community, accredited by parents rather than by a piece of paper" (Barrington 1985: 41). This form of "regulation" originally operated through referrals within the alternative childbirth community. Later on, this form of regulation was more formalized into an informed choice agreement. In such an agreement, a midwife would outline her education, background, experience, as well as the services she would provide the pregnant woman. In addition, it described the roles and responsibilities of both the midwife and the woman for whom she was to provide care and her partner. Given the midwife's qualifications and preparation, the woman and her partner would then decide whether they felt comfortable having the midwife as their birth attendant, and whether they were comfortable with their responsibilities under the agreement. Once signed, the informed choice agreement in essence became a contract between the two parties.

In addition to this informal system of regulation, midwives were also regulated by the criminal justice system. Death at a home birth, whether it was due to incompetence or not, by law would always result in an inquest. In the case of unfortunate consequences to the mother or baby as a result of incompetent practice, the criminal justice system could also be used by the parents to charge the midwife with criminal negligence causing bodily harm. Regulation through the criminal justice system was rarely ever resorted to by parents but it was used by members of the medical profession, particularly for charges of practising medicine without a licence.

To enhance their case for integration and inclusion into the HPLR legislation, midwives had to present this system of regulation as inadequate, which indeed it was. Midwifery supporter Jutta Mason (1990) described the situation midwives faced: "In order for the midwives to be of interest to the government, they had to ... prove that they had 'not enough supervision by regulated professionals,' and were not 'regulated effectively.' From the point of view of many doctors and nurses, these statements needed no proving, but within the alternative birth culture a considerable swallowing of pride was required" (4). Midwives did ultimately "choose this route" to achieve the goal of integration. As noted in the previous chapter, the alternative form of regulation sought through their initial submission to the HPLR was self-regulation. In order to achieve self-regulation, legitimacy within the health care system became an important first step.

THE HEALTH PROFESSIONS LEGISLATION REVIEW PROCESS

Regulatory Elements of the Midwifery Coalition's First Submission to the HPLR

Once it was decided to seek integration, supporting a bid for midwifery to be a self-regulating profession was not a difficult point on which to gain consensus among members of the midwifery community. In their submission to the HPLR, the Midwifery Coalition members strongly asserted that their goal was self-regulation: "We do not feel there are any acceptable alternatives to self-regulation" (Midwives Coalition, First Submission to HPLR, 1983: 13). Reference to midwives' current commitment to self-regulate in an otherwise unregulated environment lent support to the Coalition's proposal for self-regulation: "Currently, an important function of the Ontario Association of Midwives is to encourage appropriate standards of entry to practice, continuing competence, and professional discipline among midwives practising without formal regulation" (Midwives Coalition, First Submission to HPLR, 1983, 11–12). The Midwifery Coalition also supported its proposals with comparisons to the international regulation of midwifery. For example, they stated that: "the ability of the midwifery profession to set standards of ethical and professional practice and conduct is demonstrated internationally" (Midwives Coalition, First Submission to HPLR, 1983, 9).

Although the decision to recommend self-regulation was easy to make, the decision about whether the practice of midwifery should be regulated through a system of exclusive licensure or voluntary certification was a contentious one. Several members of the midwifery community voiced opposition to establishing an exclusive licence to practice. These concerns were highlighted in the Midwifery Coalition's first submission to the HPLR: "There is a tendency in the modern midwifery community in North America to be very suspicious of just how the exclusive right to practice as a health care profession really serves the public. Such a right seems often to deny to the public legitimate health-care choices. For our part, we are extremely reluctant to deny other practitioners the right to practice through our exclusive licence" (1983, 1–2). As exemplified by the regulation of the medical profession, several within the midwifery community argued that "When a profession is exclusively licensed, it can easily become entrenched in its own traditions and authority. An exclusive right to practice often means that the practitioner does not have to respond to new developments or public pressure for change. It can also mystify the skills of licensed professionals, resulting in an inflated estimation of those skills on the part of the public" (Midwifery Coalition First Submission to the HPLR, 1983). Apprehension was expressed "that a licensed health-care worker can be controlled and manipulated through the fear of losing their licence" (Midwifery Coalition First Submission to the HPLR, 1983).

Alternatively, the Coalition described certification (i.e., having a protected title but not exclusive right to practise) as having a number of advantages: "It would offer the public a regulated body of midwives,

trained in recognized schools, regulated through a College which would
ensure entry-to-practice standards, continuing competence, and professional discipline and standards. Certification also allows unregulated
midwives to exist, as long as they do not use the protected title "certified
midwife," since it does not make an offence out of practising [midwifery]
without a licence, as an exclusive right does" (Midwifery Coalition First
Submission to the HPLR, 1983, 2).

Despite the arguments that supported certification over exclusive
licensure, the Midwifery Coalition members ultimately recommended to
the HPLR that "the strongest position for midwifery is as an exclusively
licensed body" (1983, 7). Like many other professions, midwives based
this decision on the need to protect the public interest:

Despite its apparent benefits, our committee has found that certification poses a
number of serious problems. Briefly stated, certification tolerates the practice of
unskilled birth attendants ... All over the world, the midwifery profession is
recognized as having an exclusive right to practise. This is largely because of the
possibility of harm which can be done by an untrained or negligent practitioner
... Is it in the public interest to place the entire onus on the parent to evaluate
the quality of midwifery services, or should all midwives have to meet a certain
standard of training and competence? Certainly, treating midwifery as a deregu-
lated consumer service opens the door to a host of advertising and promotional
pressures, surely not welcome to women sensitive enough to the stresses of
change and expectation ... It [also] leaves the consumer [at] the mercy of myriad
promotional and pricing policies ... Moreover, the benefits that accrue to those
who seek alternatives to certified practitioners are largely illusory; only the very
few women with the time, money, or acumen to question existent services are
likely to stumble into those alternatives ... [W]hile competitive information might
benefit those well-educated and informed consumers who already have access
to, and can afford, non-regulated midwives, it would be unlikely to benefit those
lower socio-economic levels where the benefits of midwifery care are most
strongly felt. (1983, 3–4)

In deciding to recommend to the HPLR that self-regulation take the
form of exclusive licensure, the Midwifery Coalition members made a
significant shift in the way consumers were involved in the regulation of
midwifery. Midwifery consumers were not portrayed as the informed,
responsible woman suggested in the informed choice model, but as vulnerable women in need of protection. This shift in portrayal of the midwifery consumer was likely in response to the perspective of the HPLR,

whose underlying theme in the review of health professions was to better protect the public interest. Midwifery Coalition members were perhaps moulding the presentation of midwifery to suit this agenda and thus enhance midwifery's chances of becoming integrated. Jutta Mason (1990) later raised important questions about this position: "The ordinary pregnant woman was "at the mercy" of sales pitches; she needed protection ... Because of her pregnancy, her vulnerability was increased ... [E]ven if she could summon the time, the money, and the "acumen" to ask the right questions, she would still only "stumble" into an alternative. Was she blind?" (5). Simply reducing the decision to one between exclusive licence to practice and certification for the supposed better protection of the public with the exclusive licensure model, however, did not adequately address the many concerns some midwives and supporters had with the model. The same justification had been made for the self-regulation of medicine, which many argued was not in the best public interest.

Responses to the Midwifery Coalition's Submission to the HPLR

Following the first submission, the next step in the HPLR process involved providing participating groups with copies of each other's briefs as requested. Participants were prompted to review and comment on the first submissions of any of the other groups which they felt would affect their professional practice, discuss their views with each other, negotiate among themselves, and reach whatever compromises they could (Lenske 1984, *The Ontario Midwife* 1, no. 2: 6; Schwartz 1993, as cited in Fynes 1994). Midwifery Coalition member Vicki Van Wagner described how this directive from the HPLR committee gave midwifery its initial legitimacy within the health care politics arena: "The HPLR gave us an entry to sit down and talk to the CPSO and the CNO. Because the HPLR process encouraged interaction between the professions ... they couldn't say 'no' to us. They couldn't brush us off ... We were one of the groups in the HPLR and it gave us a first step of entry into those kinds of dialogues" (as quoted in Fynes 1994, 90). It also gave midwives an opportunity to make themselves and their position better known to the other participating professions, and to their reviewers (Fynes 1994).

Medical and nursing organizations expressed acceptance of the principle of midwifery as a legitimate health practice, but felt that it should either be a part of nursing or otherwise under medical control. Thus, although the issue of exclusive licensure versus certification was contentious within the midwifery community, the main concern for the nursing and medical profession was with the broader issue of self-regulation. The College of Physicians and Surgeons of Ontario (CPSO), for example, stated that midwifery practice would only be acceptable if midwives were registered practitioners who would be "restricted to practice in association with physicians" (1984). The Ontario Medical Association (OMA) also stressed a need for physician supervision of midwives because of the "immaturity" of midwifery and the "lack of proven reliability [of midwives] with the public and fellow health professions" (1984). OMA representatives suggested that, "there could be certification of advanced post-graduate training for nurses and regulation under the College of Nurses, and ... there could be delegation of medical acts making up the practice of midwifery authorized by the CPSO and carried out under physicians supervision" (1984).

Responses from the nursing profession mirrored those of medicine. The three nursing organizations, the College of Nurses of Ontario (CNO), the Registered Nurses Association of Ontario (RNAO), and the Ontario Nurses Association (ONA), all asserted that midwifery is "not a separate and distinct profession from nursing" (CNO 1984) but a specialty of nursing. The CNO specifically questioned whether there would be sufficient numbers of practising midwives to warrant the establishment of a separate regulatory body, such as a College of Midwives (Fynes 1994). ONMA President Rena Porteous noted how midwifery was likely regarded as "a golden opportunity for [nursing] to identify the nurse as a primary care giver in a particular area; at least, and it would be a start, a precedent" (personal communication 1995).

The HPLR committee took these submissions and responses into serious consideration, however they did not consider those of the medical and nursing professions to the midwifery submission to be very seriously thought out. This is best exemplified by their lack of reference to supporting research, which by way of contrast was abundant in the Midwifery Coalition's submission. Rena Porteous hypothesized that nurses perhaps thought their claim to midwifery would not be contested by a "fringe" group of practising midwives: "[The College of Nurses] probably thought that they may have to write just a little thing and that midwifery would be handed to them ... Like here it is, you're going to accept it. There were few references, if any." (personal communication 1995). Perhaps the quality of these responses were such as they were because for both the nursing and the medical profession, midwifery was not a major concern. Recall that the HPLR was to resolve several major interprofessional disputes, such as between medicine and naturopathy, ophthalmology and optometry, physiatry and physical therapy, and between registered nurses and nurse assistants. These were much more salient issues to medicine and nursing than midwifery, likely because they tended to deal with issues beyond maternity care.[1] The diffusion of medical interest was also compounded by the fact that many physicians had abandoned the practice of obstetrics due to high malpractice insurance fees,[2] and therefore many did not have significant vested interests to protect. The medical profession was also in the midst of a bitter dispute with the provincial government over the right to charge "user fees" following the federal government's ban with the passage of the Canada Health Act in 1984.

The representatives of the Midwifery Coalition also met with the HPLR committee to follow up their first submission. For the most part, the HPLR committee had viewed the leaders of the Midwifery Coalition quite favourably:

The midwives were a really terrific group of people ... Terrific in a sense that they were sincere, well-meaning, hard-working, and serious. And so they were, from my perspective, an excellent group to work with. (Alan Schwartz, personal communication 1995)

The midwives were fairly successful in convincing ... the review team that a system of midwifery could be developed ... I have a strong recollection ... of the quality of the midwifery brief – it was a very cogent brief – very convincing. (Ontario Ministry of Health Representative, as quoted in Fynes, 1994, 86)

These initial impressions would prove to be important in the subsequent decision making of the Review.

Good impressions aside, the HPLR committee had some concerns arising from the Midwifery Coalition's first submission. These included, as summarized in *Issue 4*, "formal training, the cost of integrating a new profession and whether nursing should be a prerequisite for midwifery training" (5). Following the discussion and review of the first submission, the HPLR sent follow-up questions to the Midwifery Coalition challenging them to explain more fully or to re-examine their opinions, to reconcile elements of their point of view that seemed contradictory, and to address the often differing opinions of other related groups (HPLR 1989). In their follow-up submission to the HPLR, sent June 29, 1984, the Midwifery Coalition essentially summarized their first submission, but outlined in greater detail the role of the midwife and her scope of practice, stressing their commitment to key issues. They advocated "*direct entry* midwives, providing *continuous care*, as *primary contact* professionals for *normal preg-nancy and birth*, working in *cooperation* with, but not under the supervision of the medical professional as members of the health care team" (*Issue* 11, April 1986: 6, emphasis in original).

By this time, the HPLR panel had decided that the model form of regulation for their recommended legislative package would be self-regulation exclusively. To decide which professions to include in this pack-age, the Review panel developed a list of essential criteria intended to advance and protect the public interest. The criteria addressed four basic issues: 1) whether the work of the group was related to *health*, and there-fore should be regulated by the Ministry of Health as opposed to another ministry; 2) whether the activities of the group posed a significant risk or *harm* to patients; 3) whether regulation was possible for the group in ques-tion to make this risk preventable through a body of *knowledge* that can form the basis of *standards of practice* (i.e., established education require-ments for entry to practice); and 4) whether self-regulation was practical for the group in question (i.e., the favouring of public over professional self-interest, likelihood of compliance, sufficiency of membership size, and willingness to contribute to bear the costs of self-regulation) (HPLR 1989).

As alluded to above, the main concerns the HPLR had with the midwives' case was their lack of standard educational programs and insufficient numbers for self-regulation. Different members would be needed to staff all the committees within a College (registrar, fitness to practice, com-plaints, discipline) and to staff a professional association. Midwifery Coalition members agreed HPLR's concern about the small number of midwives, as only an estimated thirty midwives were practising in Ontario at the time of the second HPLR submission. Midwives attempted to bolster these small numbers, however, with the assertion that there were "hundreds" of women in the province with midwifery training from other countries who did not work because of the legal risk, and that these midwives were committed to funding self-regulation: "Midwives unable to practise, or practising without legal recognition, have indicated that they are willing to pay high membership fees to support the cost of self-regulation. We expect a dramatic increase in the number of midwives practising when midwifery is accepted" (Midwives Coalition, First Submission to HPLR, 1983, 12).

The presentation of midwifery as a profession to the HPLR – moreover one with strong consumer support – seemed to be having the desired effect. The reorganization of midwives and their clients into two separate organizations – one representing professional interests and the other representing consumer support for midwifery – was proving to be helpful in attaining the political goals midwives and their supporters hoped to achieve. Concurrent with these interactions with other professions and the Review committee, midwives and their supporters in the MTFO strove to increase public recognition of midwifery. This was to be accomplished through the sponsorship of the Midwifery Alliance of North America (MANA) Conference in 1984 where the merger of the OAM and the ONMA was officially announced, and through the proposed Private Member's Bill to integrate midwifery. These efforts to politicize midwifery would ultimately prove successful in securing public and government support for the integration of midwifery into the Ontario health care system.

PUBLICIZING AND PROFESSIONALIZING MIDWIFERY

The Merger of ONMA and OAM at the MANA Conference

The issue of creating unity among all midwives despite differing backgrounds was one of the main objectives of many within the mid-wifery movement. Early in 1983 at a "Labour of Love" conference held in Vancouver, midwives in British Columbia passed a resolution to "work toward united vision and cooperation among midwives from varying backgrounds" (Issue 3, no. 2, Spring 1983, 1). MANA was one of the strongest advocates of unification. At the first annual meeting of MANA, held in Colorado in the fall of 1983, ONMA President and MANA Vice-President Rena Porteous made a successful bid to have the 1984 conference held in Toronto to increase the profile of the unification of the OAM and ONMA (Fynes 1994). Porteous described the symbiotic nature of the decision: "It would work both ways; it would give MANA a lot more publicity than it might have in another place in the States, and at the same time it would give us a focus for the media in Ontario, which would work very well for us at the time because we were wanting to generate greater awareness of people about midwifery as an issue at this time" (personal communication 1995).

Throughout the process of making the first submission to the HPLR committee, ONMA and OAM representatives discussed the idea of formally amalgamating their two organizations. Porteous described how, "circum-stances [arising from the HPLR] had really pushed us into the fast track of developing the relationship between the two organizations and explor-ing one another's thoughts and philosophy at a pace that wouldn't have occurred normally" (personal communication 1995). At meetings between these two groups, ONMA representatives were impressed by the political will of the home birth midwives to challenge the system and their commitment to the idea of midwifery expressed in their willingness to practise in a less than ideal legal environment. In contrast, nurse-midwives' initial enthusiasm for pursuing the possibility of implementation back in the 1970s had gradually faded and many members of the ONMA were not politically active. By merging with practising midwives, ONMA representatives undoubtedly envisaged achieving a more autonomous form of midwifery than that for which they had originally lobbied. They would also benefit from the consumer support OAM midwives had. This support would prove to be a key factor in convincing the government that midwives' desire to become integrated into the health care system was due to more than just the self-interest of a would-be professional group.

Midwives in the OAM realized, as nurse-midwives previously had, that a nurse-midwifery model would be a more acceptable form of midwifery practice to both the nursing and medical professions in the province. These midwives, however, wanted to resist making such fundamental changes to the way they practised. It could be argued that practising home birth midwives co-opted nurse-midwives into supporting their independent midwifery model; this was probably not difficult to do as it was similar to what many nurse-midwives originally desired. In so doing, however, the home birth midwives might have had a better chance to challenge the viability of the nurse-midwifery model proposed by medical and nursing organizations. Other advantages of merging suggested by OAM members in *Issue* included a larger base of members which would increase their financial base, their political support base, and organizational energy; more credibility, recognition, and access to mainstream resources; and more publicity. Advocates for merging pointed to the successful example of the merger of midwives into a single organization in British Columbia. Disadvantages mentioned included confusion in changing organizations, potential conflicting values (which seemed to be resolved through the HPLR submission process); potential disruption to client relations, and potential limitation of practice.

Because of the strength of the arguments supporting amalgamation, and the ease with which the ONMA and OAM representatives had cooperated in making the first submission to the HPLR as the Midwifery Coalition, it was decided that the OAM and ONMA would move toward an organizational merger. The merger would be officially announced at the upcoming MANA conference. This resolution was brought before the boards of each organization. The decision to merge passed easily through the OAM as it was argued, "let's not make these people who are going to argue for nurse-midwives into our enemies; let's bring them into fold so to speak" (Midwife Chris Sternberg, personal communication 1995). At the ONMA meeting which drew about fifteen members (more than the Board had seen at prior meetings for several years), the vote came out in favour of disbanding and joining with the membership of the OAM to create a new organization at the time of the MANA conference (midwife Rena Porteous, personal communication 1995).[3]

The title of the MANA conference was Creating Unity, and was held in early November 1984. Besides creating a venue for the announcement of the unification of the ONMA and the OAM into the Association of Ontario Midwives (AOM), AOM and MTFO organizers hoped that the event would "reach new audiences...such as the medical community and the feminist community" (Nimmons, *Issue* 4, 1984:8). They invited several internationally renowned experts in maternity care and prominent feminists to speak, including Dr D.J. Kloosterman, Director of the Midwifery Academy in Holland and former president of the International Federation of Gynecologists and Obstetricians (FIGO); Dorothea Lang, American College of Nurse Midwives past president, founding member of MANA, and author of "The Cultural Warping of Childbirth"; David Stewart, author of several critiques of American obstetrics and founder of the National Association of Parents and Professionals for Safe Alternatives in Childbirth (NAPSAC); Sheila Kitzinger, social anthropologist, author of many books about childbirth, and "grand dame" of childbirth educators; Mary O'Brien, feminist sociologist and author of "The Politics of Female Reproduction"; and Michele Landsberg, feminist commentator for the *Toronto Star* (and spouse of the prominent politician Stephen Lewis). The MTFO was successful in its objective of reaching new audiences as the conference drew massive attendance (between 500 and 700) from an overwhelmingly supportive crowd.

The main function of the conference for the MTFO was political. Speakers were asked to focus their presentations on the politics of midwifery (Nimmons 1984, *Issue* 4). In his address, Kloosterman provided strong support for midwifery by citing statistics from the Netherlands (where midwives not only provide home care for normal pregnancies, but also care for clients in hospitals) which showed that perinatal mortality rates for planned home births were "seven times lower than the perinatal mortality rate for hospital" (Tyson 1985:7). He argued that these statistics indicated the advantages of both home births and the presence of midwives as primary obstetric caregivers. In his concluding comments, Kloosterman strongly asserted the indispensability of midwifery: "Midwifery is indispensable, and an essential part of good obstetric care; while obstetrics, as part of medicine, deals with disease and its treatment, midwifery is the protector of health and normality" (Kloosterman, as cited in Tyson 1985: 8). At a special feature session entitled "Midwifery is a Women's Issue," organized to help consolidate the link between the midwifery and feminist community, nearly 700 people filled the hall to capacity. Midwife Vicki Van Wagner recounted the success of the event "OISE[4] was packed full. They had to turn people away. They had people in the aisles. It was hugely successful – I would say [it was] the most successful midwifery event that's ever happened in Toronto" (Van Wagner 1993, as quoted in Fynes 1994). At this session, Sheila Kitzinger described the historical persecution of midwives and criticized the fragmented care of the present medical system "which leaves a woman no guarantee that the wishes and concerns she expresses ... will actually be considered" (Worts in *Issue* 1985, no. 6: 8). She contended that "with ... woman-shaped midwifery, we can begin to erode the 'rock of obstetric power,' remoulding it according to *our* design, *our* vision" (Worts 1985, 9, emphasis in original). Mary O'Brien asserted that midwives could help to "free women from technological control and alienation in labour, and also help redefine ... the power relationship of women to men in our society" (*Issue* 1985: 9). Michele Landsberg argued that the "many petty divisions amongst women, especially in the area of motherhood vs feminism" should be put aside as "*both* the feminist and midwifery movements are about freedom of choice for women and the right not to be alienated from our own experience (childbirth) should unite us and give us the potential to make real change in our society" (Worts 1985, 9, emphasis in original). Landsberg strongly urged midwifery supporters to "use the press" to get their message across.

Together these speakers helped generate enormous support and publicity for midwifery: "It was really a very strong feeling that ... people who were interested in changing the health care system ... were uniting to say 'We need midwifery'" (Van Wagner 1993, as quoted in Fynes 1994). MTFO co-coordinator and conference organizer Holly Nimmons reported in *Issue*, no. 6, January 1985) that the task of the conference in increasing the recognition of midwifery, "inspired hundreds and will affect thousands through media attention and public awareness; the event reaffirmed the work of the MTF as essential and attainable" (4).

Stephen Lewis and the Private Member's Bill

After the Midwifery Coalition forwarded its first submission to the HPLR, a fierce lobbying strategy was initiated to bolster midwives' chances of securing protective legislation. One of the first steps in this pursuit was to solicit the support and political guidance of former NDP party leader Stephen Lewis and his staff. Coalition representative Vicki Van Wagner recounted the outcome of this meeting: "[We said] here is what we want, and Stephen Lewis said to us, 'Do you have twenty years?' And to me this was a very critical moment. We said 'yes, we don't care how long it takes, we will not go away'" (personal communication 1995). Midwife Betty-Anne Davis recalled how "Stephen Lewis ... really took us under his wing and started talking to us and telling us how to do things polit-ically" (personal communication 1995). Shortly after this initial contact, Lewis introduced Coalition representatives to Dave Cooke, the New Democratic Party Health Critic. At this meeting, Cooke became enthusi-astic about the midwives' quest for legitimacy and subsequently pro-posed to introduce a private member's bill calling for an amendment to the Health Disciplines Act to include midwifery.

Although Cooke felt that the Bill was unlikely to pass given that it would have to be unanimously approved, he nonetheless hoped that by introducing it in the legislature, debate would be stimulated on the subject of midwifery. He saw such debate as a publicity strategy "to put pressure on the whole [HPLR] process, to take midwifery seriously ... to raise public awareness and to bring the forces of support together" (Cooke 1993, as quoted in Fynes 1994). Cooke made the following argument at the press conference where he introduced his intentions to introduce the bill: "Mid-wives offer a continuity of care not found in the present system, and ... infant mortality rates are lower in countries that allow midwives to prac-tice ... Canada is one of only nine countries in the World Health Organi-zation without provisions for midwifery ... [This] bill would recognize midwifery as a separate profession, and establish a governing body and training programs for midwives" (*Issue* 3: 17). Cooke also stated that he would propose that the Ministry of Health fund midwifery services.

The First Reading of the Bill was in April 1984 with the Second Reading scheduled for the fall. In preparation for the Second Reading of the Bill, the midwives and the MTFO embarked on a massive lobbying campaign to support the Bill (Fynes 1994). The MTFO provided members with a lobby package which emphasized the important aspects of midwifery and explained the current political situation in Ontario" (*Issue* 1984: 4).

Again, they urged supporters to write to their MPPs indicating their support for the legalization of midwifery and for Cooke's Bill (Fynes 1994).

Serendipitiously, the Second Reading of the Bill in the provincial legislature coincided with the MANA conference. Following one of the sessions of the conference, hundreds of midwives and supporters marched from OISE to the legislature at Queen's Park to publicly show their support for the Bill. Midwife Vicki Van Wagner recalled the immensity of the display of support for the Bill: "There were at least five hundred midwives from around North America at the Conference ... (We) walked to Queen's Park and filled the Gallery. It was a very consciousness-raising event for the legislature and the public" (Van Wagner 1993, as quoted in Fynes 1994).

In the legislature, Cooke described the benefits of midwifery for the health care system, highlighting that it was a safe and cost-effective form of maternity care. Liberal party members concurred with Cooke's position.[5] For example, Liberal MPP Ms. Bryden added her support for midwifery as a woman's issue: "This is a feminist issue ... People who oppose the licensing of midwives are denying them ... the right to practice their profession. It is discrimination against a group that is largely women ... It is discrimination against women generally by denying them the right to choose alternative types of birthing care" (Hansard 1984: 3752). Conservative MPPs "agreed that there [were] many merits ... to the consideration of the idea of midwifery (including being) able to meet the physical, emotional and psychological needs of the mother" (Hansard 1984: 3749). Despite this demonstration of support, however, the Conservatives who had the majority of seats in the house, blocked a vote on the Bill, considering it premature given that the HPLR was already investigating changes to the Health Disciplines' Act which included midwifery.

Although the Bill failed to pass Second Reading, midwives and their supporters in the MTFO nevertheless considered it a successful part of their broader political strategy: "The vote on the bill was blocked; we never expected anything else. Private member's bills rarely get to Second Reading. But the ... debate helped educate the members of the legislature and the press and was an excellent opportunity to show the strength of our support – in the galleries, and through the petitions handed to the Minister of Health" (*Issue* 6, January 1985: 12). Moreover, midwives and their supporters argued that the fact that "all three parties spoke intelligently about an issue that two years ago could have been laughed at" was a victory that "speaks to the effectiveness of our public relations, educational and lobbying work" (*Issue* 6, January 1985: 11). They regarded it as the "first major step in the process of lobbying the government to

support [the] submission to the Health Professions Legislative [Review]."
(*Issue* 6, January 1985: 12).

The Association of Ontario Midwives

Following the MANA conference and the public show of support for the
Private Member's Bill, a steering committee was set up to begin to define
the Association of Ontario Midwives. The proposed structure for the new
organization was to combine "the successful aspects of both the OAM,
with its regional chapters and grassroots decision making, and the executive committee of the ONMA, with officers who have specifically defined
duties: president, president-elect, secretary, treasurer" (AOM 1985, 1, no. 1:
3). Thus, a board of directors was created consisting of an executive, representatives from each regional chapter, and heads of committees.
Requirements were set out stating that at least half the board must consist
of practising midwives to ensure their input on decisions affecting midwifery practice. No formal provisions were made for consumer input but
the AOM did extend an invitation to MTFO representatives to sit on committees as the OAM had done before. In addition, they created an official
liaison position between the MTFO and the AOM.

The AOM's structure was officially endorsed at the Annual General
Meeting on May 25, 1985 by sixty-two midwife members and fourteen
non-midwife members (AOM Newsletter 1985: 15). This new structure
proved to be successful in their gaining acceptance into the International
Confederation of Midwives (ICM). This was a "remarkable show of confidence" in Ontario midwives, considering that they did not yet have any
official standing in the Ontario health care system at the time.

While the publicizing and politicizing of midwifery was ongoing, the
HPLR was continuing to review all the submissions and responses to submissions that has been forwarded to it by more than seventy-five health
care provider organizations. The broad base of support midwifery accumulated, not only from the MTFO but from such key women's groups as the
National Action Committee for the Status of Women (NAC), would prove
to have a significant effect on the decision-making of the HPLR committee.

Despite some of the outstanding concerns it had with numbers and
the lack of an educational program, the HPLR decided that midwifery
would continue to be considered in the next stage of the review process.
They argued that they made this decision due to their recognition that
unregulated midwifery could potentially be harmful to the public.
Undoubtedly the increased politicization of midwifery did not hinder the

process. In September 1984, on the basis of the recommendations made by the Review panel, the Minister of Health announced the list of thirty-nine health professions still under consideration for regulation (HPLR 1989). Midwifery was included among those thirty-nine. Midwives in the AOM, however, did not rest on their laurels. They continued to reshape midwifery to demonstrate to the HPLR its commitment and capability to self-regulate.

SELF-REGULATION AND THE AOM
One recurring theme repeated by the "experts in both practical and legal fields" at the MANA conference was to "get your own structures in place or else they will be established for you." (AOM 1985, 1, no. 1: 3). In line with this directive, the AOM was encouraged to establish its own governing body, set its own standards, create its own educational systems, and discipline and regulate itself. These suggestions complemented the proposals being made by the HPLR committee. For example, AOM officials regarded one of the criteria of the HPLR, the ability to favour the public interest, as:

an affirmation of another area in which the AOM had hoped to concentrate: the establishment of standards of practice, complaints and discipline procedures, in order to be clearly able to distinguish and favour the public interest. Our willingness to cooperate with self-regulation ... would be demonstrated by our acceptance of this voluntary regulation ... It is also essential that, since the AOM currently functions both as a governing body and as a professional association, we acknowledge these functions as distinct from each other in order that they may be separable in the future; i.e., a standards committee would remain part of the governing body, while a lobby committee would be part of a professional association. (Issue 6: 17)

Thus, it was decided that the mandate of the AOM would include establishing the mechanisms of self-governance and formal training, along with: 1) acting as the professional organization representing midwives in Ontario; 2) attempting to achieve legal status as a self-regulating profession with formal direct-entry education and multiple routes of entry to midwifery programs; and 3) educating the public and other health professions about the role of a midwife. The AOM was to act both as a regulatory body and as a professional association. Membership criteria specified that each midwife must: 1) use informed consent contracts in her practice; 2) practise according to the published AOM standards; 3) engage in regular peer review; 4) have membership on one committee; and 5) complete AOM statistics forms for each client attended to and submit these on a regular basis (AOM Newsletter 1, no. 2: 1). Committees were divided into "Professional Committees" (e.g., Outreach, International, Public Relations, and Professional Advisory) and "Governing Committees" (e.g., Complaints and Discipline, Standards, and Registration).[6] The Board of Directors of the AOM was also structured in line with HPLR recommendations: "A 13-member Board, with a specified number of committees which would become statutory, was chosen because that was what it looked like [the HPLR] was eventually going to recommend, that any self-regulating profession would have to have. It was also to make those professions have half consumers, half professionals, which was not difficult. We had consumers on all AOM committees" (Midwife Michelle Kryzanauskas, personal communication 1995). Finally, in response to the concerns expressed by the HPLR regarding midwifery's ability to staff a self-regulatory body, the AOM began to focus their efforts on increasing membership: "Increasing the membership base of the AOM is essential; outreach efforts to foreign trained midwives and practising midwives who are not AOM members was identified as a priority for the AOM. All AOM members are asked to contribute to this effort" (AOM Newsletter 1, no. 2, September 1985: 7). Taking on the task of self-regulation would prove helpful in meeting the challenges of integration. One of the most significant challenges faced by the midwifery community was the inquest-turned-public-inquiry in the summer of 1985, better known as the Toronto Island Inquest.

THE TORONTO ISLAND INQUEST

The politicization of midwifery that had begun with protests and demonstrations by midwifery consumers, the ongoing HPLR process, and the attempted Private Member's Bill in 1984 peaked in June 1985. The key event of that year was the Coroner's Inquest into the death of a baby whose home birth on Toronto's Ward Island had been attended by two midwives the previous fall. The baby, Daniel McLaughlin-Harris, was born after a long yet normal labour and delivery[7] but was reported to be pale and with no muscle tone at birth. The attendant midwives, Sue Rose and Vicki Van Wagner (both of the Midwives' Collective), initiated the process to transfer the baby to the Hospital for Sick Children, continually giving the baby artificial respiration during the transfer. Despite these efforts, the baby died in hospital two days later, on October 13, 1984, of asphyxiation.

Before the inquest had even begun, the Regional Coroner for Metropolitan Toronto and Central Region, Dr James Young, decided that the inquest would not only deal with the baby's death, but publicly raise the broader issues of home births and midwifery in Ontario: "It was time to take a careful look at what was happening ... It had never been looked at publicly before, because the model of inquests is narrowly focused on a death alone. I felt that it should be an opportunity to see the issues ... an in-depth look at midwifery ... I designed the inquest with that in mind" (Young 1993, as quoted in Fynes 1994).[8] The issues to be raised by the inquest, as reported in *Issue* in January 1985, included "the present status of midwifery, the right to choose the care of a midwife either in hospital or at home, the right to choose a home birth, the safety of home births, and the integration of midwifery into the health care system" (10).

Although midwives had a sense that this was going to be yet another attempt to end midwifery and homebirths, they also regarded the inquest as an opportunity to make a public statement about the benefits and legitimacy of midwifery:

We would have tried to define it as a public inquiry as well, in the sense that for us you could not look at an individual baby's death without putting it in the wider context of the place of midwifery in the system ... We wanted to have a larger discussion. Now we didn't believe the place for [this] was an inquest ... We believed it was a very bad forum for a public inquiry ... because investigating health policy in the context of a baby dying creates an unfair bias ... [Moreover] it did not have fair rules or reasonable funding ... [but] we had to take that opportunity to assert our vision of midwifery. (Midwife Vicki Van Wagner, personal communication, 1995)

As had been done for the 1982 inquest, midwifery supporters were asked to donate funds for the legal fees incurred by the inquest, and these were to be much more exhaustive this time around.

In presenting its case, the Crown brought in expert witnesses from several medical and nursing organizations, including the Society of Obstetricians and Gynecologists (SOGC), the Canadian Pediatric Society (CPS), the Ontario College of Family Physicians (OCFP), the OMA and the CNO. A key witness was Dr Knox Ritchie, an obstetrician known to be a proponent of the "active management of labour." He testified that the mother, Alix McLaughlin, was never a low-risk candidate for home delivery as it was her first child, she was thirty-one years old, she had developed a mild case of anemia, she was eleven days over her due date, and the baby was supposedly over eight-and-a-half pounds. He argued that Daniel's death was preventable.

Official statements from the medical and nursing profession to the inquest focused more on the regulation of midwifery than on the baby death, and largely mimicked their responses to midwives' HPLR submissions. CNO representative Margaret Risk argued that midwives should be regulated by the College of Nurses, but she did not recommend the practice of home birth. Pediatrician and CPS representative Dr Graham Chance also did not support home births, but at the same time expressed concern over routine medical intervention to speed up normal labour. OMA spokesperson Dr John Milligan expressed opposition toward home birth because of the suddenness with which problems arise during labour. Family practitioner and OCFP representative Dr Rachel Edney stated that having midwives working in hospitals was an acceptable alternative to fill the gap left by a declining number of family physicians providing obstetrical care.

Alix McLaughlin, the baby's mother and long-time midwifery supporter, strongly defended the midwives' case. She described how she had spent five years reading and talking with friends about birth, and chose a home birth to avoid the usual forms of medical intervention in labour in a hospital (Hossie 1985a). Even after Dr Ritchie's claims that the baby's death was preventable, she asserted she "would do it again" (Van Wagner 1993, as quoted in Fynes 1994).

To help support the midwives' management of McLaughlin's case, the midwives' lawyers brought in expert witnesses to testify on behalf of midwifery. One of the midwives involved in the inquest, Vicki Van Wagner (1993), described how the inquest proceeded: "Three days were spent discussing the death; the rest of the time [three weeks] the CPSO, the OMA, the Canadian Society of Pediatricians ... the SOGC, all the big medical groups were called as witnesses ... What happened was that the points of view of medicine and nursing were very well represented by the Coroner's witnesses. We, the midwives, had to call witnesses to give the other point of view ... home birth is a reasonable choice; direct entry midwifery is a good idea; midwifery should be a separate profession and not governed by medicine and nursing" (Van Wagner 1993, as quoted in Fynes 1994: 116).

Testimony from Louise Hanvey, a spokesperson for the Canadian Institute of Child Health, supported the mother's conclusions regarding the high rates of intervention in hospitals. Dr Murray Enkin, a long time supporter of midwifery and an internationally acclaimed obstetrician, argued for the mother's suitability for a home birth, diametrically opposing the testimony of Dr Ritchie. Dr Enkin drew on international data to argue that home birth is as safe as or safer than hospital birth, and that maternity care in Ontario would be improved by a well-developed, medically backed up home birth program (Hossie 1985b). Queen's University philosophy professor Christine Overall also testified on behalf of the midwives. She argued that "the fact that there may be an unforseen negative outcome of one couple's choice in favour of home birth does not by itself demonstrate that all similar choices are unjustified" (as quoted in Hossie 1985b: 16).

Internationally renowned pediatrician and perinatal epidemiologist Dr Marsden Wagner of the World Health Organization was also invited as an expert witness on behalf of the midwives. By the time he was called to the witness stand, the inquest had progressed to the examination of the broader issue of midwifery and away from the specifics of the baby death. The time and financial constraints of the midwives were such that they could only afford Dr Wagner to focus on either the baby death or the broader midwifery issue. Midwife Holliday Tyson described in *Issue* (9, Oct. 1985) the difficult situation the midwives faced:

As the inquest entered its 3rd week, the midwives and parents faced time and financial constraints. Two of the three weeks had been filled with witnesses for the Crown; little time was left for evidence on the general issues surrounding midwifery to be presented. Further, the legal fees for midwives and parents had reached $80,000; it was financially impossible to support an inquest which went for much longer. A choice had to be made between concentrating on the specifics of this case, or on the general issues involved in implementing midwifery into our health care system. A number of expert witnesses would have been called by counsel to give evidence on the specific case. Alternatively, international expert witnesses could have been called in order to educate and advise the jury on general midwifery issues. The decision was made by the midwives and counsel, and by the parents and counsel, to call witnesses who would inform the jury of the general issues involving midwifery and possible routes towards change in Ontario's health care system. (11)

Consequently, the midwives decided to have Dr Wagner spend his time on the stand defending direct-entry, self-regulating midwifery as opposed to defending the midwives' management of this specific case.

In line with this request,[9] Dr Wagner pointed out the high rates of unnecessary and costly medical interventions in Ontario as compared to WHO recommendations. He argued that there was good evidence to show that if midwifery were integrated into the health care system these intervention rates would fall, as would rising health care costs. He described the situation in Canada as an "extraordinary enigma" because it denied women the basic services of midwives enjoyed by women all over the world: "We're not talking about frosting on the cake, but ... about an essential service that is not being provided" (as quoted in Tedesco 1985e). He also asserted that babies do not die just at home but in hospitals as well; he argued "that babies die and I don't see this as an absolute condemnation of midwifery" (Tedesco 1985e). He strongly urged the jury to recommend that midwifery be integrated in Ontario as a self-regulating profession.

Following Dr Wagner's testimony, the midwives presented their own vision of regulated midwifery in Ontario. AOM representative Holliday Tyson argued that midwifery should be recognized as a formally licensed, self-regulating profession. To support this assertion, Tyson presented statistics based on the care independent midwives in Ontario provided, showing a perinatal mortality rate of 2.2 per 1,000 live births compared to the national average of 9.6 (Fynes 1994, 116–17). The care midwives provide, she argued, is based on the view that childbirth is a natural, physiological function, not an illness. Because nurses are trained to deal with illness, midwives rejected arguments favouring midwifery as a specialty of nursing. In her brief to the inquest, Tyson outlined the AOM's four-phase proposal for the integration of midwifery in Ontario. The first phase, already completed, involved setting up a professional association and a committee structure for the following three phases. The second phase involved the two steps of establishing an educational program necessary for the training and licensing of midwives, and identifying and evaluating models of practice and developing a system for the ongoing assessment of the profession. The third phase involved assessing currently practising midwives and integrating them into areas targeted to have a demonstrated need for midwives (teenage mothers, Northern Ontario, birth centres, home birth, etc.). Mechanisms for self-regulation, initially intended to be carried out by the AOM but later revised to be the mandate of a College of Midwives, were projected to be established in the final phase (Ferguson 1985b, A15; *Issue* 11, April 1986: 7–8).

The midwives' final witness was Dave Cooke, NDP health critic. He argued that the integration of midwifery in Ontario would result in a reduction of the portion of the health budget allotted for doctors and institutional maternity care (Tedesco 1985c). He described how "it is seldom you can have savings and improve the system" as he asserted midwifery could. Cooke concluded by urging the jury to recommend that midwifery be legalized as a self-regulating profession in the province.

In the background to these formal proceedings, the MTFO was hard at work fundraising and managing public relations. MTFO co-coordinator and public relations organizer Holly Nimmons stated that "this case is going to make us or break us" (Nimmons, as cited in Sweet 1985, F1). She recounted how, at the outset of the inquest, the tone of articles in the press tended to be critical of the midwives and home birth: "It was being reported every day – the *Star*, the *Globe*, the *Sun*, on the TV ... The first week and a half we despaired, I remember, and then we really did some tough work" (personal communication 1995). To help ameliorate this situation, the MTFO organized a rally of midwifery supporters to send a clear message to decision-makers about the support for midwifery. The MTFO also hoped that this demonstration would help turn around the perspective of the media. More than 300 supporters turned out for the public demonstration outside the Coroner's court. Nimmons (1985) noted the significance of the event: "It was important for reporters (and consequently the general public) to see the healthy babies of home births, other midwives and the apparently intelligent, sane women and men who seek out midwives. This was not at all the image of an irresponsible, lunatic fringe!" (*Issue* 9, October 1985: 3). Portraying midwifery care as a legitimate option was the focus of these rallies. The emphasis on the alternative aspects of midwifery were minimized.

Following the rally, there was a notable shift in the tone of the media toward being more supportive of midwifery in Ontario. Midwife Holliday Tyson highlighted this shift in the media: "There is no doubt that most of the people who covered [the inquest] came in highly sceptical of midwives and people who would make these choices, and most of them went out actually feeling quite differently" (personal communication 1995). Nimmons, as MTFO coordinator, helped foster this turnaround by "feeding them facts, other facts, going out and initiating interviews to start developing support but also to refute some of the outrageous things that were coming out and being misrepresented" (personal communication 1995). Every day of the inquest, supporters also filled the courtroom to provide moral support for the midwives and parents. The MTFO also organized cables to be sent to the Minister of Health. Approximately 800 were sent, more than had ever been sent on any other single issue (Nimmons, personal communication 1995). MTFO representatives were also called to testify at the inquest to introduce the perspective of other consumers who had chosen midwifery care. They reported that consumers of midwifery care were well educated and well informed. Their decision to draw on the services of midwives was the result of thoughtful "research and conscious decision-making" (*Issue* 1985, 4). The intention of this testimony was to portray a positive image of midwifery which they felt was largely being neglected in the proceedings (*Issue* 1985).

The most important source of consumer support, however, came from the baby's parents, Alix McLaughlin and Robert Harris. Dr Rachel Edney (1993), OCFP President and witness at the inquest, emphasized the importance of the parents' support for midwifery: "I think the major thing that I can remember was the incredible … amazement that the family was still supportive of the midwives … despite the fact that they've lost their baby" (as quoted in Fynes 1994: 115). The significance of the parents' support did not evade the midwives, as indicated by the following statement by Vicki Van Wagner and Holliday Tyson in *Issue*: "The remarkable strength and conviction of the parents was central to the outcome of the inquest. In the midst of a personal tragedy, their major concern was to ensure that other parents have the choice of midwifery care and the place of birth" (8, July 1985: 7).

In the final summations made to the jury after three and a half weeks of the inquest, nearly all participants agreed on the need to legalize and regulate midwifery in Ontario. The Coroner and the Crown, however, called for regulation under the CNO, whereas the midwives had argued that midwifery be self-regulating (Tedesco 1985b). The Coroner suggested that the Health Disciplines Act (the Act under review by the HPLR) be changed as quickly as possible to set standards enabling midwives to practise in Ontario (Tedesco 1985a). Young advised the two-woman,[10] two-man jury to come up with recommendations that could be implemented to prevent baby deaths from happening in the future (Hossie 1985c).

After two days of deliberation on the contradictory evidence presented, the jury concluded that Daniel's death could have been avoided had the mother been transferred to hospital earlier. Nevertheless, they recommended that midwifery should be legalized in Ontario with an internationally accepted definition of a midwife and internationally accepted education standards, and that it be recognized and integrated as an integral part of the Ontario health care system. They recommended that midwifery be regulated under the CNO for an initial five years, after which time an independent and self-regulatory College of Midwives should be established. During this five years, specific aspects of the Health

Discipline's Act should be amended to include the practice of midwifery. This recommendation was intended to prevent "a hastily assembled college [where] there may be too little expertise available to make sound judgements." The jury also recommended that:

1 midwives' standard of conduct be set by the governing body according to internationally recognized standards and practices;
2 midwives without formal training take a training program;
3 legislation legalizing midwifery contain a clause to allow the licensing of existing qualified midwives;
4 malpractice insurance be made compulsory for practising midwives;
5 licensed midwives have admitting privileges in maternity wards of hospitals;
6 midwives' services be covered at least in part by the Ontario Health Insurance Plan; and
7 parents be given the choice of home birth (Tedesco 1985d).

Midwife Vicki Van Wagner regarded it as unfortunate that the jury felt the death could have been avoided as she "felt there was sufficient evidence to disagree with that" (as quoted in Tedesco 1985d: 2). Nevertheless, the recommendations were viewed as "a really big step forward for independent midwifery" (Van Wagner as quoted in Tedesco 1985d: 2). The AOM and the MTFO described the jury recommendation as "a major victory." "This is so, particularly because the jury urged the government to adopt the models of midwifery care developed and advocated by our organizations – self regulation, formal training, licensing of currently practising midwives, choice of birthplace, accessibility of midwifery care, and integration into the current health care system" (*Issue* 8, July 1985: 7).

Although midwives regarded the recommendations of the jury as favourable, they felt that the process of the inquest was biased against the type of midwifery envisioned by the AOM and MTFO, and threatening to the midwives involved.[11] The parents' lawyer, for example, claimed that "the issue of [her] client's baby had become an excuse to go on a witch hunt about midwives" (Martin, as quoted in Ferguson 1985a: A22). Midwives were forced to play on medicine's turf. The Coroner was a physician as well as a member of the OMA, which on record opposed the integration of midwifery into the health care system. He had a readily apparent medical bias regarding childbirth and maternity care as well as an arguably male chauvinistic attitude towards the women involved in the midwifery case, including their lawyers, the mother, other midwives, and consumer supporters.[12] To make an impact on such a medically defined and dominated process, witnesses to support the midwives' case were brought in from the "legitimate" medical community. These witnesses stressed those aspects of midwifery that were more in line with mainstream medical thinking, such as professional standards, appropriate use of technology, and cost-effective care. Consumer rallies also emphasized the legitimacy of midwifery consumers and midwifery practice. Moreover, throughout the process midwives felt the need to stress their educational background, to dress a certain way to enhance their appearance as professionals, and not appear to be the "lunatic fringe" that many considered to be. Increasingly, these more "professional" aspects of midwifery began to take on greater importance. Little by little, midwifery was becoming less of a radical childbirth alternative. Many believed it had to in order to survive.

POSTSCRIPT TO INQUEST

As noted above, the legal fees for the inquest approached $80,000 for the midwives and the parents involved in the case. Although the MTFO was successful in fundraising $20,000 there was $60,000 outstanding that remained. Because the inquest had turned into a public inquiry, the midwives and the parents made a case to the Ontario Ombudsman's office that this was an unfair financial burden to place on them. After some negotiation with this sympathetic audience, another $20,000 was raised to pay expenses. In the end, the lawyers accepted being paid only half of their costs.

THE DECISION TO REGULATE MIDWIFERY

While the inquest proceeded throughout late June and early July of 1985, the HPLR was developing the final series of questions for the remaining thirty-nine professions on the preliminary list, regarding the ability of these occupations to meet the criteria for self-regulation (HPLR 1989). Meetings were set up to explain the criteria and to assist groups in formulating their submissions.

The results of the 1985 Inquest were carefully considered by the HPLR committee when it was asked to make recommendations regarding whether midwifery should be included in the government's health profession regulations. The Inquest had made it clear to the HPLR panel that regulation was needed and that midwifery was a political hot potato.[13]

Following the inquest the AOM sent a letter to Alan Schwartz, HPLR coordinator, on August 8, 1985. They urged him to consider the jury's recommendations, which they interpreted as a clear indication of the public's recognition of the need for legalization of the profession, and of public support for choices in childbirth. MTFO members also continued their show of support for midwifery with massive letter-writing campaigns addressed to the HPLR committee and to the Minister of Health. Midwife Vicki Van Wagner recalled the following conversation at the first meeting between the AOM and HPLR following the inquest: "Alan Schwartz ... sat me down [and] said, 'The jury said you were at fault. How can you possibly tell me this profession should be [self] regulated?' ... And we said look at these recommendations ... They're exactly what we've been proposing" (personal communication 1995). Van Wagner felt that the arguments midwives made at this meeting satisfied Schwartz: "We had to talk him through all of the rational, coherent reasons that [we] disagreed with the jury's findings, and [I] believe that [we] convinced him that it wasn't just midwives defending midwives ... It was based on good arguable medical reasons ... [I] believe that at that point he felt satisfied that he could go to [Minister of Health] Murray Elston and argue that [we] were a credible profession that he could recommend" (Van Wagner 1993, as quoted in Fynes 1994: 126).

Over and above the concerns about the regulation of midwifery raised by the inquest, the HPLR committee had some outstanding concerns of its own. These mainly had to do with the lack of a standard educational program and with the small numbers of professionals, which would make it difficult to self-regulate their profession in an "unprejudiced" manner.[14] These were the issues that midwives were asked to address in their third submission to the HPLR.

The AOM responded to the concerns of the HPLR in their submission presented to the HPLR in October 1985. The submission focused on three areas: 1) midwives' potential for complying with the rules of self-regulation (highlighting the AOM's complaints and discipline procedures); 2) a proposed educational program; and 3) a description of a four-phase integration proposal (a revision of their previous presentation to the inquest intended to circumvent the implementation of the jury's recommendation for regulation under the CNO for a five-year interim period). Although the concerns over the numbers of professionals remained, Schwartz "came to see that [midwives] weren't uncommitted to working in a professional context" (midwife Vicki Van Wagner, personal communication 1995).

Following this submission, the Review's recommendations regarding midwifery were presented to the Minister in a series of briefings in November and December 1985. Recalling his decision to recommend the integration of midwifery, Alan Schwartz argued that there were several reasons on which to base the integration of midwifery: "We could see that midwives would provide a service that many people wanted, that they could provide this service in a safe and rational way at many stages of the birthing process and that this could be done in a way that would be less expensive for the system. Other than tradition or territorial protection, why on earth would you not go forward. It was pretty tough to argue that going forward was a mistake" (personal communication 1995). In these briefings, the HPLR committee told the Minister essentially to "pick his poison" as either choice would result in political fallout. Deciding not to regulate would likely result in significant political fallout from midwifery supporters. On the other hand, in deciding to regulate midwifery, which was what the Review recommended, a lot of work to bring midwifery up to par with other health professions would be needed: "We ... recognized that the profession of midwifery was in a unique position. Midwifery's questionable legal status had prevented it from evolving naturally, and unlike the other professions that would be newly regulated, it functioned primarily outside the official health care system. Critical issues relating to the very nature of the profession and its role in the health care system would require resolution" (HPLR 1989: 11).

Specific areas in need of development included professional standards and a standard educational program. Because of this need for substantial professional development, the HPLR committee recommended that if the Minister decided to integrate midwifery into the health care system, a "Task Force" be created to investigate and make recommendations on those areas necessary to bring midwifery up to par for inclusion in the larger HPLR package: "The HPLR group at the time recommended to the Minister of the day, Murray Elston, that the status of midwifery be changed in significant ways and that because of the nature of the particular issues surrounding midwifery, it be hived off from HPLR and then brought back into HPLR once these distinct issues had been dealt with" (Alan Schwartz, personal communication 1995). In the end, the HPLR was not the one to make the final decision; it put the options before the Minister who, with Cabinet approval, would ultimately have to decide.

On January 26, 1986, Minister of Health Murray Elston announced that he formally accepted the Review's recommendation that the government begin steps toward the regulation of midwifery, and announced the "government's intention to establish midwifery as a recognized part of the Ontario health care system."[15] Elston based his decision on the following argument: "The practice of midwifery is well established throughout the world. Indeed, Ontario is one of the few western jurisdictions where it is not regulated. In many other jurisdictions, the practice is already viewed as a safe and integral element of health care ... [A] small but growing number of people have expressed a wish to have available the services of a competently trained midwife ... I believe Ontario citizens are entitled to the same choices" (Hansard 1986: 3372). Elston also announced the establishment of a ministerial-appointed Task Force on the Implementation of Midwifery in Ontario (TFIMO) which was to recommend a framework for "how midwifery should be practised in Ontario and how midwives should be educated" (Hansard 1986: 3373).

Although Elston based his decision to integrate midwifery into the Ontario health care system on the equity and accessibility argument, the assumed cost-effectiveness of midwifery care also fit well with the government's agenda to rationalize the health care system. That is, the government could be seen as responding to consumer demand for midwifery while at the same time potentially saving health care dollars. Rarely are governments blessed with such a palatable cost-cutting measure. Given their previous endorsement of midwifery, both the NDP and Conservative parties lent their support to this Liberal government initiative.

Elston's announcement meant that discussions within the midwifery community about whether it should become integrated into the mainstream maternity care system or not became a moot point as the government had already decided that midwifery *would* be integrated and regulated; the only question that remained at this point was *how*. The AOM and MTFO's pursuit of integration was achieving success but this pursuit was in turn increasingly changing the face of midwifery. The extent of these changes would be directly addressed by the newly appointed Task Force.

SUMMARY

The challenges that faced the midwifery community in the early 1980s – the first Coroner's Inquest, the CPSO statement against home births, and the ongoing HPLR – continued in full force in the subsequent few years. But as Arms (1975) and Burtch (1994) noted of trials against midwives in the United States and Canada, these events not only represented challenges, they could also be used as platforms on which midwives could openly promote themselves, the legitimacy of their work, and the right of women to choose their care. It is telling of the political sagacity of midwives and their supporters in Ontario that they were able to turn these challenges into opportunities. This is particularly so of the inquest-turned-public-inquiry in the summer of 1985. Midwives and their supporters also successfully organized some of their own "showcase" events (Bucher

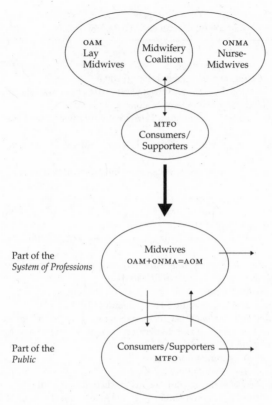

Figure 3
Continued professionalization of midwifery community organizations

1988), including the organizational merger of the OAM and ONMA at the
MANA conference, and the proposed Private Member's Bill. The organization of the midwifery community was becoming even more professionalized (see figure 3). Throughout this process, the activities and strategies
not only of the midwives but most notably of their consumers and supporters were integral to successfully meeting these challenges, and state
officials were beginning to take notice.

The strategies that midwives and their supporters employed had
successfully managed to achieve integration within the HPLR package
which was being based on a self-regulatory model. But because midwifery's unique circumstances resulted in it being delegated to a special
Task Force, there was the potential that midwifery was not going to get
the same treatment as the rest of the professions still being considered
by the HPLR. Challenges and opportunities were still to be met with the
Task Force.

Table 1
Midwifery legislative and integration timeline (1983–1994)

1983	Creation of the MTFO
	CPSO's Home birth Statement
	Midwifery Coalition's first submission to HPLR
1984	Official merger of the OAM and ONMA into AOM at the MANA conference
	NDP health critic's private member's bill
1985	Inquest into death of McLaughlin-Harris baby following home birth on Toronto Island
	HPLR recommendation to minister of Health to include midwifery in regulatory package
1986	Minister of Health announces decision to integrate midwifery and appoints the TFIMO
1987	TFIMO submits final report
1988	Creation of the midwifery coordinator position within the ministry of health
1989	Appointment of the IRCM
	Final Report of the HPLR including a draft Midwifery Act submitted to Minister of Health
1990	First Reading of the RHPA and Midwifery Act in the provincial legislature
	[*Change of Government from Liberal to NDP*]
	CDC submits final report
1991	First, second, and third reading of RHPA and Midwifery Act
	AOM secures liability insurance for practising Ontario midwives
	Royal Assent of RHPA and Midwifery act (makes the practice of midwifery officially legal in the province)
	MIPP Committee submits final report
1992	MOPP Committee submits final report
	Midwifery Assessment program begins at Michener Institute
1993	Creation of the Transitional Council of the College of Midwives of Ontario
	Amendments to PHA to allow midwives hospital admitting privileges
	Midwifery Education program begins at Ryerson, McMaster, and Laurentian Universities
	Proclamation of RHPA and Midwifery Act
	OMP program begins public funding for midwifery services
1994	Midwives secure hospital admitting privileges

CHAPTER SIX

Dilemmas of Regulation

In the previous chapter, I outlined how the provincial government, upon the advice of the Health Professions Legislation Review, decided that midwifery would become integrated as a regulated health profession in the province of Ontario. But because of the midwives' unique situation of operating outside of the formal health care system, a thorough investigation was needed in terms of how midwifery would be integrated in the province. The Task Force on the Implementation of Midwifery in Ontario (TFIMO) was struck to do just such background work.

THE TASK FORCE ON THE IMPLEMENTATION OF MIDWIFERY IN ONTARIO

Mandate and Members

The formal terms of reference of the Task Force on the Implementation of Midwifery in Ontario were outlined as follows: "The Task Force on the Implementation of Midwifery in Ontario will provide advice to the Minister of Health on matters of particular interest to him [sic] within the areas of education of midwives, requirements for entry to practice, scope and standards of practice, governance of the profession, locations of practice, patient access and whether midwives should operate as independent practitioners or as part of an organized service" (TFIMO 1987: 29). The Task Force essentially took midwifery out of the HPLR process because the task of bringing midwifery up to par with the professional criteria the HPLR developed for the regulation of all health professions was considered to be too large a task for the HPLR to handle. The work of the Task Force, however, was still intricately linked to the HPLR process.

Ultimately, the Task Force's recommendations had to fit within the regulatory context created by the HPLR.

Initially, Minister of Health Murray Elston considered having HPLR Coordinator Alan Schwartz chair the committee, but Schwartz was fully occupied with work emanating from the HPLR: "I was dealing at the time with over 40 health care groups. The task of determining precisely how midwifery should be integrated, everything from the educational requirements to the relationship of midwifery to the hospital system was too much for me to undertake on my own. It would have taken too much energy away from the broad thrust of HPLR and was inconsistent with the main focus of my mandate" (Alan Schwartz, personal communication 1995). Out of a consultative process internal to the Ministry of Health, it was decided that Mary Eberts, a feminist lawyer, would be appointed Chair of the Task Force. Eberts was known to the Liberal government for her strong feminist perspective and her work on women's rights in relation to the Charter. HPLR Coordinator Alan Schwartz "thought it was important that the Task Force have a large representation of women" and that the Chair "should be a strong, relatively high-profile person with credibility in the ... community of women that would be interested in this issue" (personal communication 1995). Mary Eberts recalled that "[the Liberal government] clearly did want a feminist; that was one of the things that they talked to me about" (personal communication 1995).

Schwartz was appointed as Vice-Chair "to maintain a good liaison with the health professions legislation review" (Hansard 1985: 3373) and to "ensure that [the Task Force's] work would be coordinated with the work of the review" (HPLR 1989: 11). The other members of the Task Force were Dr Rachel Edney, a family physician with an obstetrics practice and former president of the Ontario College of Family Physicians, and Dr Karyn Kaufman, associate professor at McMaster School of Nursing and former American-trained nurse-midwife. Edney was considered a champion of natural (or low-tech) birth and had previously expressed support for midwifery at the 1985 inquest. She recalled that it was politically important for a pro-midwifery physician to be appointed: "My understanding was that [the government] wanted a physician that had some understanding of midwifery and ... I suspect one that they already knew had some sympathy with the idea" (Edney, personal communication 1995). Kaufman was an associate of Dr Murray Enkin on the extended-role nursing project at McMaster University where nurses, through the delegation of specific medical acts, practised similarly to midwives albeit within the hospital setting.

Concerns were initially expressed within the midwifery community regarding the appointment of these Task Force members, mainly because no practising midwives or consumers were appointed. These concerns were soon allayed, however, upon consultation with Alan Schwartz. He asserted that all members tended to be pro-midwifery and the government chose them precisely because of these sentiments. Midwife Vicki Van Wagner recalled Schwartz' justification for the choice of Task Force members: "What Schwartz argued was…"Listen, in some ways it may be more powerful for you to be on the outside. This way the practising midwives would not be compromised by having to be involved and [would] appear objective … and the Task Force would have [more] credibility" (personal communication 1995).

The Work of the Task Force

Once appointed, the Task Force undertook a lengthy consultative process involving international investigations: written submissions; oral presentations; public hearings; and several meetings among stakeholder groups (midwives, nurses, physicians, and hospital representatives), other organized groups (women's groups, church groups, ethnic groups, and trade unions), consumers and the general public. As described in the Task Force report, it "gathered information about how midwifery [was] practised outside and inside Canada, how Ontario midwives and other health care providers envision midwifery care being integrated into the health care system, and how the public perceived its needs" (TFIMO 1987: 33). Chair Mary Eberts recalled little involvement from the Ministry regarding the process the Task Force took, which meant it had "a tremendous amount of flexibility to shape [its] own mandate" (personal communication 1995).

One of the first steps of the Task Force was to conduct an initial round of consultations with key stakeholder groups. Task Force member Karyn Kaufman recounted that these initial consultations informally told groups how the Task Force was going to proceed "We want you to know we're here – we're up and running. This is the nature of our mandate. This is the question we've been asked to address. Tell us where you are on this issue right now. We're telling you [these are the kinds] of things we're planning: we're going to travel; we're going to ask questions; we're going to meet with other groups; we're going to have public hearings. And as we move along, and we think we're getting to the point of having some sense of things, we will do another round of consultations, because we have no intention of dropping the Report out of nowhere" (personal communication 1995). Mary Eberts later described these consultations as negotiations rather than inquiries, because since midwifery was clearly going to be implemented the various stakeholders needed to get beyond the issue of *whether* midwifery was to be implemented and focus on *how* this was going to happen.

Following the initial consultations, written submissions were requested by the Task Force from interested parties asking their position on midwifery, including the advantages they thought midwifery care might bring to the overall maternity system; overlaps between midwives and other health care providers; midwifery education; place(s) of practice; costs; professional liability; and what it considered to be the major obstacles to implementing midwifery in Ontario. Additionally, public hearings were held across the province in October and November of 1986, enabling groups and individuals to follow up their written submissions. In total, the Task Force received more than 500 written submissions and approximately 180 individuals and representatives of interested organizations made oral presentations at the public hearings (TFIMO 1987).

While the Task Force pursued these initiatives, the AOM and MTFO pursued its own agenda as they had done during other challenging events: "The work of the next year will involve making presentations to the government task force from both the AOM and MTF, inviting international experts to make statements and to carry on our public education and press work, in order to present our position on the most effective kind of midwifery care in Ontario" (*Issue* 10, Feb. 1986: 4). Both organizations urged midwives and midwifery supporters alike to get involved: "*Every midwife and midwifery supporter must take advantage of this opportunity to be part of the creation of midwifery in Ontario.* Presentations should come from individuals and the many groups who support our positions ... Each MTF and AOM chapter should begin to coordinate local support groups and individuals to make presentations when the public hearings are held in their areas ... *You need to let [the Task Force] know what kind of midwifery care will benefit you*" (*Issue* 11, April 1986: 12, emphasis in original).

THE SUBMISSIONS AND HEARINGS

In their submission to the Task Force, the AOM outlined two elements of their position: the philosophy and orientation of midwifery (the midwifery model); and an implementation plan intended to create a midwifery system in accord with this philosophy. The midwifery model was described as including fully informed choice – including choice of birth attendant, style of birth, place of birth, and access to midwifery care –

and quality care – involving continuity, personal attention, preventive care, education and counselling, and a caregiver who is an expert in normal birth. Mechanisms outlined for implementing this model included self-regulation, formal direct-entry training; integration of currently practising midwives; and community-based care with the midwife as primary caregiver and full member of the health care team. Self-regulation was recommended to be phased in according to the AOM's revised four-phase strategy. This involved 1) establishing a provisional governing body for midwifery; 2) sharing administrative personnel, space, and equipment with other professions to keep the administrative and financial aspects of self-regulation more manageable; 3) and developing the number of registered midwives gradually to ensure safe, standardized practice. During these stages midwifery practice and educational programs would be implemented.[1]

In addition to this submission from the AOM, the Task Force received another thirty submissions from individual midwives and midwifery associations, including MANA, the Midwives Association of Canada, the Midwives Association of British Columbia, and the Alberta Association of Midwives. These submissions were expressly supportive of the AOM submission (TFIMO 1987: 250).

The submission of the MTFO also echoed the elements of the AOM submission: "The Midwifery Task Force said, "Not only do we want midwives, we have some clear ideas about why we like [the AOM] model, and that vision of midwifery care" (Midwife Holliday Tyson, personal communication 1995). During the public hearings many consumers detailed their personal experiences with midwifery care to help illustrate the reasoning behind their support of the model of midwifery care proposed by the AOM (TFIMO 1987: 258). Chair Mary Eberts described the strong impression these consumer presentations made on the Task Force: "One of the really positive aspects of the Task Force was the strong consumer support manifested at all the hearings. They were great hearings. We had moms and dads and babies and little kids and some wonderful personal witnessing by people because of the happiness that they had having births with midwives" (Eberts, personal communication 1995). The more than 200 submissions received from consumers were strongly supportive of the implementation of an independent, self-regulating profession of midwifery, responsive to public needs and wishes (TFIMO 1987, 262).

Support for the AOM submission also came from a broad range of over twenty women's groups, from left-wing, feminist groups to more right-wing and conservative women's groups. The feminist-oriented Toronto

Women's Health Network, for example, described that: "Central to our ability to have control over our bodies and lives is the ability to make choices on issues such as birth control, sexuality, sexual orientation, pregnancy and childbirth. In the same way that we advocate universally available safe and effective birth control, including the option of abortion, we support a woman's right to give birth with the professional of her choice, in the setting of her choice, in the manner of her choice" (TFIMO 1987: 259). Many feminist groups in Ontario had come to the realization, due largely to the active solicitation of support from midwives and consumers, that midwifery ideology and practice, specifically its focus on women's choice and control, was congruent with their own ideology (cf., Rushing 1993). In fact, several feminists subsequently became involved in midwifery (either becoming consumers, supporters, or midwives) because of this congruence. At the same time, midwifery, unlike other women's health initiatives such as abortion, was also compatible with the beliefs of more conservative women's groups. That is, although feminist and conservative women's groups varied widely in politics and philosophy, all were supportive of the implementation of midwifery in Ontario: "One of the most important things about the process of the Task Force was the incredibly large amount of support for midwifery; and so you have midwives presenting, clients presenting, but you also have church groups, women's groups, anti-choice groups, pro-choice groups ... My favourite memory from the Task Force [is having] the OCAC [Ontario Coalition for Abortion Clinics] and REAL Women [a pro-life group] agreeing about midwifery[2] ... to me that is so symbolic: the diverse, contradictory, tension-filled meaning that midwifery has for women" (Midwife Vicki Van Wagner, personal communication 1995).

In addition to making formal submissions, both the AOM and MTFO inundated the Task Force with information to support their submission: "What we did was [take] an aggressively proactive stance. Every week, more or less, we said, 'What are we sending them this week?' ... They were appointed to do their homework but we just continued to do our homework, and continued to send them things in case they hadn't found this particular study or that particular piece of information about midwifery. ... We buried them in paper ... We decided that we would just be incredibly proactive in providing them with information that we wanted them to have...to support the kind of midwifery we were proposing" (Midwife Robin Kilpatrick, personal communication 1995).

Throughout the process of the Task Force, midwifery community leaders also made a concerted effort to control the presentation of midwifery to

the Task Force and the media. One of the underlying themes of this controlled presentation was to present midwives as legitimate health care
professionals and not a radical bunch of counterculture women:

Midwifery has its countercultural roots ... Would people go to meet with
government officials dressed like hippies? ... Many of us who were involved with
it would say ..."Why would we threaten [the officials] by doing that? This isn't
about how we dress, this is about midwifery." (midwife Vicki Van Wagner,
personal communication 1995)

We used to make jokes about dress code – I think there was this whole sense of
we have a body of knowledge and information and experience that won't be
taken seriously unless we present it in a professional way. And it wasn't that we
were going to change what we said about what we believed, but put it in a
package in a context that they would hear ... I remember doing a presentation
and thinking "Well, I want to wear something that won't make them think about
what I'm wearing because I want them to listen to what I'm saying." (midwife
Jane Kilthei, personal communication 1995)

At the same time that there was this enhancement of the professional
aspects of midwifery, some felt that there was a downplaying of its spiritual and emotional side. Midwife Jane Kilthei, for example, remembers
how one presentation that got into the "spiritual aspect of midwifery"
was not making a connection with the members of the Task Force; "it
wasn't working" (personal communication 1995). By controlling the presentation of midwifery by midwives and midwifery consumers, the AOM
and MTFO hoped that they would make a good "professional" impression
on the Task Force.

Other submissions to the Task Force were received from the stakeholder
groups in the health care system – medicine, nursing, and hospitals. The
submission from the medical and nursing professions largely reiterated
what they had proposed throughout the HPLR process. Submissions from
the medical professions included those from the CPSO, OMA, OCFP, SOGC,
and the Medical Reform Group (MRG). With the exception of the OMA,
all groups supported or accepted the integration of midwifery into the
health care system.[3] Although many physicians favoured the idea of
nurse-midwifery, either because they were familiar or more comfortable
with it, self-regulation and formal direct entry education were generally
believed to be acceptable alternatives. Concerns regarding liability
encouraged many within the medical profession to be less opposed to the

idea of self-regulation; they felt that if midwives were to be integrated into the health care system, they should be responsible for their actions: "[Doctors] had the impression that some ... midwives were pretty irresponsible, wild-eyed people and ... that they were doing loony things for which these doctors would be left holding the bag ... [They] didn't want to be in a position where they were the ones with the insurance and the deep pockets and the place in the system that caused them to be sued" (Task Force Chair Mary Eberts, personal communication 1995). Submissions from the nursing profession, as represented by the ONA, RNAO and CNO, however, maintained their original position that midwifery be recognized as a specialty of nursing regulated under the CNO.

Submissions from the hospital sector were received from the Ontario Hospital Association (OHA) as well as from fourteen individual hospitals across Ontario. The OHA submission also included results from a survey of eighty Ontario hospitals regarding the issue of midwifery. The majority of hospitals indicated considerable support for the integration of midwifery into the Ontario health care system. Four hospitals expressed their interest in participating in pilot projects of midwifery care. Midwives, it was thought, would play a positive role in helping hospitals develop family-centred maternity care. There were concerns expressed, however, regarding the payment of midwives and the coverage of midwives under liability insurance, but in the end most hospitals felt that these issues could be resolved with further study. Although most hospitals expressed the view that midwives should be regulated under the CNO, the OHA reserved comment.

International Consultations

In addition to local consultations made through submissions and public hearings, the Task Force members supplemented their investigation with an examination of midwifery internationally. They undertook an extensive literature review of midwifery world wide, with the assistance of the AOM. During July and August of 1986, Eberts, Kaufman, and Edney also consulted with midwifery experts in the US, the UK, Denmark, and the Netherlands. These countries were chosen so that a range of midwifery options could be examined. Task Force members requested a list of contacts in each of these countries from midwives in the AOM.

The knowledge of what has and has not worked elsewhere acquired from these international consultations guided the Task Force's thinking about what should and should not be attempted in Ontario. Midwife

Vicki Van Wagner also stressed the importance of the international consultations in highlighting how midwifery "is happening everywhere and isn't such a radical thing that we need to be so afraid of" (personal communication 1995). It was through these consultations that issues such as autonomy, self-regulation, and continuity of care were highlighted as essential principles of midwifery. In-depth examination of the structure of midwifery in the US, which is marked by a division between nurse and non-nurse midwives, was viewed as an unfortunate obstacle to "full public acceptance and appreciation of midwifery care" (TFIMO 1987: 46). There, nurse-midwifery had secured some legitimacy within the system largely at the expense of non-nurse midwives. This division diffused public support for midwifery generally as one group was often pitted against the other. This division between nurse and non-nurse midwifery was regarded as an undesirable model for Ontario. This decision laid to rest proposals for a similar nurse-midwifery model made by some within the medical and nursing professions.

Task Force Recommendations

A strong theme in the presentations to the Task Force, especially from consumers and midwives, was the need to recognize the emotional and familial significance of childbirth, and to think of childbirth not just in medical terms but also in human terms (TFIMO 1987: 25). This theme made a strong impression on Task Force members. Consequently, the search for new ways to humanize the birth experience while emphasizing skill through the integration of midwifery became part of the Task Force's agenda.

RECOMMENDATIONS OF THE TASK FORCE ON THE
IMPLEMENTATION OF MIDWIFERY IN ONTARIO, 1987

1 Self regulation
2 Multiple routes of entry to practice, including direct entry
3 Primary care attendants at both hospital and home birth
4 Public funding

When the TFIMO presented its 426-page report to the Minister in October 1987, the recommendations were highly supportive of the kind of midwifery that midwives wanted; indeed, they mirrored some of the key elements of the Midwifery Coalition's First Submission to the HPLR four years earlier (see chapter 4). It recommended that midwifery should be an autonomous, self-regulating profession fully integrated into the health care system and funded by the government. Midwives could enter practice from multiple routes, including formal direct entry at the baccalaureate level (discussed further in chapter 9), and would be able to practise both in hospitals and at home (discussed further in chapter 7).

Self-regulation was recommended, as it had become clear that the prototype model of regulation proposed by the HPLR was self-regulation; and given that midwifery was to be included under HPLR legislation, it too would have to be self-regulating. When the HPLR officially announced their final list of twenty-five professions under its legislation, including midwifery, on April 3, 1986, it argued: "The leaders of the profession have demonstrated an ability to distinguish between the public interest and professional self-interest, and to favour the former ... The efforts of the Association of Ontario Midwives and of individual midwives to obtain recognition and to draw up standards of practice and protocols for education and peer review indicate that widespread compliance with self-regulation is likely" (TFIMO 1987: 135).

Although self-regulation was prescribed, because midwifery was a new and inadequately regulated profession, the Task Force had to address several transitional problems before midwifery could become fully self-regulating. For example, although the Task Force recommended the establishment of a new governing body for midwifery, a College of Midwives, it noted that establishing a separate College for midwifery was problematic for several reasons: "College business must be performed before there are any licensed practitioners available to serve on the Council. Somebody must perform the functions necessary to license practitioners: examine credentials, set and administer examinations, and establish and apply licensing requirements" (TFIMO 1987: 138). For this reason, the Task Force recommended that an interim college be established. It was also recommended that this interim College include thirteen members: one obstetrician; one general practitioner whose practice includes obstetrics; one neonatologist; one nurse whose field of practice in maternal/newborn nursing; one hospital administrator; one childbirth educator; five consumers, representatives of women's health organizations, ethnic and visible minority women, francophone women, and women from northern Ontario; and two lawyers who practise in the fields of administrative law and corporate law. Representatives of currently practising midwives and foreign-trained midwives were recommended to provide liaison and advice to such an interim council. Once there was a sufficient number of licensed midwives, it was recommended that the College be composed of a majority of elected members. Because of the small numbers of midwives that were projected to be governed under the College, the Task Force also recommended that the Ministry of Health subsidize the establishment and ongoing operation of the College until the profession had sufficient numbers to bear the full costs of College operations. It also recommended that in order to keep costs down, the College of Midwives share administrative services, office facilities, and staff with one or more governing bodies of unrelated health professions.

Given that these recommendations were so supportive of the model of midwifery the AOM and the MTFO proposed, it was viewed most favourably by these two groups.[4] By the time the Task Force had published its recommendations, the medical profession had resigned itself to accepting the self-regulation of a direct entry form of midwifery. The nursing profession, however, viewed the recommendations as yet another lost battle. Commenting on the recommendations of the Task Force for community midwifery rather than the nursing model proposed by the nursing profession, Task Force member Alan Schwartz emphasized: "A community-based model was more in keeping with what we believed was required and needed. It was more responsive to what we were hearing was the void that needed filling. The medical and nursing models were less responsive to this void in our view" (Task Force member Schwartz, personal communication 1995). This comment highlights the importance that consumer input had on the Task Force decision making process.

Effects of the Task Force on Midwifery

Throughout the process of the Task Force, the input and recommendations of midwives to the committee proved to be influential. Although in separate organizations, midwives and consumers were still working together toward a common goal of integrating midwifery into a favourable regulatory model. Over time, however, there was a sense that the midwives active in the AOM were taking the lead, with the MTFO following suit. Some consumers felt that the leaders of the MTFO were largely being directed by the AOM midwives. Specifically regarding the model of midwifery proposed to the Task Force, it was largely developed by midwives within the AOM, and endorsed by the MTFO. The professionalization of midwifery was becoming increasingly evident. This was also exemplified in the way the AOM leaders exerted control of the presentation of midwifery, limiting it to those aspects that were deemed "professional" or otherwise conducive to the political process of integration. Thus, although midwives had a significant impact on the Task Force, the midwifery community was continually being shaped by what midwives and others viewed as acceptable. While the inclusion of midwifery was changing the Ontario health care system, midwifery itself was also in various subtle and not so subtle ways being transformed.

This reshaping of midwifery into a profession was serving to potentially increase the social distance between midwives and the women they provided care for. It also served to exacerbate dissent within the midwifery community arising from the initial decision to seek integration. Those midwives and supporters who expressed concern with the integration process back in 1983 were becoming more and more uncomfortable with the professionalization of midwifery throughout the Task Force process.

Following the Task Force, the AOM continued to carefully control the image of midwifery being portrayed publicly. Anticipating an increase in media inquiries into midwifery following the release of the Task Force report, the AOM drafted press protocols to guide members in their dealings with the media to standardize responses to particular questions. These protocols were highlighted in the AOM newsletter: "We propose that any requests for interviews, appearances, etc. be reported and discussed with the President or head of the Legislation Committee. This will ... provide an opportunity to discuss the important issues to be covered in an interview ... We do not want to discourage members from speaking with the media ... We must remember, however, that any statements affect all of us, and we must recognize the responsibility we have to represent our Association professionally" (AOM newsletter 3, no. 4, December 1987: 17). Some midwives felt that it was "like somebody had to be a watchdog over anybody who was going to speak publicly about midwifery – a Big Brother's watching you kind of attitude squashing anything that seemed a little bit too far out, to make sure that nothing undermined the efforts of the AOM" (Midwife, personal communication 1995). Midwife Betty-Anne Davis commented that although she did not disagree with the image of midwifery being portrayed, she nevertheless felt it was having an impact on what midwives were becoming: "Part of the problem here is at one point the image you are presenting you start to own and you start to lose the original reasons why you were doing this birth in the first place – to give the woman what she wants and what is really best for her, instead of what "looks good" in the eyes of the medical profession, the media, etc." (personal communication 1995).

Concurrent with these deliberate attempts to control the presentation of midwifery in the media was an increased tendency for the AOM to hold its meetings predominantly in Toronto rather than in other Ontario centres. This exacerbated some of the feelings of alienation and dissent within the midwifery community. One midwife argued that by this point "everyone else wasn't as in love with the process as the small group was" (personal communication 1995).

In response to this rising feeling of discontent within the midwifery community, a special AOM workshop addressing the "Dangers of the Professionalization of Midwifery" was held in February 1989. The fears of professionalization expressed at this conference centred around midwifery becoming more distant and bureaucratized – more like medicine. Long-time midwifery supporter Jutta Mason highlighted several dangers of professionalization for midwifery. These included: 1) the subversion of the straightforward language developed by the women's birth network into the style of media and government reports; 2) the identification of the midwife as a different kind of medical expert; and 3) the overshadowing of the intimate project of reworking our own knowledge about our bodies and our capacities by the quest of the midwives for legitimacy in the "land of monopoly medicine" (Mason 1989). The focus of the alternative childbirth community, she argued, had already shifted from the broader issue of women's control in childbirth to the narrow focus of the legitimacy of midwifery. That is, midwifery was now being viewed as an end in and of itself, rather than a means to an end of greater female control of pregnancy and birth.

Those leading the integration process, however, argued that midwifery was different and would not become professionalized in the same manner as medicine: "For the medical profession the crux of professionalism is autonomy – "the right to act as I think best." For midwives it is different. It is the ability to be responsive to our clients' needs and to the needs of the community ... You have to respect the midwife and her right to practice in order to protect any woman's right to make choices" (Kilthei, AOM newsletter 5, no. 1, April 1989: 26–7.) Self-regulation under the legislative context recommended by the HPLR was considered preferable to the current state of regulation under criminal law, "with all the fear and harassment that entails inquests and court battles" (AOM newsletter 5, no.1, April 1989: 26). Regulated midwifery, it was argued, would mean accessible, quality midwifery care: "It means access for poor women, immigrant women, and teenage mothers to midwives ... It also means access of the midwife to the system, so that she can better provide safe care – primary care in hospital, and access to hospital back-up in out-of-hospital births. We seek the status that comes with legislation and regulation because it means we can use our skills, rather than being expected to put our hands in our pockets as we cross the threshold of a hospital" (Kilthei, AOM newsletter 5, no. 1, April 1989: 27). Midwifery leaders added that the HPLR made it inevitable that midwifery would be regulated: "Both the nursing and medical professions sought to control midwifery practice. Consumers, through the Midwifery Task Force (MTF), and midwives, through the Association of Ontario Midwives (AOM), both realized that if we did not take up the issue of regulation and become active participants in the HPLR we would be excluded and midwifery would be defined and controlled by others" (Kilthei, AOM newsletter, 5, no. 1, April 1989: 27). Thus, the issue was not whether there would be regulation but who would control it and what kind of regulation it would be. In making this argument, midwifery leaders hoped to respond to the concerns of some midwives about the integration process. They felt that the "dangers of professionalization" could be minimized only through the continued involvement of midwives in the regulation-defining process.

POST-TASK FORCE COMMITMENTS OF THE GOVERNMENT

Following the presentation of the Task Force report, midwives continued to lobby the government to implement the Task Force recommendations. Another MTFO letter-writing campaign was aimed at the Minister of Health, Elinor Caplan, and the Minister of Colleges and Universities, Lyn Macleod. TFIMO Chair Mary Eberts also approached the AOM and MTFO about organizing a lobby group of influential women to put some pressure on Caplan to help ensure the Task Force report did not get shelved.

The AOM's and MTFO's continuing efforts succeeded, perhaps because of continued government support. Following the publication of the TFIMO report, the government asserted its strong commitment to midwifery by acting on the Task Force recommendations. The first indicator of its commitment was the organization and sponsorship of an international interdisciplinary conference entitled "Birth: The Future is in Our Hands" held in the fall of 1987. Although the conference was not exclusively focused on midwifery, midwives were presented at the conference by then-Minister of Health Elinor Caplan as legitimate professionals about to be integrated into the health care system. Their integration was lauded as one of Ontario's latest initiatives in improving maternity care. Minister of Health Caplan described the purpose of the Conference: "The Conference was organized to raise the consciousness of existing providers about midwifery, what the role was going to be, and it was to permit the kind of discussions and interactions to both allay fears and also to gather acceptance. It was also to show the support of the Minister and the government and to send the message out that this was going to happen and to ask for help and assistance in bringing this about" (personal communication 1995). Task Force Chair Mary Eberts described the conference as another indication of the government's support for midwifery: "It was really [the government's] first stage of outreach about midwifery and its validation ... This was the Ministry kind of getting its muscle behind midwifery and saying we think this is a good idea ... It was the first time that [stakeholders] were actually getting together to do something about midwifery" (personal communication 1995). Midwives fondly referred to the conference as their "coming out party" (Kilpatrick 1995).

Another show of government support came with the creation of the Midwifery Coordinator position within the Ministry of Health, first filled by former TFIMO member Karyn Kaufman. The position was created in 1988[5] in order to act on the TFIMO recommendations and to help shepherd the integration process. Minister of Health Elinor Caplan described the reasoning behind the creation of the position: "The Ministry had to have a point person, somebody that would direct the implementation because we had a time line and many different pieces ... of things to prepare the Province for the implementation of midwifery [i.e., legislation, education, etc.] ... So it was really important that all of those pieces come together and converge so that everything needed to be coordinated ... So we brought in Karyn Kaufman" (personal communication 1995). Kaufman felt she had been chosen because she had both clinical as well as political experience (derived from her work on the Task Force). She provided much needed continuity to keep up the momentum for the midwifery integration project.

As Midwifery Coordinator, Kaufman was also a welcome liaison between the AOM and the government, providing midwives with updates about the process of implementation and decisions facing the midwifery profession. This helped the AOM to more fully prepare for the integration process. Midwife Michelle Kryzanauskas emphasized the importance of the Midwifery Coordinator to the AOM: "The Midwifery Coordinator was an extremely important person to the AOM ... [She] was the person the Ministry employed to liaise with us and assist us in approaching or being

approached by the government, and in fact worked fairly closely with us
... She offered advice and timelines" (personal communication 1995).

In 1989 the government furthered its commitment to midwifery by
appointing a thirteen-member Interim Regulatory Council on Midwifery
(IRCM) which was to develop the midwifery implementation strategy and
practice standards, and to act as the regulatory body for midwifery. The
IRCM was to follow the regulatory context created by the HPLR in its final
report presented to the Ministry of Health in January 1989.

FORMALLY REGULATING MIDWIFERY

Final Report of the HPLR

During the tenure of the Task Force, the HPLR had decided what form of
self-regulation it would use as its model for all health professions. The
Review identified several inconsistencies and problems with the existing
system of licensure and certification: "The existing system, in which a
small number of health professions are 'licensed' (their members have an
exclusive licence or monopoly over the provision of services that fall
within their scope of practice) and others are 'registered' (their members
have an exclusive right to use certain titles), does not effectively protect
the public from unqualified health care providers" (HPLR 1989: 3). Instead
of licensing a profession's scope of practice, the HPLR chose to license
potentially harmful "acts" or procedures which could be performed only
by qualified health professionals authorized by their Professional Act to
perform them. Restricting the use of professional titles was also recommended to enable the public to distinguish regulated professionals from
unregulated health care providers.

In its final report to the Ministry of Health in January 1989, the HPLR
prepared a draft Midwifery Act with the assistance of Karyn Kaufman
(in her capacity as Midwifery Coordinator) and representatives from the
AOM. The Act expanded on the recommendations of the Task Force and
included definitions of midwives' scope of practice (see chapter 7), College
structure, committee composition, and regulation and by-law making
powers. It was recommended that the College Council be composed of
between eight and ten midwives and between four and five public members. College committees were to include an executive committee, a registration committee, a complaints committee, a discipline committee, a
fitness to practice committee, and a continuing competence committee all
to include both midwife and public members. The recommendations of

the HPLR and the draft Midwifery Act would provide the regulatory framework for the subsequent development of midwifery standards and policies by midwifery regulatory bodies.

The Interim Regulatory Council of Midwifery

MEMBERS AND MANDATE

The membership and terms of reference of the Interim Regulatory Council of Midwifery (IRCM) were drafted by the Midwifery Coordinator, Karyn Kaufman, following the Task Force recommendation that an interim body be set up to begin drafting regulations. The IRCM's mandate was to provide recommendations to the Minister of Health and to prepare the way for a statutory College of Midwives. It was also to act in the interim as a regulatory body for midwifery until the Midwifery Act was proclaimed law.

Kaufman's next step was to choose members for the IRCM. Names of nominees were solicited from consumer groups, midwifery groups, and other professional groups (*The Gazette* 1, no. 1, Sept. 1990: 5). Kaufman described the recruitment process: "It was talking to various groups and trying to come up with the constituency groups that needed to be represented on the IRCM, get names put forward (a nomination process), present those to the Minister and then the Minister's office makes the final decision" (personal communication 1995). More than forty names of nominees were forwarded to the Minister of Health, Elinor Caplan, who then made the final decision. Caplan (1995) described the process of choosing the members of the committee: "They were all Minister's appointments and we had a number of recommendations of individuals that were active both from the Task Force, from consumer groups ... I tried to select individuals who had a history and commitment to midwifery, and I had a personal commitment to midwifery so I tried to choose people very wisely that would expedite, and be thoughtful, and use good judgement" (personal communication 1995).

In the end, the membership on the IRCM generally followed the recommendations made by the Task Force and the HPLR. The thirteen members of the IRCM officially appointed by the Lieutenant-Governor in Council on May 19, 1989, included Mary Eberts, lawyer and former chair of the Task Force as Chair; Patricia Hennessy, an administrator from Sudbury as Vice-Chair; Murray Enkin, pro-midwifery obstetrician from Hamilton; Catherine Oliver, family physician from Toronto; Susan Phillips, family physician from Kingston[6]; Ina Caissey, maternal-child nurse from Timmins; Patricia Legault, maternal-child nurse from Kitchener; Winifred

Hunsburger, childbirth educator from North York; Dianne Pudas and Jesse
Russell, both midwifery consumers from Thunder Bay; Anne Rochon Ford
and Wendy Sutton, midwifery consumers from Toronto; and Victoria
Mummery, a midwifery consumer from London. IRCM members were not
chosen to represent any particular organizations but rather were to come
as informed individuals.[7]

Liaison Committee. As was stipulated in both the Task Force report and
in the HPLR report, midwives could not be appointed to the Council until
they were licensed. Midwifery Coordinator Karyn Kaufman described
the reasoning behind that decision "We felt that there was a very real
potential conflict of interest if you appointed practising midwives to that
group ... and so [we really needed to] make it clear that this had to be
a group that looked at the public's best interest with the advice and input
of midwives so the IRCM didn't make decisions that were irrelevant to
midwives. They had to have input, but they had to be seen to be somewhat impartial, or at least more broadly representative than just midwives themselves" (personal communication 1995). Although midwives
were officially excluded from the IRCM, a Liaison Committee between
the AOM and the IRCM was established to ensure midwives had input
into the policy and standard development process. The terms of reference of the Liaison Committee were as follows "The role of the Association of Ontario Midwives Liaison Committee is to provide input and
feedback regarding proposals and policies developed by the IRC. Members will provide information on the current practice of midwifery, the
AOM's background in providing voluntary regulation, standards of practice, and educational standards, and will provide AOM documents relevant to regulatory functions. Members will also relate relevant
information regarding current AOM activities" (AOM Newsletter 6, no. 3,
November 1990: 4).

Although midwives felt affronted at being excluded yet again from an
important midwifery decision-making body,[8] the Liaison Committee was
seen as a good compromise. Midwives also took consolation in the fact
that official IRCM members were very supportive of midwifery.[9] Although
officially independent of midwives, the IRCM partly became "a third
party confirmation that what [midwives] were doing was really important" (IRCM member Wendy Sutton, personal communication 1994). The
Liaison Committee was also welcomed by IRCM members. Midwife
Robin Kilpatrick recounted that IRCM members "may have felt rather

awkward having to [develop policies] without midwives" (personal communication 1995).

In order to deal with the increasing complexities of the integration process, the AOM decided that Liaison Committee members would be required to attend all meetings of the AOM legislation and education committees as well as meetings with representatives of the government and other professions. Thus, midwifery representatives on the Liaison Committee included the executive of the AOM and the chairs of each AOM committee. This included AOM President Edythe Johnson, President Elect Bobbi Soderstrom, secretary of research and statistics committee Chair Eileen Hutton, membership committee Chair Jane Kilthei, standards committee representative Michelle Kryzanauskas, complaints and hearings chair Rena Porteous, education committee Chair Elizabeth Allemang, legislation committee Chair Robin Kilpatrick, and Liaison Committee Chair Vicki Van Wagner. By and large, Liaison Committee members were the core group of midwives who had been highly involved in the AOM and in the implementation process from the beginning. The selection of Liaison Committee members resulted in some feelings of discontent from some midwives who felt excluded from the integration process. Although the AOM board attempted to address this issue, they maintained their decision: "The Board [of the AOM] wonders how to get more people involved especially those who live a long distance from Toronto. Participation on this team would not just require attendance but other work as well. There is a difficult balance to be found because although this Committee wants to be more inclusive it needs to be realistic about the level of understanding about the issues which only regular attendance and participation might develop" (6, no. 2, August 1990: 11).

Liaison Committee members were not official members of the IRCM and were not allowed to vote. However, given that the decision-making of the Council operated largely on a consensus basis, midwives had a strong say in the development of policies at the IRCM. Midwifery Coordinator Karyn Kaufman confirmed the openness with which Liaison Committee members were included in the IRCM process: "I would say that at the table it was pretty much indistinguishable who was an appointed member and who was from the liaison committee. It really functioned as a large group ... I think it was a very open process; very much an exchange" (personal communication 1995). IRCM member Murray Enkin concurred that "midwives had every bit as much say, probably more than the official members because they had the experience" (personal communication 1995).[10] The influence of the Liaison Committee was especially striking in the regulation development process of the IRCM.

REGULATION DEVELOPMENT PROCESS

The regulation development process of the IRCM often began with AOM documents drafted during the interim period between the TFIMO and the IRCM. These regulations and policy statements were used as background and revised in order to fit within the context created by the HPLR process. Within this context, however, there was a fair bit of freedom in the development of policies. Midwife and Liaison Committee member Bobbi Soderstrom described the role of AOM documents at the IRCM: "[AOM documents] were used [by the IRCM] as a base or beginning document, to say 'Okay, here is what the midwives have been doing prior to legislation, what additions, deletions and changes would we want in order to make it fit appropriately within the regulatory body'" (Soderstrom, personal communication 1995).

This trend of relying on AOM documents was especially true of the work of the standards committee. Both during and following the Task Force consultation process, the AOM worked diligently to revise their standards of practice. The aim of these efforts was to develop the rules by which midwives would be governed before they were developed for them.[11] As described by midwife Vicki Van Wagner, advice from the international midwifery community as well as outcomes of the HPLR process helped delineate the types of governing principles that midwives would need to develop: "Looking around at all of the other places and looking at the other professions in Ontario, we always took those as our two reference points: midwifery elsewhere, what are they doing? The other professions here, what are they doing? The CMA has a code of ethics; should we have a code of ethics? British midwives have a code of ethics; of course we should have a code of ethics" (personal communication 1995).

By the time the IRCM had begun, the AOM had developed a core collection of professional practice standards – the AOM "Blue Book" called *Guidelines to Standards of Practice*. Midwife and standards committee member Michelle Kryzanauskas described how these documents provided the basis from which IRCM Standards were developed: "The AOM's standards book was adopted by the IRCM in principle. The documents in the standards book were then independently stylized and prepared for the regulated system" (personal communication 1995).

Throughout the policy development process, the IRCM, like the Task Force before it, not only consulted widely within the consumer and midwifery community, it also sought input from established maternity care providers. To help midwifery become fully integrated into the health care system, the IRCM made a concerted effort to keep all lines of communication open with other stakeholder groups, keeping them informed of IRCM developments so that their recommendations would not be seen as "coming out of the blue." Proposed IRCM policy documents "were shopped around to different professions and to different interest groups [to get] feedback from them" (IRCM Chair Mary Eberts, personal communication 1995). In addition, all IRCM meetings were open and representatives from stakeholder groups were often invited to attend. The IRCM also initiated several meetings with stakeholder groups (ONA, CNO, OMA, CPSO, etc.) with regards to specific policy implementation issues.

Although the term of the IRCM was originally to end by December, 1991 (one-and-a-half years after its official formation), their work ended up taking three-and-a-half years. During this time, the Regulated Health Professions Act (RHPA) and all the separate professional acts drafted by the HPLR, including the Midwifery Act, passed through their first reading in the Ontario Legislature in June 1990. Because of the change in the provincial government in the fall of 1990, the acts did not proceed through to Second Reading. Under the new NDP government, the RHPA and Midwifery Act were reintroduced and passed through First Reading on April 2, 1991 and Second Reading on May 29.[12] When the Act passed Third Reading and Royal Assent on November 21, 1991, the practice of midwifery officially became legal, even though it was not yet completely integrated into the health care system. The task of integration continued with the creation of the Transitional Council of the College of Midwives of Ontario when the IRCM officially dissolved in January, 1993.

The Transitional Council of the College of Midwives of Ontario

The Transitional Council of the College of Midwives of Ontario was officially appointed on February 14, 1993 by Order-In-Council as the direct precursor to the College of Midwives of Ontario. Its official mandate was to prepare for the proclamation of the Midwifery Act and the Regulated Health Professions Act (RHPA), expected to take effect at the end of 1993. With the transformation of the IRCM into the Transitional Council, the task became writing regulations to fit within the framework of the pending RHPA, rather than just making recommendations to the minister. That is, the Transitional Council was not a ministerial advisory body like the IRCM, but a direct precursor to the statutory, self-regulatory body, the College of Midwives of Ontario. Thus, it had the power to write midwifery regulations. Midwife and Transitional Council member Michelle Kryzanauskas detailed the differences between the IRCM and Transitional Council: "On the IRCM we were making recommendations, we were getting ready; we were taking the AOM documents and giving them a change towards the regulated system. When the Transitional Council adopted them they indeed became the documents that would govern midwives" (personal communication 1995). The other difference between the IRCM and the Transitional Council was that there was more work to be done to get ready for proclamation, in a shorter space of time, and with fewer members.

The change in membership from the IRCM to the Transitional Council was also notable. The first major difference was that midwives were now official members of the Transitional Council, although they were clearly a minority.[13] Vice Chair of the IRCM, Patricia Hennessy, described the recommendations made by the IRCM regarding Transitional Council membership: "We were first advised by the Ministry of Health that the Transitional Council would be made up of twelve members, three of them midwives ... The IRCM responded by requesting that the number of midwives be increased to five ... [to] reflect the level of representation of midwives throughout the IRCM consultation process, and we reminded the Ministry that their input and commitment has been necessary and fundamental to our work and achievement" (*The Gazette* 3, no. 2, August 1992: 6). The ministry later accepted this recommendation. The five professional representatives were: Katsi Cook, an Aboriginal midwife, Brenda Hyatali, a midwife from Trinidad; and Robin Kilpatrick, Michelle Kryzanauskas, and Vicki Van Wagner; the latter three were currently practising midwives who had previously served on the liaison committee.

It is interesting to note that these three midwives were chosen because of their "distance" from the professional association. That is, although all three midwives were active members of the AOM, none of them had been members of the AOM executive. Recent membership of the AOM executive was regarded by the Ministry appointment committee as representing a potential conflict of interest:

There is a general policy that the professional association works on behalf of the interest of the profession; the regulatory bodies are there to protect the public. And if you've been heavily involved with a professional association ... it takes time to divest yourself of that approach to things ... We said people should not hold positions on the Executive or the Board of Directors of professional associations ... for at least two years ... Now in the case of midwifery, I mean, this became a night-mare. Because (a) the profession is so small, (b) anyone who was really interested in doing some work had been very active with the AOM, (c) their whole Council, the AOM Council is humungous ... So we had a lot of difficulty with some of that in terms of trying to appoint people that were "clean" from the professional interest. (Ministry of Health staff Bogna Andersson, personal communication 1995)

This policy fostered yet another organizational affirmation of the distinction between clients and midwives' interests.

Although midwives now had official representation on the Transitional Council, MTFO members did not. MTFO and IRCM member Dianne Pudas recalled how "we know many people applied to be on the Transitional Council and not one person who had applied ... using MTFO in their résumé was selected" (personal communication 1995). Pudas felt that it was almost as if the MTFO was viewed as a "special interest group" (personal communication 1995). Ministry of Health midwifery implementation coordinator Margaret Ann McHugh described the basis for the Ministry's exclusion of MTFO members from the Transitional Council:

There wasn't a directive that said an MTFO member couldn't be on the Council. But anyone who was seen as too close to midwives, that is too close to professionals were not seen to be able to ... but you have to think it's not just about midwifery. It's about every profession. Those people massively supporting chiropractors also can't sit on the chiropractic council as public members. Because you are not representing the interests of the profession and they are not supposed to be representing the interests of the profession. They are supposed to be there representing the interests of the public. (personal communication 1995)

Transitional Council Chair Mary Eberts took issue with this position:

Generally speaking ... the government has a distrust of the vested interests of consumers. The NDP government and I believe the Liberal predecessor took the position that any old friendly person of good will would make a good lay nominee to a governing body and that they didn't want to set up the dynamics of having people accountable to certain constituencies ... The idea of the poor soul who's at sea without a constituency trying to stand up to a bunch of professionals is just ludicrous ... It drove us wild because the whole NDP "get involved in grass roots community organization" thing was contradicted by their insistence that the organized consumers would not be represented. (personal communication 1995)

Despite this official exclusion, MTFO representatives continued their involvement in an *ex officio* manner on several of the Transitional Council committees, just as they had done on the IRCM. AOM midwives who were not officially members of the Transitional Council did the same.

The committee structure of the Transitional Council reflected the recommendations of the HPLR regarding statutory committees of a self-regulating college. Statutory committees included a qualifications and registration committee, which was to develop the registration process for midwifery, and a standards and professional relations committee, which was to develop, maintain, and educate other professions about the standards of practice for midwifery.

Funding for the work of the Transitional Council was heavily subsidized by the Ministry of Health. Vice Chair of the IRCM Patricia Hennessy described how government support for self-regulating professions worked:

In Ontario, the self-regulating health professions are expected to be self-supporting. Interest-free loans are being provided by the Ministry to transitional councils for new colleges where necessary to allow time for the registration of members and collection of fees. Since the initial size of the midwifery profession is expected to be relatively small, however, the Ministry has considered an alternative form of financing the College of Midwives until it can become self-financing. Grants would be provided for operating costs not covered by members' fees, decreasing proportionately as membership numbers increase. (*The Gazette* 3, no. 2, August 1992: 6)

The Transitional Council was also given office space in a government building and computer software.

The College of Midwives of Ontario

Upon proclamation of the Midwifery Act on December 31, 1993, as part of the Regulated Health Professions Act (RHPA), the Transitional Council of the College of Midwives officially became the College of Midwives of Ontario (CMO). The major function of the CMO was to administer the Midwifery Act in the public interest (*The Gazette* 1, no. 3, March 1994: 1). Also included in its mandate under the RHPA, the CMO was to 1) regulate the practice of the profession and govern the members in accordance with the legislation, regulations, and by-laws; 2) develop, establish, and maintain standards of qualification for persons to be issued certificates of registration; 3) develop, establish, and maintain programs and standards of practice to assure the quality of the practice of the profession; 4) develop, establish, and maintain standards of professional ethics for the members; 5) develop, establish, and maintain programs to assist individuals to exercise their rights under the RHPA; and 6) provide protection to the public by regulating the profession (College of Midwives document, August 1994).

Some of the members of the new Council of the College of Midwives changed from the Transitional Council. Midwife Michelle Kryzanauskas was elected as the first president of the new college with public member Pat Israel as vice-president. Four public members (including Chair Mary Eberts) and one midwife member of the Transitional Council resigned and were replaced by two midwives and one public member. Midwife Robin Kilpatrick also resigned from the College Council to assume the position of College Co-Registrar with midwife colleague Elizabeth Allemang (both from the Midwives' Collective). The position of registrar was a shared position because of the AOM's stipulation that midwifery administrators continue to be in practice. This was to prevent a "professional class of midwives" (Kilthei, AOM Newsletter 5, no. 1, April 1989: 28). The College Council thus had a total of nine members: five midwives and four public members.

With the proclamation of the RHPA and the Midwifery Act, the core attributes of the regulation of midwifery became identical to the regulation of other health professions, including nursing and medicine. This is because midwifery now fell under the same omnibus legislation as other health professions – the Health Professions Procedural Code of the RHPA. Under this code, a core set of regulations is applied to all professions covered under the RHPA, addressing such matters as advertising, annual fees, the appointment of non-council members to committees, the composition of statutory committees, the election of council members, notice of open meetings and hearings, professional misconduct, and record-keeping (*The Gazette* 3, no. 2, August 1992: 5). One important stipulation under this code is that public representation on college councils should be no less than 40 per cent. College President Michelle Kryzanauskas stated that unlike other professions, this stipulation was not problematic for midwifery: "Midwifery really fits well into the RHPA. We didn't have to change much at all … Anything that had to do with sharing [with] and involving the consumers of your profession, we already had it all done … So we came to be in the RHPA in a much different fashion than other professions. We came with our consumers on board promoting and supporting us" (personal communication 1995).

Though midwifery managed to reach the proclamation stage, as a self-regulating profession it was still plagued with the problem of having few practitioners (less than seventy). This represented a continued challenge to midwives' ability to sustain the self-regulatory organization of the profession. However, as it had for the Transitional Council, the Ministry of Health continued to fund the newly established College until there were sufficient numbers of midwives to fund themselves.[14] Midwifery Implementation Coordinator Margaret Ann McHugh described the reasoning behind the government's continued financial backing of midwifery: "It is impossible for [midwives] to run a professional college with 70 members. They would have to be charging each member $20,000 a year to support the Council. And the Ministry, since they are paying the midwives, would be paying it out of one pocket and putting it in the other. We either would have to pay the midwives as individuals to support it or pay to support the College" (personal communication 1995). This would prove to be yet another in a long list of examples of government support for the midwifery integration project in the province.

SUMMARY

One of the major challenges that midwives overcame through the integration process was the possibility of their being regulated by another profession, such as nursing or medicine. Clearly, midwives had to present a viable case for self-regulation and this was particularly difficult in light of the small size of their profession and the lack of a recognized educational program. Nevertheless, exceptions were made and these were largely due to ongoing state and state-appointed committee support, which in turn was partly in response to vociferous consumer support, particularly during the Task Force process. So the nexus between midwives, consumers, and state support was critically important in this achievement.

Attaining self-regulation is even more significant when examined in a comparative context. As highlighted in chapter 2, self-regulation has been very difficult if not impossible to achieve for midwives in other jurisdictions, as exemplified by the cases of midwifery legislation in Britain (Donnison 1977; Witz 1992), Australia (Robinson 1996/97; Willis 1989) and most recently the United States (DeVries 1982, 1985, 1986, 1996; Sullivan and Weitz 1988; Tjaden 1987). Other health professions have also had considerable difficulty in securing self-regulation (Larkin 1983; Willis

1989). Lack of self-regulation has resulted in serious negative consequences for the midwifery profession, such as significant medical control, limited scope of practice and limited access to its client population. In achieving self-regulation, Ontario midwives hope to avoid some of these negative consequences of regulation and integration that are so well documented. As we shall see in the next chapter, they have largely been successful.

Midwives are now no longer controlled by others through the criminal justice system. Hence, they are less vulnerable to the legal harassment of inquests and criminal trials. In this way, midwives have secured protection through integration. At the same time, however, the regulation of midwifery has altered significantly from its initial development (as discussed in chapter 5) when women and families decided who they sought as a midwife. In fact, midwifery clients who were members of the MTFO are unofficially excluded from participating in the regulation of midwifery. Moreover, it is seen as somewhat inappropriate to have consumers as "lay" representatives on the College council. This lack of consumer involvement in the regulation of midwifery at the organizational level may or may not be paralleled at the interpersonal level between individual midwives and clients. That is, one question to be asked is whether midwifery self-regulation might be bad for midwifery consumers.

Midwife Vicki Van Wagner emphasized that the autonomy that midwives achieved through self-regulation is an important component of client autonomy: "The autonomy of midwifery and the autonomy of women are very interconnected ... Midwives need autonomy to give women autonomy" (personal communication 1995). According to this argument, midwifery self-regulation and consumer control are not necessarily mutually exclusive. Nevertheless, the establishment of a bureaucratic organization to regulate midwifery in place of midwifery consumers (even in their interest) serves to distance midwives from their clients. Midwives are now not only accountable to the women they care for, they are accountable to the self-regulatory body that licenses and sets standards for them. Moreover, in this specific case, midwifery autonomy has been achieved through a process that has simultaneously curtailed consumer input. The separation of midwifery's self-regulatory body from its professional association also epitomizes the distinction between midwives' interests and those of their clients.

Not only does self-regulation represent a change that may have negative consequences for the midwife-client relationship, a great deal of "self"-regulation is actually state-regulation conducted by midwives within the self-regulatory body. This has long been noted to be true of the regulation of other health care providers (Allsop and Saks, 2002). That is, although self-regulation of midwifery is conducted by midwives (the development of standards, etc.), the RHPA strictly defines the boundaries of regulation which in turn are ultimately under the control of the Minister of Health. Self-regulation may also not be the "big prize" midwives anticipated it to be. Other health occupations often considered "marginal," such as massage therapy, have also achieved self-regulation under the RHPA. Moreover, several elements of self-regulated midwifery were challenged as the integration process more fully unfolded.

In sum, the achievement of self-regulation represents a significant change for midwifery that will have positive and negative consequences for both practitioners and clients. The form with which midwifery is regulated, however, is but one aspect of the integration project undertaken by midwives and their supporters. In examining the quest to sustain the midwifery model of practice and the evolution of midwifery training in the following chapters, a similar theme of paradoxical outcomes of integration will also be revealed.

CHAPTER SEVEN

Defining Themselves before Being Defined

Midwives don't deliver babies. They help women give birth.
(*Toronto Star*, Nov. 21 1984: D1)

Although members of the midwifery community sought changes to the regulation and legitimacy of midwifery care through the integration process, they wanted to preserve the model of midwifery and expand midwives' scope of practice. In this chapter, I describe how the model of midwifery practice evolved during the late 1970s and early 1980s. During the HPLR process, midwifery leaders began to formally document the core principles of this model of practice, which included continuity of care, informed choice, and choice of birthplace. This model of midwifery practice faced several challenges during the integration process; some arose from forces within midwifery itself, others from external forces. The first challenge came with the development of practice standards by the AOM in response to the HPLR's concerns. Following this, both the Task Force and the IRCM represented potential threats to the model, but in fact both government-appointed committees upheld and, in fact, enhanced the model of practice. With each revision, the scope of midwifery practice was expanded to offer more women access to midwifery care in a greater choice of birth settings. Other more serious challenges to the model of practice involved the institutionalization of mandatory practice standards, negotiations about attaining malpractice insurance, and hospital privileges. This examination reveals that the model of midwifery practice has been maintained but some of the broader consumer-oriented aspects of it, including the principle of client choice, have been constrained by such factors as hospital policies and professional standards to which midwives must now adhere.

THE EVOLUTION OF MIDWIFERY PRACTICE
PRIOR TO INTEGRATION

As noted in chapter 4, many midwives were originally assistants to physicians who would attend home births. These "midwives" emerged partly in response to the discontinuation of the back-up assistance VON nurses provided, and partly because of their own desire to promote the idea of home birth (often because of their own positive home birth experience). These birth attendants would come to a woman's home once her labour became established or when the labouring woman needed support (Tate 1988). She would be in attendance at the home birth to coach the woman through the labour, offering advice and reassurance and comforting measures such as massage and relaxed breathing. The physician arrived when the birth seemed imminent.

Midwifery care focused on serving the emotional and physical needs of the woman, providing her with care options and following her lead in how she wanted to give birth. The emphasis was on women's control in childbirth. Midwives' work was in direct response to the needs of their clients (Driver, *Issue* 8, 1985). Providing information to the woman which she would then use to make choices regarding her care was a basic component of midwifery care. Informed choice and client-centred care were the two pillars of early midwifery practice.[1]

Although midwifery practice was originally limited to childbirth, midwives later began to do prenatal care, holding their own clinics independent of physicians (Barrington 1985).[2] Appointments were scheduled throughout a woman's pregnancy often in either the woman's house or the midwife's. These appointments were informal, lasting approximately an hour. This allowed sufficient time for midwives and their clients to delve into important social and emotional issues arising during pregnancy. It was believed that "spending this time helps to establish a trusting relationship" (Tate 1988: 1). Many midwives also taught childbirth education classes, and some did prenatal massage and yoga. Through these classes, parents would become "more confident and informed" (Tate 1988: 1) and, it was assumed, more likely to have positive birth outcomes. At first, midwives provided little postpartum care, as it was mainly being done by the woman's physician. Soon after, however, midwives began to continue their care for the women they assisted and their babies up to six weeks postpartum. Continuity of care throughout a woman's pregnancy and immediately following became an integral component of the care midwives provided.

Midwives' childbirth assistance was also not restricted to home births. Some women who were not yet comfortable with a home birth but who wanted the care midwives provided requested their services at a hospital birth. Midwives' services in hospital largely mimicked their assistance at home births – they acted mainly as labour coaches. Labour would be monitored at home and once active labour was well established, the midwife would accompany the woman to the hospital. Once in the hospital, however, the midwife's role was severely limited due to her lack of official status. At home midwives were sometimes able to "catch" the baby with the approval of the physician attending home birth. In the hospital, a midwife was required to transfer care of her client to the physician in charge (either the back up obstetrician or another physician the woman was receiving care from, such as her family physician). This limited the continuity of care that midwives could provide.[3]

It was not until physicians discontinued attending home births, largely in response to the directives from the CPSO in 1982 and 1983, that midwives' scope of practice at home births expanded to that of primary caregivers. Their status in hospitals, however, remained as highly skilled labour coaches and patient advocates. This pattern of primary care at home births and labour coach at hospital births was also the predominant pattern for midwifery in areas where midwives did not have the support of sympathetic physicians. Midwives in these areas had no choice but to be primary caregivers at home births.

Because of the way midwives practised – providing several long prenatal appointments, childbirth education classes, continuous attendance during childbirth, twenty-four hour on-call attention, and six weeks postpartum care – the number of clients midwives served was generally much smaller than in a typical physician's practice. Midwife Ava Vosu described how she "personally attended only a few births a month because midwifery should be based on friendship and trust, which are difficult to maintain if a midwife takes on too many cases" (*Toronto Star*, June 17, 1982, E14). Client loads varied markedly from one midwife to another but tended to be higher in urban centres than in rural communities due in large part to a higher demand for midwifery services in the city: "While some rural midwives with intimate practices catch only one or two babies a month ... the average in Toronto is four to six primary care births a month" (Barrington 1985, 47). Being on call twenty-four hours a day, seven days a week was also likely a factor that had an impact on midwives' case loads.

At first, many midwives practised independently, sometimes making arrangements with other midwives to provide backup care in the event that they were not available (because of personal emergencies, simultaneous labours, etc.). As client loads increased and midwives were increasingly unavailable when they were needed, some midwives began to practise in pairs. One midwife would be the primary attendant and the backup midwife would come just for the birth to provide assistance to the primary midwife, such as monitoring the baby's heart rate and providing labour support while the primary midwife delivered the baby (Tate 1988). In the case of the primary midwife's unavailability, the backup midwife would assume primary care. Barrington (1985) described some of the positive features of the "pairing" of midwives, which were not just practical but also political: "Working in pairs allows the primary midwife a nap during a long labour. As well as four hands and two brains, it can double the number of past birth experiences to draw on if a problem arises. Generally, one midwife or the other will recognize a problem situation. Second opinions are invaluable to midwives working in the current political climate" (46). This practice arrangement, with two midwives that the client would come to know, helped ensure continuity of care. At the same time it helped prevent "burn out." Later some midwives formalized these backup arrangements and began to work in practice groups. This was far easier for midwives in urban centres to organize as there were few midwives to draw on for back up support in rural areas, let alone establish group practices.

In sum, early midwifery practice was characterized by having a woman-centred focus on normal birth, continuity of care, and choice of birthplace, but not as being primary caregivers in hospitals due to their alegal status. Although midwives sought to change the legitimacy of their service, especially in hospitals, they strove to maintain the underlying philosophy of care – client-centred care, informed choice, continuity of care, and choice of birthplace.

FORMALLY DOCUMENTING THE MODEL
OF MIDWIFERY PRACTICE

Midwives' Submissions to the HPLR

The first opportunity for Ontario midwives to formally articulate their model of midwifery practice was in the Midwifery Coalition's submission to the HPLR committee. One of the twenty-two questions asked by the HPLR in its first round of submissions addressed the definition of the scope of midwifery practice. In responding to this topic, the members of the Midwifery Coalition drew upon the international definition of the midwife adopted by the International Confederation of Midwives (ICM), the World Health Organization (WHO), and the International Federation of Obstetricians and Gynecologists (FIGO) which states:

The midwife's sphere of practice demands of her the ability to give the necessary supervision, care and advice to women during pregnancy, labour and the post-partum period, to conduct deliveries on her own responsibility and care for the newborn and infant. This care includes preventative measures, the detection of abnormal conditions in mother and child, the procurement of medical assistance, and the execution of emergency measures in the absence of medical help. She has an important task in counselling and education, not only for women and their families but also within the community. The work involves antenatal education and preparation for parenthood and extends to certain areas of gynecology, family planning and child care. She may practice in hospitals, clinics, health units, domiciliary conditions or any other service. (TFIMO 1987: 85)

Within this broad scope of practice, Coalition members highlighted the principles of continuity of care throughout a woman's pregnancy, and choice of birthplace.

Although midwives' proposed scope of practice entailed a broad range of care, it was limited to those women considered to have a "low-risk," or "normal" pregnancy: "[Midwifery's] specific focus [is] on normal pregnancy and childbirth ... The midwifery profession is specially trained to monitor and assist throughout the normal childbearing cycle" (Midwifery Coalition First Submission to HPLR, December 1983: 9). Informed choice was emphasized as an integral component of "Parents are seeking out caregivers who familiarize them with their options and support them in making informed choices appropriate to their own needs" (Midwifery Coalition First Submission to HPLR, December 1983: 10).

Thus, the essential attributes of midwifery practice emphasized by Midwifery Coalition members in their submissions to the HPLR were its focus on normal birth, continuity of care, choice of birthplace, and informed choice. Keeping these elements of midwives' scope of practice intact throughout the integration process became the primary theme of all subsequent activities of Ontario midwives. They were to be confronted with several challenges in their task of maintaining and promoting this model of midwifery practice.

CHALLENGES TO THE MODEL
OF MIDWIFERY PRACTICE

The HPLR and the Development of Professional Standards

Several challenges to the model of midwifery practice formally conceptualized by the Midwifery Coalition arose as a result of the HPLR process.
One of the first came in response to the HPLR's emphasis on the need for
practice standards. Midwives in the OAM had earlier recognized the need
to more clearly articulate their standards of practice, following the 1982
Inquest and the 1983 CPSO statement on out-of-hospital births (TFIMO
1987: 30). Midwives felt that through the development of standards, they
would be better able to justify the type of care they provided, basing it
on internationally accepted standards and research. In the consultations
midwives had with the HPLR committee and other professions during the
ongoing review process, the need to develop standards came to be of
critical importance to the AOM's integration project: "There was a lot of
awareness in terms of writing briefs that standards of practice were an
issue ... that it would be an expectation from the government and from
other professions" (Midwife Jane Kilthei, personal communication 1995).
Standards identified as in need of development ranged from contraindications for home birth and other risk screening and consultation protocols
to lists of the essential equipment midwives should carry.

   The development of standards, however, was regarded by some within
the midwifery community as a significant challenge to midwifery's ideals
of informed choice and woman-centred care. Vocal opposition to the
imposition of practice standards was expressed by several midwives and
consumers. They argued that standards limited midwifery practice, and
in turn limited the choices midwives could offer their clients. In *Issue*
(1981a), for example, one midwife noted that "the more [we] define our
parameters, the less we will be sensitive to the uniqueness of each situation" (1). Midwifery supporter Jutta Mason also highlighted how midwifery consumers' "choices are never made in a vacuum" (personal
communication 1995):

Women were required to evaluate their desires regarding place of birth and the
circumstances they wished to build for themselves, against a standard of political
expediency. *You want to give birth to your breech baby at home? Now is just the wrong
time for that. If something happened, the whole campaign could go down the drain, just
because of your insistence on staying home for this birth.* Women found themselves

being located on a grid of risk factors by their professionalized midwives, according to pre-established score sheet ... Midwives were eager to share information with their clients, so that each woman could learn how to continuously evaluate her own capacities within this grid of greater or lesser deviation from the norm of a healthy pregnancy ... Any choices that didn't imperil a woman's position on the grid of "safe care" were acceptable. (Mason 1990, 20)

Discussions about the contraindications for home birth were especially sensitive. Some midwives expressed grave concern that they would not be able to offer clients the option of a home birth if it was contraindicated by specific standards.

The counterargument to these concerns, persuasively presented by midwives promoting integration, was that if midwives did not develop standards, the nursing and medical profession would do so for them. This, it was argued, would create even greater and more rigid constraints on midwives and the women they served. Midwives would keep their model of practice in mind (one providing greater consumer choice than medicine or nursing could offer) when creating standards of practice:

At this point in our growth towards a legally regulated system of midwifery, the development and clarification of standards of practice is vital to the survival of the art of midwifery in Ontario. The models of care and practice protocols which have evolved in response to women's needs and our philosophy of normal childbirth, continuity of care, and informed choice must be reflected in our standards or our midwifery model could be lost in paper regulations. Not only must our standards reflect our practice accurately, but we must be able to defend them, in light of the obstetrical literature, international midwifery practice and community standards. ... Politically the reality is we had better define our practice before it gets defined for us. (Van Wagner, AOM newsletter 3, no. 1, March 1987: 6)

In the end, the OAM proceeded with the development of standards and created a committee specifically to develop voluntary standards of midwifery care. As with other OAM (and later AOM) committees, consumer representation from the MTFO was encouraged to foster consumer involvement in the development of standards. Midwife and Standards Committee chair Michelle Kryzanauskas recalled how: "consumers worked hand in hand with midwives on those standards committees right from the start" (personal communication 1995). Ultimately, however, the official adoption of standards could only be voted on by practising midwives according to the constitution of both the OAM and AOM.

The AOM Board also recommended that all practising midwives provide their clients with a copy of the AOM Risk Screening Protocols[4] to ensure that clients were kept informed of the developing standards of midwifery care. This essentially informed clients of the limits of what midwives could do for them.

Adherence to standards developed by this committee and endorsed by the Association became a criterion for membership. Because the OAM and the AOM were voluntary organizations, midwives who disagreed with the standards of practice had the option of ceasing to be members or not joining in the first instance. Many, however, remained or became members but continued to challenge the trend towards standardization. One example of the midwives' challenge of AOM standards was in regards to the issue of allowing women who had had caesarean sections to have a normal vaginal delivery at home – the home VBAC (vaginal birth after caesarean) issue.

INFORMED CHOICE AND THE HOME VBAC ISSUE

The issue of midwives attending women who had had a previous caesarean section at home was a contentious issue for midwives:

When women choose to give birth at home when planning a vaginal birth after a previous cesarean delivery, it presents several difficult dilemmas for midwives. With our fundamental belief in both informed choice and the right to maternity care in all circumstances, it is very difficult for midwives to refuse to attend women in labour even when their decisions are not sanctioned by current medical opinion or practice. However, the current legal status of midwives leaves them extremely vulnerable to criminal charges … For a midwife to willingly attend a home VBAC would call into question her ability to "risk screen," to practice within her scope of practice, and [to] maintain midwifery standards. There is no international standard to use in her defence, and at least yet, no medical literature to support VBAC at home. This leaves her extremely vulnerable: Personally – to charges of practising medicine without a license and criminal negligence; politically – the whole movement would be at risk, at a time when midwives are misunderstood and struggling for recognition of their role and skills. In our view a case involving VBAC at home would be extremely damaging to the future of midwifery and choices in childbirth in our country. (Midwives' Collective of Toronto, *Issue* 12, Summer 1986: 4)

When the AOM drafted its first policy statement on "contraindication for home birth" in 1986, previous uterine surgery (i.e., caesarean section) was included on the list. Some midwives argued, however, that the AOM position on home VBACS should be based on research and not come from taking a politically safe position. Consequently, the AOM Standards Committee struck a subcommittee in mid-1987 to review the AOM's position on including "previous uterine surgery" on the home birth contraindications list.

The VBAC subcommittee contacted many international experts and reviewed available literature on VBACS. All those contacted unanimously endorsed VBAC at home but were unable to provide any statistics or documents to back up their endorsement. Midwife and VBAC supporter Chris Sternberg suggested the following points for the VBAC subcommittee to consider: 1) the probability of emergency caesarean section being required seems to be the same for VBAC and non-VBAC births, and 2) it could be argued that a VBAC in hospital is more dangerous than a VBAC at home due to an increased risk of ending up with another caesarean section which had attendant risks. (AOM Newsletter 3, no. 3, Sept 1987). The VBAC subcommittee concluded from this review that: "'previous uterine' surgery" should be removed from the Contraindications list and added to Risk Screening Protocol #3. It must be noted that this decision was made not because we can defend home VBAC, but because we have no information that clearly contraindicates home VBAC" (AOM Newsletter, Sept 1987: 7). Thus, the decision to attend a VBAC woman at home was one that would require peer consultation but essentially could be made at the discretion of the primary midwife and her backup. Clients would have to be duly informed of the risks of a home VBAC. The AOM decided in favour of informed choice. The subcommittee nevertheless did not encourage the practice of home VBACS arguing that "the political risks [of home VBAC] are great and extend to the whole midwifery community" (AOM Newsletter 3, no. 3, Sept 1987: 7).

Tensions between informed choice and the need to standardize practice in anticipation of integration were being experienced by the midwifery community before any formal implementation occurred. The practice standards that the midwives developed served to help satisfy the HPLR and other participating professions but also created more rigidly defined boundaries around the choices available to both midwives and their clients. Moreover, the development of midwifery standards, which were created in part from the obstetrical literature and medically dominated "community standards" that midwifery arose in reaction to, inherently contradicted midwives' earlier position. These contradictions were exacerbated by the perceived need for midwifery as a corporate entity and midwives individually not to do anything to "rock the boat" during the HPLR process.

Although the HPLR was the first government recommendation-making body challenging midwives' ideal model of practice, it was not the last. As the Review handed the decision of *how* to integrate midwifery to the Task Force on the Implementation of Midwifery in Ontario, the Task Force then became the next major challenge to the model.

The Task Force on the Implementation of Midwifery in Ontario

As noted previously, part of the mandate of the Task Force was to make recommendations regarding midwives' scope of practice. In its submission to the Task Force in 1986, the AOM outlined its own proposals for midwives' scope of practice. Once again they based their submission on the international definition of midwives' scope of practice. They argued that any model of midwifery care must be planned in order to achieve the maximum continuity of care for clients. Specific acts proposed to be within the midwives' scope of practice included antepartum care (i.e., conducting a general physical assessment, completing prenatal examinations, and ordering and interpreting screening and diagnostic procedures); intrapartum care (i.e., monitoring and managing of normal labour and delivery); and postpartum care (i.e., physical examination of mother and newborn and contraceptive counselling and prescription). The AOM also outlined a list of medications that midwives should be able to prescribe and administer, including analgesics and anaesthetics. The ability to prescribe and administer medication meant that midwives would not necessarily have to transfer care of a client who required or requested medication to a physician. This was designed to help ensure the greatest continuity of care possible.

It was also argued that a model of midwifery care should ensure that clients were seen as active participants in their own care (i.e., informed choice), and that their choices of birthplace be respected and supported by enabling midwives to practice in both hospital and community settings. A hospital admitting privileges model was proposed to be better than a rotating-shift, hospital staff model in ensuring both client choice of birthplace and continuity of care. Midwives also made a strong argument for preserving the option of home birth. Home births, it was argued, were not going to disappear, and so they should be made a safe option for the consumer by enabling trained midwives to attend with proper backup from a supportive medical profession.

Consumer submissions, both individual and through the MTFO, strongly supported the AOM proposals. Consumers argued that midwives should be unsupervised primary caregivers able to practise in various settings and offer choice of birth setting. They also strongly endorsed the principle of continuity of care.

The submissions of stakeholder groups to the Task Force also addressed the issue of midwives' scope of practice. All medical organizations were supportive of midwives in hospitals, but as staff and not as independent practitioners with hospital admitting privileges. Home births were not considered acceptable by most medical organizations who made a submission to the TFIMO, with the exception of the more left-wing Medical Reform Group (MRG). Home births were considered to be riskier than hospital births for both mothers and infants. The MRG argued that home births were safe and questioned the evidence on which other medical organizations based their position. When pressed at the hearings, many representatives of medical organizations agreed that parents should have the right to choose.

Submissions from the nursing profession strongly supported many elements of a midwife's scope of practice included in the international definition, but maintained that midwifery should be a specialty of nursing governed by the College of Nurses. The CNO did not express support for the practice of home birth, but stated that it would not discipline a midwife for attending a home birth if she had fully informed the family about the risks it entailed. Both the RNAO and the ONA argued that midwives should be specialized nurses acting within institutions rather than in independent practice.

Many Ontario hospitals also accepted the international definition of midwifery, although some wished to limit midwives' practice to the hospital setting. Nevertheless, 45 per cent of the OHA members surveyed saw a place for homebirth and were willing to provide backup support for home births (TFIMO 1987).

With these submissions in mind, the Task Force recommended that Ontario enact a Midwifery Act in which the midwife's scope of practice is consistent with the international definition of a midwife. The Task Force defined a midwife's main activities as: 1) carrying out examinations necessary to establish and monitor normal pregnancies; 2) advising on and securing the examinations necessary for the earliest possible diagnosis of pregnancies at risk; 3) providing education and preparation for childbirth, including advice on exercise and nutrition; 4) caring for and assisting the woman during labour and monitoring the condition of the fetus during labour by the appropriate clinical and technical means; 5) conducting spontaneous vaginal deliveries; 6) recognizing the warning signs of abnormality in the mother or infant that necessitate referral to a physician; 7) taking necessary emergency measures in the absence of a physician; 8) examining and caring for the newborn infant; and 9) caring for the woman during the postpartum period and advising her on infant care and family planning (TFIMO 1987).

In order for a midwife to carry out these functions, the Task Force recommended that provision be made for delegating medical acts to midwives, but that these be used sparingly so that it did not result in creating midwives with more technological competence than of clinical midwifery skills. Although midwives were defined as specialists in "normal" pregnancy and childbirth, the Task Force asserted that they should not be excluded from assisting women whose care must be managed by a physician, as these women could benefit greatly from midwifery care.

In making these scope of practice recommendations, the Task Force attempted to create a collaborative relationship between midwives and physicians. In line with this aim, it recommended that standards for midwifery practice include criteria for consultations with, and referrals to physicians, to be developed jointly by the governing body for midwifery and the CPSO and SOGC. These standards were to differentiate between consultations for advice, consultations for treatment, and transfers of care. The Task Force also recommended that midwives' clients visit a physician twice during their pregnancies to "maintain some communication between medicine and midwifery." (Task Force member Karyn Kaufman, personal communication 1995).[5] Interestingly, this recommendation was not supported by the medical community: "The concern ... within the medical community ... was that if a physician was involved at all and sort of seeming to bless the midwives' care, then that person could incur liability for midwifery decisions...so the fate of that recommendation was that physicians said, 'No.' They really didn't want to be involved except on clear indications for consultation when it was an identified problem" (Task Force member Karyn Kaufman, personal communication 1995). This lack of a requirement for contact with physicians is important because it meant that although midwives were limited to "normal" pregnancy and birth, "normality" was not being defined by physicians but by midwives. This situation is unlike that in Britain where at one point in time, physicians were the first point of contact. There it meant they were in the position to define "normality," and hence what women midwives could and could not provide care for. This form of medical control was avoided in Ontario, but this independence also meant that midwives had a greater responsibility to identify potential problems.

The Task Force also recommended that midwives be allowed to perform the activities delineated under their scope of practice in a variety of settings, including hospitals, birthing centres, community health centres, boards of health, medical practices, and private midwifery practices. Within each of these settings, however, midwives would be required to adhere to a model or framework of practice for midwifery in Ontario outlined by the Task Force. This included ensuring that: 1) continuity of care be provided ideally by one midwife but more practically by a group of midwives sharing a woman's care in order to prevent midwifery burnout, the need for personal time off-call, and professional development; 2) the midwife's responsibilities included counselling, education and emotional support; 3) the midwife be given access to both institutional and community settings; 4) the midwife have arrangements with physicians for consultations and referrals and for ordering medications, tests, and procedures; 5) the midwife practise autonomously within her scope of practice; 6) the midwife focuse on low-risk pregnancies and normal childbirth; and 7) the midwife's practice be responsive to consumer needs and preferences (TFIMO 1987).

With respect to the home birth issue, in the words of member Rachel Edney, "after looking at all the issues, we [the Task Force] *felt* that home birth should still be allowed" (personal communication 1995). In its report, the Task Force stated how its position on home births was based on the research evidence: "Several recent reviews of the scientific literature on home birth have concluded that the evidence does not prove that home birth presents inordinate risks to all women and infants; indeed, there is some evidence that morbidity (illness) is greater among women and infants delivered and cared for in hospital" (TFIMO 1987: 14).

Therefore, the members asked not *if* home births should be allowed, but given that a small, yet persistent segment of the population would always choose to give birth at home, and that planned home births can never be eliminated, *how* should it be made as safe as possible. Framing the question this way meant that medical and nursing organizations, who were united in their opposition to planned home births, were hard pressed to disagree with the Task Force's intention to make home births as safe as possible: "That put it in a different context than having to fight for home birth per se. It was a fight for good care" (midwife Vicki Van Wagner, personal communication 1995). The Task Force recommended that safety could be accomplished by 1) ensuring that a trained attendant (i.e., a midwife) can assist in home births; 2) having the governing body for midwifery prepare a home birth protocol covering assessment of risk and contraindications to home births; and 3) having the midwifery governing body develop a standard of practice with regard to the care of women who choose to give birth at home despite contraindications.

Subsequent consultations focused on ensuring adequate transport for emergencies arising at home birth. The idea of flying squads (ambulance services designed specifically for home birth emergencies) was proposed but discounted on the grounds of excessive cost given the small number of home births. A more viable option proposed was that midwives be allowed to provide treatment en route in the current ambulance system. In order for this proposal to work, midwives' scope of practice would need to be expanded to include activities related to emergencies, including maternal and neonatal resuscitation.

With respect to hospital births, the Task Force recommended that midwives should have admitting privileges similar to those of physicians. This was to ensure that midwives could offer continuity of care and choice of birthplace to their clients: "More than 99 per cent of babies born in Ontario are delivered in hospitals. It is therefore impossible to integrate midwives into the health care system without allowing them access to hospital birthing facilities. If midwives cannot attend hospital births, their clients will be forced to choose between giving birth at home and giving birth in hospital with a caregiver (a physician) not of their choosing. Far from advancing the policy of encouraging women to give birth in hospital, excluding midwives from hospitals will encourage women to stay at home" (TFIMO 1987: 100).

Because the Public Hospitals Act (PHA) made no provision for the appointment of midwives to hospital staff, the Task Force recommended that the PHA be amended. The necessary amendments to the PHA identified by the Task Force included: one to empower a hospital board to pass by-laws that provide for the appointment and functioning of a midwifery staff; another to permit a patient to be admitted and discharged on the joint order of a midwife and a member of the medical staff; a third to permit a midwife to write a history, make a physical examination, and make and record a provisional diagnosis; and finally one to make provision for a midwife who is unable to perform her duties in the hospital. These amendments would leave the ultimate decision-making as to whether or not they would like to appoint midwives in the hands of the hospitals. The Task Force felt that making such by-law changes compulsory would create a counterproductive, hostile environment between midwives and hospital administrators. At the same time it would leave a midwife seeking hospital privileges little recourse when denied privileges from a hospital.

Thus, the Task Force recommendations regarding scope and model of midwifery practice strongly resembled the submission made by the AOM. In fact, the Task Force marked the first official endorsement of the expansion of midwives' scope of practice as stipulated by the AOM in its conceptualization of the ideal model of midwifery practice. But as mentioned previously, the Task Force only had advisory status. The litmus test was whether or not the government would act on these practice recommendations as it had on the regulation recommendations. Before that, the scope of practice recommendations of the Task Force would have to be integrated into the broader HPLR recommendations.

Fitting into the HPLR Mould

While the Task Force process was ongoing, the HPLR chose to define the scopes of practice of the regulated health professions in a consistent way. As highlighted in chapter 6, the HPLR committee had decided that instead of licensing a profession's scope of practice, it would instead license potentially harmful *acts*, that is, procedures which could be performed only by health professionals authorized by their Professional Act to perform them.[6]

In the summer of 1988, the HPLR invited the AOM to participate in discussions regarding midwives' scope of practice. Together the AOM and the HPLR committee prepared a general statement of midwives' scope of practice and licensed acts of the midwifery profession in keeping with the HPLR model. These statements were to become the basis for statutes of the Midwifery Act. Regulations which dealt with the details of midwifery practice (such as the medications and substances midwives could prescribe) were to be worked out at a later time. As an outcome of these consultations, midwives' scope of practice became defined as follows: "The practice of midwifery is the assessment, monitoring and provision of care during normal pregnancy, labour and the post-partum period and conducting spontaneous normal vaginal deliveries" (HPLR 1989: 243). Proposed "licensed acts" midwives could perform included: 1) managing labour and conducting spontaneous normal vaginal deliveries; 2) performing episiotomies and amniotomies; 3) repairing the perineum, excluding the anus, anal sphincter, tectum, urethra and periurethral area; 4) administering medication for such purposes as are specified in

regulation; and 5) administering by injection or inhalation such substances for such purposes as are specified by regulation (AOM Newsletter
4 no. 4, December 1988: 24).

The AOM regarded this definition as favourable for midwifery. They
felt that the bulk of the work in hammering out midwives' scope of practice, however, would come with the drafting of specific midwifery regulations. It was anticipated that negotiations regarding scope of practice
would prove challenging, especially with the medical profession. Even at
the initial scopes-of-practice discussions, some physicians expressed
concern about the definition of "normal" birth. Midwives in the AOM,
along with the newly appointed Midwifery Coordinator, Karyn Kaufman,
began to work on writing the model regulations in the fall of 1988,
consulting widely to help allay other stakeholders' concerns.

When the HPLR submitted its final report in January 1989, it included
a draft Midwifery Act. The definition of scope of practice essentially read
as above. "Performing invasive instrumentation, including manual and
digital instrumentation beyond the labia majora during pregnancy, labour
and the post partum period" was added to the initial list of licensed acts
a midwife could perform (HPLR 1989, 243). Although the draft Act did not
include a list of regulations detailing midwives' scope of practice, it did
describe the regulation-making powers of a midwifery regulatory body.
Among these were the powers to develop governing standards of practice
for the profession in respect of its scope of practice and to specify medications and substances that might be used or administered in the practice
of midwifery (HPLR 1989). Making recommendation on what these regulations should look like became one of the tasks of the Interim Regulatory
Council on Midwifery (IRCM). Before undertaking this task, the IRCM felt
it necessary to revisit the midwifery model of ensure this would be a
central theme for subsequent standards and policy development.

The Midwifery Model Revisited – The Interim Regulatory Council

One of the first official decisions made by the IRCM, including its Liaison
Committee with the AOM, as it began its mandate in the fall of 1989 was
to adopt the international definition of midwifery. This indicated the
IRCM's support of the principles of continuity of care and choice of birthplace. Shortly after this, the IRCM recommended that "out of hospital
birth be encouraged to promote normal childbirth," signifying its support
of the option of home birth. This support for home births was later outlined in the IRCM's statement on home birth: "A number of expectant

parents choose to give birth at home. The Interim Regulatory Council on Midwifery (IRCM) believes that midwives must continue to support this option and that for families seeking this option, normal birth at home must be encouraged and supported."

These aspects of the model of midwifery practice were subsequently synthesized in the IRCM's statement on the philosophy of midwifery care in Ontario:

Midwifery care is based on a respect for pregnancy as a state of health and childbirth as a normal physiologic process ... Care is continuous, personalized and non-authoritarian ... Midwives respect the woman's right to choice of care-giver and place of birth in accordance with the Standards of Practice of the College of Midwives. Midwives are willing to attend birth in a variety of settings, including birth at home. Midwives encourage the woman to actively participate in her care throughout pregnancy, birth and postpartum period and make choices about the manner in which her care is provided. Midwifery care includes educa-tion and counselling enabling a woman to make informed choices. Midwives promote decision-making as a shared responsibility, between the woman, her family (as defined by the woman) and her caregivers. The mother is recognized as the primary decision maker. Fundamental to midwifery care is the understand-ing that a woman's caregivers respect and support her so that she may give birth safely, with power and dignity.

This statement highlighted the midwifery view of birth as a normal life event, and emphasized the importance of the principles of informed choice, continuity of care, and choice of birthplace to midwifery practice.

Following the articulation of the philosophy of midwifery care, the IRCM created a specific subcommittee, the Model of Practice and Payment (MOPP) Committee, to link the tenets of midwifery philosophy – continu-ity of care, informed choice, and choice of birthplace – to a model of mid-wifery practice to be integrated into hospitals and health care funding.

MODEL OF PRACTICE AND PAYMENT COMMITTEE

The Model of Practice and Payment (MOPP) Committee was created in October 1991 to make recommendations to the IRCM regarding models of practice and practice sites and funding mechanisms for midwives and midwifery practices. The Committee was chaired by IRCM member Wendy Sutton and included three other IRCM members, Pat Legault, Susan Phillips, and Diane Pudas; an MTFO representative, Sue Haffie; and an AOM representative, Vicki Van Wagner. Recommendations made in its final report released in June, 1992, were based on a series of meetings between November 1991 and June 1992 with several stakeholder groups, and with reference to several documents, including those of the AOM (*The Gazette* 3, no. 2, August 1992: 1).

The MOPP committee proposed a practice model which was to integrate the principles of midwifery philosophy as follows: "We recommend that within the midwife's scope of practice and according to the standards of practice as set by the College of Midwives the midwife [or team of midwives] will *follow the woman* throughout the full course of care from pregnancy to post partum and attend birth in the setting chosen by the woman" (MOPP Report, June 19, 1992: 3, emphasis mine). To enable the midwife to "follow the woman," the committee recommended that all midwives must be capable of and willing to provide care in all settings. This was recommended to avoid a midwifery system where some midwives specialized in out of hospital births, while others restricted their practice to the hospital setting. Such a system was seen as restricting women's choice of birthplace, especially in settings where it is unlikely that women would have access to a choice of midwives.

Within this practice model midwives were expected to provide continuity of care according to the following definition:

Continuity of midwifery care is achieved when a relationship develops over time between a woman and a small group of no more than four midwives. Two of these midwives will be identified and act as the client's primary care midwives throughout the course of care. One or both of these midwives will normally be present for the birth ... Midwifery services must be made available by the same small group of care givers from the onset of care (ideally, at the onset of pregnancy), during all trimesters, and throughout labour, birth, and the first six weeks post partum ... There must be 24-hour on call availability of the primary care midwives known to the woman. (MOPP Report, June 19, 1992: 4)

The Committee also recommended that two midwives attend all births regardless of setting.[7] This recommendation was to help ensure that the midwifery model of practice did not differ by practice setting (the hospital setting was a special concern). "Continuity of care" was becoming more and more diffuse, from one midwife to a pair of midwives to a "group of no more than four" midwives. Sustainability of midwives (i.e., prevention of burnout) was becoming increasingly important, some might argue to the detriment of continuity of care.

To help support the proposed model of midwifery care, the Committee recommended that the expectations of a midwife under this model be written into College regulations. This protective measure would help midwives resist the pressure from the mainstream maternity care system to compromise certain aspects of the midwifery model, such as choice of birthplace. The public, health professionals and administrators would be advised that it is an expectation of the midwives' regulatory body that she must practice according to the regulated model. These recommendations were accepted by the IRCM and were subsequently written into regulation by the transitional council. Thus, the model of midwifery practice was not just outlined as a guideline for practice but became a regulated expectation of midwives. This measure of protection would prove to be necessary as negotiations over access to hospitals and negotiations over the funding mechanism for midwifery care got under way. But these more external challenges were not the only challenges facing the MOPP/IRCM model of midwifery practice. The informed choice principle was still vulnerable to the development of standards within the IRCM as it had been before by the development of AOM standards.

The Fate of Informed Choice – Mandatory Professional Standards and Code of Ethics

In developing standards of practice for midwifery, the IRCM not only referred to AOM documents for background (as described in chapter 6), it also referred to its own model of midwifery practice as a guide. It could be argued that several of the standards developed by the IRCM, however, limit the informed choice and choice of birthplace principles of the midwifery model of practice in much the same way that AOM standards did. In the IRCM document "Indications for Planned Place of Birth",[8] for example, several references are made to the limits of women's choices of birthplace:

When the midwife is providing primary care, she will support the woman's choice, after the client has carefully considered the information and recommendations. Notwithstanding this, birth should be planned to take place in hospital in the circumstances of multiple birth, breech presentation, preterm labour prior to 37 weeks of pregnancy, and documented post-term pregnancy of more than 43 completed weeks. Other situations in which hospital birth should be planned would be assessed prenatally, with appropriate consultation as detailed in *Indications for Mandatory Consultation and Transfer of Care*.

In the document "Indications for Mandatory Consultation and Transfer of Care," risk factors for four periods of midwifery care – the initial history and physical examination, the prenatal care period, labour and delivery, and postpartum period (separately for mother and infant) – were put into three categories: 1) those risk factors that required a midwife to discuss care with the midwife or midwives or physician(s) sharing primary care; 2) those risk factors requiring a midwife to consult with a physician; and 3) those risk factors requiring the midwife to transfer to a physician for primary care. This document was based largely on the format of the AOM document "Guidelines to Scope of Practice of Midwifery." Within each period of maternity care, a woman's choice of caregiver was limited, depending on her risk factors. The main difference, however, was that for the AOM, these guidelines were voluntary, whereas for the IRCM these standards were to become mandatory for all practising midwives in the province.

Members of the IRCM were aware of the limitations these policies placed on informed choice, and in order to help ameliorate this situation created an "escape clause," as the AOM had done previously. This was clause 12 of the IRCM Code of Ethics which stated that: "A midwife may not refuse to attend a client in the course of labour."[9] In a subsequent policy document developed by the IRCM entitled "When the Client Requests Care Outside Midwifery Standards of Practice" the IRCM advises that when a client refuses to follow the advice of her midwife regarding compliance with regulated midwifery standards, the midwife should advise the client of the standard, consult with another midwife or physician and document the consultation and advice given to the client. This document reiterates the escape clause in the code of conduct stating that "*In the course of labour or urgent situations*, the midwife may not refuse to attend the client in keeping with the Code of Ethics of the College of Midwives" (emphasis in original). In non-urgent situations, however, midwives are required to take the following actions: "*In other situations*, should the client continue to request care outside midwifery standards of practice the midwife should: a) clearly communicate to the client that she is unable to continue to provide care; b) inform the client that a letter … will follow which confirms the termination of care by a date that provides her with a specific amount of time to find another caregiver" (emphasis in original). As midwives cannot abandon a client, the principle of informed choice and the woman's ultimate control was upheld, at least during labour, by the standards developed by the IRCM. This clause was subsequently written into regulations by the Transitional Council and the College. This made the midwifery profession unique among health professions in making the client the ultimate decision-maker in the contractual relationship between midwife and client. Clients nevertheless must contend with the persuasiveness of midwives' newly developed professional power.

Thus, the model of midwifery practice developed by the AOM evolved through the Task Force process, was detailed by the HPLR, and was further elaborated upon by the IRCM. Although each of these committees represented a potential challenge to the model of practice envisaged by midwives, all of them supported, promoted and expanded upon the model. As previously noted, other challenges still faced the IRCM model of midwifery care. Similar to the Task Force and the HPLR, the IRCM did not have any official decision-making power vis à vis the government; it was simply an advisory committee making recommendations to the Minister of Health. Ministry of Health Midwifery Implementation Coordinator Margaret Ann McHugh[10] described what this meant for the model of practice: "There was nothing in the legislation that legislated the model of practice. And everything else were only suggestions. That was all the weight they had. Any report, anything the IRCM did the Minister would just write a letter and say 'thank you very much for your advice.' It was advice. It didn't have any force of legislation behind it so there was a constant challenge to the model of practice" (personal communication 1995). In light of this situation, McHugh stressed the importance of the commitment of successive Ministers of Health to midwifery: "Both the Ministers that I worked primarily under, which were Francis Lankin and Ruth Grier, were committed to the model. So in essence when it got to the top you could count on them to support the model" (personal communication 1995).

Despite this important support from key officials within the state, the midwifery-friendly model of practice was nevertheless to be more directly challenged by the actual integration process. Several structures had to be changed in order to allow midwives to practise according to the scope of practice as outlined in the HPLR draft Midwifery Act. This included the Ambulance Act which allowed midwives to continue to care for their clients in ambulances; the Ontario Drug Benefit Act and the PHArmacy Act which allowed midwives to independently write orders for and administer medication and other substances which they needed for their clients; and the Laboratory and Specimen Collection Centre Licensing Act which allowed midwives to request and interpret laboratory tests. The most challenging aspects of the integration process to the model of midwifery practice, however, proved to be the negotiations to secure midwives access to hospitals and determining how they would be funded (discussed in the subsequent chapter). In preparing for these challenges, the Transitional Council of the College of Midwives exercised its regulation-making authority by quickly adopting the MOPP/IRCM model of midwifery practice into College regulations. This would help ensure the model had regulatory clout as opposed to just being a vulnerable form of "advice."

Negotiating Access to Hospitals for Midwives

Access to hospitals was essential for the choice of birthplace component of the midwifery model of practice. Throughout the HPLR and Task Force process, representatives from both the nursing and medical profession thought that for safety reasons, the practice of midwifery should be restricted to the hospital setting and that midwives should be staff of the hospital.[11] Although the Task Force had recommended that midwives have admitting privileges in order to support women's choice of birthplace, many of those in the nursing and medical profession maintained their earlier position that midwives should be hospital staff. Many physicians and representatives from medical organizations (save the MRG) expressed vocal opposition to the idea of midwives being able to admit to hospital, a privilege which is restricted to the physicians.[12] Nurses' concerns about non-nurse midwives in hospitals was more complex. On the one hand, some had concerns that a midwife with hospital privileges would be yet another "boss" in the hospital that they would have to serve. On the other hand, many nurses worried that if midwives became hospital staff, this would displace labour and delivery nurses from maternity wards.

In trying to achieve the privileges model, midwives realized that one of the main things they needed as a prerequisite was to secure professional liability (malpractice) insurance. If they could not secure professional liability insurance as independent practitioners, they would have to become hospital staff in order to have coverage. The importance of professional liability insurance for acquiring hospital admitting privileges was emphasized in the MOPP committee report (June 19, 1992): "A strong system of individual liability insurance is the best answer to any concerns hospitals may have about their indirect liability for actions taken by midwives who hold privileges in their institutions" (13). Securing professional liability insurance would also be necessary in order to be considered seriously by the key decision-makers at the negotiations around government funding.

SECURING PROFESSIONAL LIABILITY INSURANCE

The importance of malpractice insurance was highlighted during the 1985 Toronto Island inquest when the jury recommended that malpractice insurance be compulsory for midwives. The experience of the inquest for the midwives also made it clear how costly such legal proceedings can be, both for midwives and for the parents involved. The inquest had cost upwards of $80,000 for the midwives and parents. The AOM felt it important to at least examine the possibility of securing professional liability insurance to protect themselves and their clients from such devastating court costs.

In the AOM's submission to the Task Force, it documented how in 1986 it had investigated the possibility of obtaining insurance coverage from a private company. The company informed them that the premium for practising obstetricians was $12,176 and for family practitioners doing obstetrics was $9,459; however, they could not specify an appropriate fee for a midwife. Midwives argued that such insurance premiums would be prohibitive given that many midwives' incomes were not much higher than these quoted premiums. The AOM concluded that it would continue its investigation into the malpractice issue, but that it could not make any initial suggestions at the time. The AOM still felt that midwives should carry malpractice insurance in the interests of public protection even though it was difficult to arrange in a climate of financial crisis and government constraint. It asserted that any insurance premium for midwives should reflect the fact that midwives' scope of practice is limited to normal childbirth. Moreover, it should be taken into account that the increased rate of malpractice litigation against physicians had not been paralleled by a similar increase against midwives in the UK and the US. The AOM also added that the way midwives practice in Ontario, with its focus on effective communication; informed choice; and establishing a close, non-authoritarian relationship between midwife and client (factors highlighted by experts in preventing malpractice suits), must also be taken into consideration in setting premiums.

The Task Force agreed with the arguments made in the AOM submission but felt that the decision to make insurance mandatory was a separate issue from whether or not it was available. The Task Force decided that malpractice insurance should be mandatory for midwives for four reasons. First, given that the Task Force was recommending a midwife be a primary caregiver and that she be primarily responsible if something went wrong, she should carry liability in order to be truly accountable for her actions. Second, unless midwives were insured, many physicians

would not feel free to consult with midwives for fear that their own liability would be increased. This, the Task Force argued, would not create
an environment conducive to communication and consultation between
physicians and midwives. Third, the existence of malpractice insurance
should not be a factor in a woman's choice between a physician and a
midwife (i.e., between an *insured* physician and *uninsured* midwife).
Finally, the Task Force felt that without insurance a midwife's practice
options would be unduly limited (i.e., she would not be able to work in
hospitals). If, on the other hand, the lack of availability of insurance
deterred midwives from being self-employed or practising home births
due to prohibitive premiums, the Task Force felt that it would be "necessary for the government to consider taking extraordinary action to assist
midwives to obtain insurance" (TFIMO Report 1987: 107).[13]

With respect to the availability of insurance for midwives, the Task
Force consulted with representatives of the insurance company Reed
Stenhouse Limited. These representatives informed the Task Force that
insurance for midwives was likely to be attainable. Nevertheless, they
identified some overriding concerns: "Insurers will be concerned about
such things as midwives' education, their relationships with physicians,
and their places of practice. Attendance at home birth may be particularly
troublesome. Another problem will be the small size of the profession,
because there will be fewer practitioners amongst whom to spread the
risk" (TFIMO Report 1987: 108). The Task Force was also told that a self-
insurance program through midwives' governing body would be helpful
because it would ensure that only duly registered midwives obtained
coverage. For this reason, the Task Force recommended that midwives,
through their professional association, should take steps to develop a self-
financed insurance program as soon as possible.

Following the Task Force recommendations, the AOM continued their
investigation of attaining malpractice insurance. In the September 1988
AOM Newsletter, it was reported that the AOM had struck an ad hoc
committee on Insurance, headed by midwives Holliday Tyson and Bobbi
Soderstrom. Following the Task Force recommendation, Tyson investigated the possibility of self-insurance through the AOM. The AOM identified several advantages to self-insurance, including the protection of
community midwives, cheaper rates, and autonomous control. A major
disadvantage, however, was that self-insurance would be too big a project
to fund given that one settlement against a midwife could be well over
one million dollars.

Concurrently, midwife Bobbi Soderstrom, on behalf of the AOM, investigated the possibility of private insurance. She contacted an insurance broker who would contract with insurance carriers on behalf of the AOM. This broker, Soderstrom postulated, envisaged midwifery as "a good investment in the future" and a new future market area for insurers (personal communication 1995). He developed a portfolio for the AOM, including its model of midwifery practice, that he then used to help attain interest from insurance companies. The broker successfully secured initial interest from three insurance companies. Soderstrom explained that it was then incumbent upon her "to convince the potential insurers that [midwives] would in fact be a good investment" (personal communication 1995). Throughout the negotiations with these three insurers, AOM representatives Soderstrom and Tyson attempted to secure the best possible insurance package, one which would maintain the model of practice (including home birth) at an affordable rate.

In the end, the AOM was able to secure an arrangement with Wray Brokers and Guarantee Company for $1 million coverage for individual members early in 1991 with "affordable" premiums[14] (AOM Newsletter 7, no. 1, March 1991: 33). Soderstrom described the agreement to which the AOM and this insurance company agreed: "We did get a policy which suited our needs in that it provided us with insurance well before the legislation and included the understanding of the kind of services we offered including the choice of home birth. The company we used felt that the way midwives practised made [us] a low risk group to insure. The fact that midwives spend a lot of time with their clients is expected to contribute to making them less likely to be sued" (personal communication 1995).

Although malpractice insurance coverage was not mandatory for membership in the AOM, the association nevertheless strongly encouraged all of its members to purchase the insurance for two main reasons:

[First, w]e have found a broker and a company sensitive to and respectful of home birth. This may not be a common finding in today's climate. It is important that our enrolment grows so that they are motivated to continue working with us. We will only be in a position of bargaining power to keep improving our policy when we have increased enrolment. [Second, v]ery soon we will all be required to carry insurance in order to practice. It has been the expectation of other health professionals, health service administrators and government that we would not be able to find a company which would insure us on our terms, including attendance at home births. Many health professionals and advisors have pointed out that midwives, not having their own professional insurance policy will need to be insured by hospitals and/or other places of work; these policies will not cover attendance at home births. Therefore, midwives may be unable to attend women giving birth at home. Here, perhaps, is the most important argument for purchasing insurance immediately. We have managed through hard work and good fortune to negotiate a policy which promotes both professional autonomy and our client's choice of birthplace. It really depends on our enrolment for its success. The alternatives would not be ours to control and will not have been developed to serve the values which are so important to us as midwives and the clients we serve. (AOM Newsletter 8, no. 1, March 1992: 44)

Thus, the AOM managed to attain malpractice insurance for their model of practice. That midwives were able to secure insurance coverage is remarkable given that the practice of midwifery (by midwives) was not officially legal in Ontario until November 1991. It is also striking that the insurance carrier accepted the midwives' practice of home birth, given the general societal trend in opposition to it. The acceptance of home birth was likely due in part to the persuasiveness and research-based arguments made by AOM representatives that home births are not as risky as generally believed. The carrier also covered midwives despite their "lack" of formal education. AOM representatives emphasized the AOM's educational guidelines, membership review process, and standards to help allay these concerns.

Midwife Vicki Van Wagner emphasized the importance of securing liability insurance especially since several medical representatives thought that midwives would never be able to secure liability insurance: "From the very beginning of the Task Force, doctors were often sitting back and saying this is academic, this will never happen, they will never get insurance ... Much to all the physician organizations' surprise, we managed, by the time of regulations, to negotiate coverage with a reputable insurance company" (personal communication 1995). Perhaps this is partly why physicians never made a concerted effort to obstruct the midwifery integration project – they felt that the midwives would be thwarted by their inability to secure malpractice insurance, which was a necessary element for full integration into the health care system. If indeed this was the case, this passive "strategy" on the part of some in the medical profession was not successful. Indeed, after securing professional liability insurance, the negotiations for hospital privileges became easier.

SECURING HOSPITAL ADMITTING PRIVILEGES

The issue of attaining hospital admitting privileges for midwives was controversial in light of the initial positions of the nursing and medical professions. However, the initiation of a review of the Public Hospital Act (PHA), the act which makes provisions for hospital admitting privileges, by the provincial government in 1989, was regarded as the opportunity for midwives to achieve their goal. Midwife Jane Kilthei described how the AOM became involved in the PHA review: "The Liberal Government implemented a committee to review the Public Hospitals Act, which was like this ancient piece of legislation, to look at it being a piece of legislation that would drive hospitals to be more fiscally responsible, but also for it to be more multidisciplinary in terms of looking at all professions equally rather than just physicians being the gate keeper. That process started and then they invited the AOM to put forward names of people to sit on that committee ... That was the beginning of the process of being aware that midwives would have to be dealt with" (personal communication 1995).

On September 30, 1989, the AOM prepared its first submission to the PHA steering committee based on discussions with Karyn Kaufman as Midwifery Coordinator and presentations from the Ministry of Health Legal Services. In this submission, AOM representatives highlighted the changes that would be necessary in order for midwives to function fully within the health care system once midwifery legislation was passed, specifically addressing admitting and discharging privileges: "The Task Force on the Implementation of Midwifery in Ontario stated that midwives should provide primary care in a variety of settings including hospital, and that midwives would be able to continue caring for a client in the event of a transport from a home birth. This makes it clear that midwives will need hospital privileges" (AOM Newsletter 6, no. 1, January 1990: 14). The AOM's main argument for attaining hospital admitting privileges was to ensure continuity of care, especially in the case of a home birth transport.

With regards to the issue of hospital governance, the AOM submission proposed that a Professional Advisory Committee replace the Medical Advisory Committee "with multidisciplinary representation to consider issues previously referred to the Medical Advisory Committee" (AOM Newsletter 6, no. 1, January 1990: 14). This would help ensure that midwives, through representation on the Professional Advisory Committee, have a say in the granting of privileges.

The IRCM's hospital subcommittee also submitted a series of proposals for midwifery care in hospital to the PHA Steering Committee in June

1990. These recommendations paralleled the AOM submissions, and included the following: "a) A midwife may assess whether a woman is in normal labour, and may admit her to hospital. She will then, within her scope of practice, be the primary caregiver for that woman. b) A midwife may assess whether a newborn infant is normal, and may admit him/her. She will then, within her scope of practice, be the primary caregiver for that newborn" (*The IRCM Gazette* 2, no. 1, March 1991: 4). These recommendations were made to ensure continuity of care for midwifery consumers by permitting community midwives to accompany and care for their clients in hospital. The IRCM also supported "the creation of a Professional Advisory Committee" and recommended that midwives "form a hospital department with representation on and direct accountability to the Professional Advisory Committee" (*The Gazette* 2, no. 1, March 1991: 4). In these midwifery departments, it was anticipated that midwives would be in charge of reviewing applications and credentialling midwives seeking to join the hospital staff.

In its report (1991), the PHA steering committee recommended that regulated health professions not employed by a hospital should be given "the right to apply for access to the hospital's resources appropriate to their scope of practice" (PHA Steering Committee Report Recommendation #7.01). With specific reference to midwives, the report made the following statement: "Midwives ... will need admitting privileges because a midwife's scope of practice is defined as '... the assessment, monitoring and provision of care during normal pregnancy, labour and the postpartum period and conducting spontaneous, normal vaginal deliveries.' Since the majority of deliveries in Ontario currently occur in hospitals, the privileges required by midwives, when appointed to the clinical staff of a hospital will likely include admission, care and discharge" (PHA Steering Committee Report, 103). The Steering Committee also recommended the establishment of a Professional Advisory Committee to replace the Medical Advisory Committee, reflecting the diversity of health professionals who would be able to have hospital privileges. These recommendations were favourable for midwives' efforts to achieve hospital privileges.

Following the publication of the Steering Committee Report, the PHA review process continued with public hearings scheduled across the province in the summer of 1992. At these hearings, the AOM reiterated its previous position. It also expressed support for the Steering Committee recommendations for the opening up of hospital privileges for other health professions, and the establishment of a Professional Advisory

Committee. They added that instead of having the decisions regarding the granting of appointments and privileges left up to management, such decisions should be made by a profession-specific committee. Midwives would also need to have regulatory authority to write orders in keeping with their scope of practice. One of the main concerns expressed by the AOM about the recommendations made by the Steering Committee was with reference to the refusal to grant privileges:

As a new profession applying for hospital privileges, the "human resource grounds" for refusing privileges proposed for the new Act can be very broadly interpreted and may well be used in some institutions to prevent change ... Using a human resource plan that assumes institutional and physician-based models of care, may not see the long-term benefits of granting midwives privileges [i.e., lower rates of interventions and decreased hospital stay] ... The government needs to be proactive in encouraging hospitals to grant midwives admitting privileges and will need to explore what kinds of incentives are appropriate. (AOM Newsletter 8, no. 4, December 1992: 2)

The IRCM also prepared a submission to the public hearings on the Public Hospitals Act largely reiterating the points made by the AOM above. Specifically regarding the process of enabling the "first generation" of midwives to obtain hospital privileges, the IRCM recommended that this "be dealt with specifically in the legislation" for the following reasons: "Given some of the historical resistance to midwives, we cannot allow this issue to be dealt with on an ad hoc basis, community by community or hospital by hospital. We recommend that this issue be the subject of further consultation between the College of Midwives or the body which [precedes] it, i.e., the Transitional Council, the Association of Ontario Midwives and the Midwifery Task Force of Ontario" (IRCM Submission to Public Hearings on Public Hospitals Act, August 18, 1992). The IRCM also recommended that "legislation include not only the right of midwives to apply for privileges but also provisions to ensure that the public has access to midwifery care in hospitals to the extent that it is available" (IRCM Submission to Public Hearings on Public Hospitals Act, August 18, 1992).

Although the initial recommendations of the PHA review had several positive elements for midwifery in hospitals, they did not come to fruition. The review dissipated in response to many concerns, including intense medical opposition to changes in hospital governance. This left midwives in a precarious situation: without access to hospitals, midwives would not be able to fully perform within the scope of their practice as stipulated under the Midwifery Act: "[Midwives] were the ones that probably had the biggest stake in the revision of the Public Hospital's Act because it was rewriting the statute to allow midwives to have admitting privileges. Hospital privileges were key to midwives practising in the system" (Midwife Robin Kilpatrick, personal communication 1995). Consequently, both the IRCM and the AOM pressed the government to pursue amending the regulations of the PHA to permit midwives to apply for hospital privileges until such time as the statutes of the PHA would be reopened for revision.[15]

The recommendation for special access to hospital privileges for midwives was regarded by some Ministry of Health officials as potentially "opening the flood gates" for other professions, such as chiropractors and psychologists, to request admitting privileges. Some argued that the hospital employee model might be less cumbersome to implement. Both the AOM and IRCM, however, pushed for hospital admitting privileges for midwives arguing that the employee model was not in line with the model of midwifery practice now written into the Transitional Council's regulations. Hospital representatives also expressed apprehension with the employee model due to concerns over increased hospital liability with midwives as employees. Midwife Robin Kilpatrick explained the reasoning behind hospitals' concerns with a staff model: "Midwives would be working outside of the hospital providing at least half their clients with care outside of the hospital. How would the hospital manage that one? How would they deal with that in terms of liability, which is one of their biggest concerns?" (personal communication 1995).

The AOM and IRCM countered concerns of the "opening of the flood gates" by asserting that a valid argument could be made that access to hospitals for these other professions, unlike midwifery, was not essential for them to fully perform within their scope of practice. OHA representative Ron Sapsford and Midwifery Implementation Coordinator Margaret Ann McHugh described the argument that was made:

[Midwifery] was an exception, and the only exception. Mostly because the scope of practice had been defined. It has always been defined with the thought of active hospital privileges ... Of all the professional groups, midwifery ... was the only one that had a very specific and clear need for access to hospitals ... All the rest of the professions didn't have the same compelling argument. (Sapsford, personal communication 1995)

Most chiropractic services don't go on in hospital and most psychological services aren't done in hospital. Yes, there are occasions where they might want to admit someone to a psych ward but they don't need it to carry on their business day to day. Midwives actually need admitting privileges to practice. (McHugh, personal communication 1995)

Both the AOM and the IRCM also argued that if hospital admitting privileges were not available, this would *de facto* limit regulated midwifery care to home births. This assertion was strongly endorsed by Midwifery Coordinator McHugh: "The major argument was that we should not end up with a profession whose job it was to deliver babies who were not allowed to do that in a hospital setting in a Province where 99 per cent of the babies were born in hospital settings. It would be sort of 'why bother?' It could also be construed as putting some people at risk" (personal communication 1995).

These arguments made a strong case for setting up the conditions within the current PHA structure by which midwives could obtain hospital admitting privileges. Midwifery Coordinator McHugh stated that "this was where it became important to have the Minister and the Deputy Minister going along" (personal communication 1995). On January 9, 1993, the Ministry advised the IRCM that it would be going ahead with amending the regulations of the current PHA in consultation with several of the stakeholder groups (AOM, OHA, OMA, CPSO, Transitional Council, CNO, ONA and RNAO). These amendments would enable midwives to independently admit, discharge and write orders in hospital, both on an outpatient basis (e.g., ordering an ultrasound) and for inpatients (labour and delivery and postpartum), within the scope of practice as defined under the Midwifery Act. Although this regulatory approach would enable midwives to obtain hospital privileges, it would not change the role and function of the Medical Advisory Committee as stipulated in the statutes of the PHA (OHA 1994). This situation was described in the AOM Newsletter: "Because the actual statute (the PHA) is not being amended at this point, and because the credentialling functions of the Medical Advisory Committee (MAC) are in statute, midwives will have to apply for hospital privileges through the Hospital Board via the MAC, just as physicians and dentists do now" (9, no. 2, August 1993: 14). Thus, because changes were to be made in regulations and not in statutes, midwives would be under the auspices of the Medical Advisory Committee and ultimately under the supervision of physicians.

At the same time that the regulations of the PHA were being changed by the government to permit midwives to practise in Ontario hospitals, the consultation process among stakeholder groups proceeded with the task of revising the prototype by-laws hospitals would need to use in credentialling midwives. The IRCM had earlier drafted proposals for the credentialling of midwives based on the existing PHA and the prototype by-laws for hospital privileges. The proposals were then forwarded to the OMA, OHA, and College of Physicians and Surgeons (CPSO). IRCM recommendations included that applications for hospital privileges should be made by midwives to individual Medical Advisory Committees for a particular hospital to obtain privileges. Requirements for midwives making an application could include: proof of registration with the College of Midwives; proof of liability insurance; three letters of reference, including one from a physician active in obstetrics; and a résumé setting out training, qualifications, and experience (*The Gazette* 3, no. 1, Jan. 1993: 5). The IRCM also recommended that newly credentialled midwives be supervised by a family physician with hospital obstetric privileges, until such time that a midwife could undertake this supervision.

Changes to the prototype by-laws addressed the application process midwives would have to go through in order to obtain hospital admitting privileges – criteria for appointment and reappointment, term, staff categories and duties, appeals, and reporting structure. These changes generally followed the recommendations made by the IRCM. Most of the changes created a structure for midwives in hospitals similar to that of other physicians seeking privileges. For example, midwives could admit clients to hospital without having to be under a physician. In addition, by-laws stipulated that midwives would have a similar reporting structure to that of physicians – that is, to other physicians. Upon being granted privileges, midwives, like new physicians, would initially be under the direct supervision of another physician. This responsibility structure was justified on the basis of the small number of midwives and their limited experience in the hospital setting:

During the initial years in which midwives are applying for hospital appointments, there will likely be insufficient numbers of midwives within any particular hospital and limited experience of midwives in hospitals to establish a separate department of midwifery. It is recommended, under these circumstances, that midwives become members of the existing departments of obstetrics and paediatrics or family medicine. The chiefs of the departments to which the appointments are made, and ultimately, the Chief of Staff, will be responsible for the supervision of the quality of midwifery care provided in the hospital. (OHA 1994: 22)

Thus, although midwives enjoyed a similar structural position to physicians in hospitals, they were not self-regulatory within the hospital structure as physicians were. In cases where there were several midwives with privileges, however, the prototype by-laws did make provisions for the appointment of a head of the midwifery staff: "This position would be responsible for the general supervision of the midwifery staff, within a medical department. This would allow midwives to manage their practice in the hospital, but within the overall clinical management system of the hospital. The Head of the Midwifery Staff would report to the designated departmental chief" (OHA 1994: 23). Ultimately, however, the practice of midwifery in hospitals falls under medical supervision and the accountability structure of the hospital (OHA 1994).

A notable exception to this structural and procedural similarity of midwives and physicians is that midwives would not have the same right to appeal a refusal for hospital privileges as physicians do under the PHA.[16] "The appeal process for physicians regarding appointment and privileges is provided for in the *Public Hospitals Act* itself. Until the *Public Hospitals Act* is amended, midwives do not have the right to appeal decisions of the hospital board with respect to the granting of privileges" (OHA 1994: 22, emphasis in original). Moreover, because the statutes of the PHA stipulate that membership on the MAC be restricted to members of the medical staff and head of dentistry, the regulations could not be changed to include midwives on the MAC (OHA 1994). Midwives' position in hospitals, therfore, is structurally and procedurally subordinate to the medical professions.

Furthermore, because these prototype by-laws are just recommendations, they may represent the best-case scenario. That is, there is nothing requiring hospitals to use these by-laws or allow midwives to have admitting privileges for that matter. As midwife Robin Kilpatrick described, this is left to the discretion of individual hospital boards: "Individually each hospital has its own decision making powers, so that all the regulation change to the Public Hospitals Act does is *enable* them ... It doesn't mean they *have* to give midwives privileges" (personal communication 1995, emphasis in original). The OHA, however, strongly encouraged hospitals to include midwives: "[We encourage] hospital boards to be leaders in seeking input from women and families about their interest and support for midwifery services, and, where there is support, to establish midwifery

within the maternal and newborn services offered to the community"
(OHA 1994: 2). Moreover, although the OHA recommended that hospitals
include midwives as non-voting members on the MAC in an "ex-officio"
capacity, this again was ultimately left to the discretion of individual hospitals. Hospitals can, and some have, integrated midwifery in a less subordinate fashion than the structure outlined in the OHA prototype by-laws
and some have denied privileges to midwives altogether.

   Despite its shortcomings of significant medical supervision and control,
the privileges model for midwives – and hence the core principles of
choice of birthplace and continuity of care of the IRCM model of midwifery
practice – ultimately prevailed. The day-to-day working under the supervision of physicians in hospitals may, however, pose a significant challenge to the autonomy of midwives as well as the alternative form of care
they currently provide. This situation is viewed as a necessary, yet hopefully temporary "evil" by midwives to enable them to serve their clients
in their choice of birthplace until such time as the PHA is opened for
revision and midwives' position vis à vis hospitals can be renegotiated.

   The tensions in midwifery care arising from hospital practice are not
limited to the concern with supervision by physicians in hospital
(whether direct or indirect). Midwives now have responsibilities to the
hospital and are accountable to hospital policies:

Privilege implies you have a broader responsibility to the organization – peer
review, quality assurance programmes, participation in the internal affairs of the
hospital ... committee work, and so forth. So that in return for the privilege to
practice there is an obligation to satisfy the needs of the hospital as an organization
providing care. (OHA Spokesperson Ron Sapsford, personal communication 1995)

Hospitals do have the ability to put varying restrictions on midwives. I mean
certainly midwives are bound by their College regulations, but hospitals can
impose over and above those other criteria about when a midwife can consult or
transfer care, or the ability to work directly with various groups. (Midwifery
Coordinator Karyn Kaufman, personal communication 1995)

This has caused concern from within the midwifery community for two
reasons. First, midwives may have to practise according to hospital policies that they originally criticized through their social movement. Second, midwives now have to deal with what sometimes are competing
lines of accountability between their clients and the hospital facility they
work in: "My whole role in the hospital is totally different now that I am

a primary caregiver. My thinking is different than when I would go in there as a labour support person ... I could challenge ... I had no allegiance to the hospital. I had allegiance to my client and that was it. Now I have a responsibility to the hospital ... [Nevertheless] I would not go back to the old system because of what I saw at hospital births" (Midwife Chris Sternberg, personal communication 1995). These concerns are difficult to reconcile.

At the same time that the Midwifery Act was proclaimed (December 31, 1993), the regulatory amendments to the PHA also came into force. Shortly after, midwives who had attained registration within the newly established College began to secure admitting privileges in their local hospitals, enabling them to provide their clients with choice of birthplace. To help maintain the model of midwifery care within the hospital setting, the AOM drafted a document entitled "Midwifery Friendly Hospital Policies". In it, the AOM described such things as continuity of care, informed choice, and appropriate use of interventions and hospital services. Midwife Robin Kilpatrick described the reasoning behind the development of this document: "The midwife-friendly policies document was written up ... trying again to outline what midwifery practice is, [such as] ... Midwives' clients expect rooming in. Midwives' clients will not accept being separated from their babies. Midwives don't do routine shaves, routine enemas. Midwives don't do these things. So if you as a hospital think that you want midwifery or when midwives come to you, here are the ways midwives practice" (personal communication 1995). For example, under the section "Non-authoritarian Relationships with Caregivers", it is documented that: "Midwives recognize that childbearing belongs to the woman and that she is central in the course of care. No routine policies or procedures will be carried out on her or her baby without her permission" (Midwifery Friendly Hospital Policies, 2). At the same time as presenting standard elements of midwifery care, the AOM document did concede to its members that: "We will have to prove our competence and earn the trust of both physicians and nurses. They will be watching us very closely. Like new physicians, we will have one year of supervised (associate) practice and will report to the Chiefs of Obstetrics and Paediatrics. It is important to directly address many of the outstanding concerns of hospital staff ... We will need to play by their rules on some things until they learn to trust our judgement" (Midwifery Friendly Hospital Policies, 4).

The first midwife-assisted hospital birth came soon after proclamation on January 28, 1994, with the birth of Rebecca Rutherford to Anita and

Paul Rutherford attended by Peggy Cannon and Carol Cameron at the Markham Stouffville Hospital. This historic event not only marked the first time in Canada that regulated midwives caught a baby in a hospital without a physician, it also marked the beginning of the ongoing, day-to-day challenges midwives face to their model of practice in the hospital setting.

SUMMARY

The model of midwifery practice developed by midwives through the AOM, with consumer input through the MTFO, and revised through the Task Force and IRCM committees, faced several challenges throughout the integration process. These included the development of standards, the securing of professional liability insurance, and the attainment of hospital admitting privileges. In the face of these challenges, the core attributes of the midwifery model of care identified by the leaders of the midwifery integration project (i.e., informed choice, continuity of care, and choice of birthplace), have largely been maintained. Indeed, the model of midwifery practice that was finally implemented was strikingly similar to those the leaders of the midwifery integration project had initially proposed to the HPLR in 1983. Remarkably, midwives have also acquired an expanded scope of practice by becoming integrated as primary caregivers for births in both home and hospital.

Like the achievement of self-regulation discussed in the last chapter, the maintenance of midwives' model of practice and the expansion of their scope are truly unique outcomes compared to other professional projects. As outlined in chapter 1, professions seeking integration often succumb to forces that limit their scope, subordinate their practitioners, and medicalize their mode of practice (Coburn and Biggs 1986; Larkin 1983; Willis 1989). For example, Coburn and Biggs (1986) detail how chiropractors in Canada underwent a significant shift away from chiropractic's alternative roots to a more medicalized specialty limited to musculoskeletal disorders of the spine. Although an argument can be made that Ontario midwives are limited to "normal" births, they never sought to expand their scope in the direction of high-risk births. This was always considered to be the domain of obstetrics. They also managed to maintain their "alternative" roots, primarily with respect to the legitimation of home birth and the focus on women-centred care.

Comparing this midwifery professional project to those undertaken in other jurisdictions reveals similar unique outcomes. Many of those projects have resulted in a practice limited in setting – almost exclusively in hospital – and with subordinate status – often as staff. Midwifery integration in Arizona, for example, resulted in extensive medical control over the type of services midwives could provide (Sullivan and Weitz 1988). Ontario midwives are primary care providers who are not limited to hospital births, but are also not limited to home births as they previously were (albeit under precarious legal circumstances). Moreover, they do not require their clients to be referred by physicians as do many midwives from other jurisdictions. So despite the cultural context being more similar to that existing in the UK, the US, and Australia, the practice of midwifery in Ontario ended up being much more like their ideal type in the Netherlands.

The maintenance of the "core" attributes of a strongly consumer-oriented midwifery model and the achievement of an expanded scope of practice speaks to the crucial and influential involvement of midwives and consumers throughout the process, but also to the strong support provided along the way by state officials and bureaucrats. Midwife Vicki Van Wagner described how the model of midwifery care for which midwives fought was in the interests of childbearing women:

It is a big challenge to midwives … It's not in your personal or professional interest to handle all these settings … You have all the protocols, equipment and issues for home births. You have to feel fully confident and competent in that setting. In the hospital or in a birth centre, a whole other set of rules … Some of us are dealing with more than one hospital, and the rules and regulations in each place are slightly different. To be flexible enough as a practitioner to work in many sites is a big challenge … It's really in the interest of women who wanted choice. The consumer organization said to midwives, "We need you to have the flexibility so that I can change my mind and say I thought I wanted to go to a birth centre, but after all I'd rather be at home," or, "Yes, I thought I wanted a home birth, but actually I don't feel safe with that choice, I want to be in the hospital." (personal communication 1995)

While the legislated model of practice potentially suits the interests of consumers more than it does the interests of midwives, it is important to note that the promotion of a consumer-oriented model could also be viewed as an important strategy used by midwives to maintain consumer support for the integration project – support which was crucial in the government's decision to integrate midwifery. Thus, it could be argued that the consumer orientation of the midwifery model was also in the immediate if not the long-term interests of midwives as they sought integration. Implementation of this women-centred model required significant state support to overcome the various legislative barriers to integrating it, particularly in the context of the Ontario hospital system.

Despite this maintenance of the "core" attributes of the model of practice at the level of legislation and regulations, the midwifery model has became bound and constrained throughout the implementation process. This has created a potential chipping away of the solidarity between midwives and their clients. This is shown most clearly with respect to the fate of the principle of informed choice. Midwives are now not only accountable to their clients, they are also accountable to mandatory Standards of midwifery care regulated by the College of Midwives. There is always a potential for conflict between these accountabilities, especially regarding a client's choice of home birth when it is contraindicated by College standards or a midwife's professional opinion. In a hospital birth, midwives are additionally accountable to the policies and procedures of the hospital in which they have privileges, over and above their accountability to their College and their clients. Thus, the further they were along the integration process, the more structurally mediated the relations between midwives and their clients became – by the College, by the hospital, and by the government. All these served to increase the social distance between pregnant women and their midwifery care providers.

In this way, the challenges to the midwifery model of practice have not ended with the proclamation of legislation and official integration, but the structural conditions created as a compromise to meet these challenges may continue to affect the way midwives practice. That is, legislation is one thing, actual practice another. Perhaps it is in their everyday work, particularly in the hospital, that midwives will face the "embedded" power of doctors, hospital administrators, and nurses (Alford 1975). Although midwifery self-regulation could help sustain the model of practice, the compromised nature of "self"-regulation entails a number of "fault lines" that potentially limit the College's capacity to maintain the ideal practice model. Given these structural conditions of practice, midwives will have to continue to resist co-optation and strive to deliver women-centred midwifery care.

Besides these concerns with how the model plays out at the "micro" level of everyday practice, another important concern was the price paid for the "success" of midwives' achievement of self-regulation and their "ideal" model of practice. I have already noted the increased profession-alization of midwifery as indicated by the separate organizational repre-sentation of midwives and clients, self-regulation, and development of standards of practice. As we shall see in the next chapter, the model of practice and accessibility to midwifery services in general were also to be challenged by negotiations dealing with public funding.

CHAPTER EIGHT

Ensuring Equity of Access through Public Funding

Tied to the issue of maintaining the model of practice discussed in the previous chapter is the desire of midwives and their supporters for midwifery services to be publicly funded. Public funding was sought not only in orders to ensure equity of access to midwifery for childbearing women, but also to ensure equity of access to childbearing women for midwives. That is, public funding would help ensure a level professional playing field between midwives and physicians, whose maternity care services were covered under publicly funded Medicare. But public funding was not only viewed as a positive achievement in and of itself; the form that public funding would take was seen to have a critical impact on the way midwives practised. So funding was not only tied to the issues of access and equity, it was also tied to the midwifery model of practice. Public funding was also an issue that would connect the midwifery community to the provincial government even more directly than the issue of regulation; regulation can be delegated as it is in a self-regulatory model but public funding for services would require ongoing state involvement.

In this chapter, I trace the evolution of the funding for midwifery services from its roots in the private sphere to the accomplishment of public funding that came about with the passage of the Midwifery Act in 1993. The negotiations about the funding mechanism for midwifery is a particular focus in light of its potential impact on practice in the years following midwives' official integration. Yet again we see the influential nexus between midwives, their consumer supporters, and the state in the efforts to secure public funding in a manner consistent with the midwifery model of practice.

PRIVATELY FUNDED MIDWIFERY CARE IN ONTARIO

Very early in the home birth movement, birth attendants/midwives did not charge for the services they provided. This was either because they were providing care for a friend, or because they wanted to get more experience as home birth attendants and in exchange would offer their services for free. As the demand for midwifery services grew, some midwives, especially those with young families to support, began to charge fees. At first the fees were quite modest [one early midwife recalled sharing a fee of $150 (Sternberg, personal communication 1995)], often just covering the costs of a baby-sitter for the midwives' children when she was suddenly called away for a birth. As birth attendants increasingly came to see themselves as midwives and as primary caregivers for women, their fees increased proportionately. These costs were borne directly by clients; that is, clients paid midwives directly for education, support, and maternity care services. Midwifery services were not only not covered by public health insurance, private medical insurance also did not cover midwifery care (Giacomini and Peters 1996).

It could be argued that direct payment for services reinforced the client-centred focus of this early form of midwifery care. Direct payment may also have resulted in more of a balance of power between the woman and her midwife. At the same time, however, direct payment made midwifery services inaccessible to many childbearing women. As noted in chapter 5, midwifery clients were well-educated women, the majority with post-secondary education, many with the means to pay directly for midwifery care. Although this well-informed and politically astute consumer base may have been an essential element of the success of the midwifery integration project, limiting midwifery care to this group of women was regarded by many as inequitable. Some midwifery practitioners attempted to increase accessibility to their services by developing a sliding-scale of fees depending on the woman's ability to pay. For example, in 1986 a range from $400 for low-income clients to $700 for high income clients covered a full course of care including pre- and post-natal visits as well as care at birth (Fooks and Gardiner 1986). Some midwives even continued or went back to their earlier practices of accepting payment in kind, such as in exchange for babysitting services or fruits and vegetables to better ensure accessibility. Curiously, this practice is similar to what has been described about traditional lay midwifery. Despite these attempts, some midwives still felt that the accessibility of midwifery care was limited. Moreover, one of the consequences of attempts to equalize access was that midwives made a very poor living practising midwifery. For midwives working out of one of the busiest practices in downtown Toronto, the average gross income in 1986 was $20,000 (Fooks and Gardiner 1986) and this changed little until 1994 (Mickleburgh 1994); other practices fared much worse.[1]

MAKING THE CASE FOR PUBLIC FUNDING

Seeking public funding was one of the less controversial elements of midwives' decision to become integrated into the Ontario health care system (see chapter 4). It was generally agreed by those within the mid-wifery community that public funding would be one of the more positive features of seeking integration. Indeed, it was assumed that with integra-tion would come public funding; this, however, is not necessarily the case.[2] The case for public funding, therefore, was mentioned briefly in the Midwifery Coalition's first submission to the HPLR, but it was not high-lighted as one of its key elements. To be fair, the Coalition's first submis-sion was to respond to key questions set out by the HPLR, none of which pertained specifically to public funding, and this was not considered to be part of the mandate of the Review Committee. This lack of prominence of the funding issue was also reflected in the responses to the Coalition's submission by the medical and nursing professions. The only discussion of funding came from the Ontario Medical Association which asserted that midwifery would be an unnecessary duplication of services.

The issue of public funding did, however, figure prominently in the Private Member's Bill introduced in the legislature by NDP Health Critic David Cooke as well as in the jury recommendations at the Toronto Island Inquest (see chapter 5). Coverage of midwifery services under the pro-vincial health insurance plan was included in the AOM's plans for the integration of midwifery care submitted to subsequent rounds of the HPLR: "One of the goals of the AOM and the MTF in seeking legal recog-nition of midwives has been to make midwifery care accessible to the general public ... Obviously OHIP coverage is ... essential in integrating midwifery as a real choice into maternity care in Ontario" (AOM Response to the McLaughlin-Harris Inquest, 19).

Public funding was also an issue to be addressed by the Task Force on the Implementation of Midwifery in Ontario, but here too, it seems to be largely assumed that this was not a contested issue. For example, in the AOM's written submission to the Task Force, there is no specific section addressing the issue of public funding.[3] Perhaps this is implicit in the recommendation of "the midwife as a full member of the health care team." The issue was not so much *whether* to fund midwifery services publicly but *how* such public funding would be organized:

Midwives in private practice could be privately paid by their clients, as they are now. But if midwifery services are to be accessible to all women who want them, other pay schemes will have to be devised. If midwifery services are to come under OHIP's current fee-for-service scheme, it is the Association of Ontario Midwives' position that midwifery care must be considered a single service, compensated by a flat fee. Alternatively, midwives could be salaried as they are in the Netherlands and paid through provincial health insurance. They would be required to attend a minimum number of births. (AOM Submission to the Task Force, Sept. 1986: 29)

Midwives, therefore, began to articulate that they sought a particular form of funding to support the model of practice rather than undermine it. Having a flat fee per birth or a salary based on a certain number of births, it was argued, would help maintain midwives' holistic, low intervention-based perspective on pregnancy and birth, which was essential for continuity of care, and would avoid the pressure "to do more" which was inherent in the physicians' fee-for-service system.

Curiously, there was little information pertaining to the funding issue in the submissions of other professions to the Task Force. The Medical Reform Group (MRG) strongly supported that midwifery be "fully publicly funded" and that this should be in keeping with the principle that midwifery be viewed as an alternative mode of maternity care rather than a supplementary add-on to existing services. The College of Family Physicians (CFPC) also indicated that midwives should be paid under a model that recognized their role, but that also acknowledges the role to be played by family physicians. None of the nursing organizations specifically addressed the issue of public funding for midwifery services.

As noted previously, the Task Force ultimately recommended that funding for midwifery services should be provided by the provincial government. When Minister of Health Murray Elston made the announcement to integrate midwifery into the health care system in January 1986, no specific statement was made regarding the funding of midwifery services. Nevertheless, the Task Force argued that unless midwifery services were paid for by the province, midwifery would never be fully integrated into the health care system:

In announcing the decision to recognize midwifery as a regulated health profession and to integrate in into the overall health care system, the Minister of Health did not explicitly address whether midwifery services will be paid for by the province or by users. Virtually every individual consumer and consumer organization, as well as medical and nursing organization, told the Task Force that the province should pay for midwifery services. This was also the view of midwives and midwifery organizations. Consumers and midwives said every women is entitled to the important, basic health care service that midwives provide and that midwifery care should not be denied to less affluent women. They claimed that any apparent increase in the provincial health care budget due to midwifery services would be balanced by long-term savings resulting from midwifery. We think midwifery will not be fully integrated into the health care system unless midwifery services are paid for by the province. (Task Force Report 1987, 98)

The Task Force also argued that government funding of midwifery services was an effective mechanism for ensuring that the recommended framework of practice was upheld.

Therefore, like the AOM submission, the Task Force asserted that the issue was not whether or not to fund, but *how* to fund midwifery care. Neither the government, the midwifery community, nor the Task Force wanted a fee-for-service funding model. The government felt that with a fee-for-service system, it would be difficult to control the overall costs of midwifery care.[4] Moreover, the government believed that including midwifery services in OHIP would increase the pressure on the Ministry of Health from other professions to include their services as well. As mentioned above, members of the midwifery community also did not want fee-for-service because it tended to compartmentalize care, which was contrary to their model of care. The Task Force agreed with these concerns and also highlighted that: "Payment on the basis of fee-for-service also necessitates the preparation of fee schedules. The preparation of a fee schedule for midwifery care would involve difficult comparisons with the fee schedule for obstetrical services rendered by physicians. We think this could easily be a continuing source of friction between midwives and physicians" (Task Force Report 1987, 99). The Task Force felt that a global fee would also necessitate comparisons with physicians' services and it would also make timely and cost-effective transfers of care difficult. It ultimately recommended that midwifery funding be provided on the basis of global, program-based budgets from which midwives would be paid a salary; that midwives be prohibited from obtaining payment for their services directly from clients (similar to the ban on physicians extra-billing), but that they be allowed to charge fees for childbirth education classes.

Although there was no formal response by the government to the funding issue specifically, the government-appointed Midwifery Coordinator forged ahead with several of the implementation issues identified in the Task Force report. During the Task Force, however, the Legislative Research Services branch of the Government of Ontario commissioned a "current issue" paper on the implementation of midwifery in Ontario (Fooks and Gardiner 1986).[5] One of the key issues identified in the paper was the cost-effectiveness of midwifery care. Specifically, it asked, "Is the addition of midwives an unnecessary cost to an already strained system or could the use of midwives lead to a more cost-effective allocation of human and fiscal resources? (5) One of the first studies it reviewed to help address this question was conducted in Quebec by the Interministerial Committee on Midwives in 1983 which was summarized as follows:

On the assumption that midwives would be primary providers for normal low-risk births only, they began by calculating the direct costs of normal pregnancies and hospital deliveries. They found that this cost, based on 1981 data, was $2167.90: $511.90 for the fees of the general practitioner attending and $1656.00 for hospitalization expenses ... Assuming that midwives received the same salary as nurses, which was $483.80 per week, and that they attended two deliveries per week or 104 per year, then the cost of their professional services would be $241.90. Assuming also that the hospitalization expenses remained the same, the total cost of a midwife attended pregnancy and delivery was $1897.90, which was $270 less than a comparable physician attended birth. (7)

The authors did note that a case could be made for lower hospitalization costs in light of the indirect impact of midwives' model of practice. For example, it was argued that, "[m]idwives tend to rely less on technological monitoring, drugs and other intervention and there is evidence that midwives' clients require less postpartum care and recovery time" (7).

Another study cited in this report was of a US-based rural nurse-midwifery program (Reid and Morris 1979). The service was introduced to address the increasing lack of prenatal care for women delivering at the hospital studied. Following the introduction of nurse-midwifery care, overall expenditures for perinatal care dropped by over 50 per cent largely a result of a sharp decline in hospitalization expenditures.

The third study reviewed was also based on US data comparing the costs of a certified nurse-midwifery practice and a physician practice in

Salt Lake City (Cherry and Foster 1982). The methodology involved a matched cohort analysis of normal maternity clients comparing the charges generated for their care. Important differences in procedures were noted, including: a greater proportion of midwifery clients delivering without anaesthesia (52 per cent versus 18 per cent for physicians); a lesser proportion of midwifery clients using electronic fetal monitoring (64 per cent versus 89 per cent for physicians); lower charges for pharmacy and IV for midwifery clients; and a shorter length of postpartum stay (mean of 1.5 days for midwifery clients and 2.0 for physicians). In terms of dollar figures, the average hospital bill for midwifery clients was $114 less than for physicians' clients.

After reviewing these studies, the authors of this Ministry commissioned report concluded: "Available research indicates that midwives can provide important cost savings when compared to conventional hospital-based obstetrics. Relying on midwives as the primary caregivers for normal low-risk births could also potentially free the more highly specialized expertise of obstetricians to concentrate on high-risk and complicated cases, resulting in a more effective overall allocation of medical resources" (10). Curiously, neither this report nor the three studies reviewed therein were included in the reference list of the Task Force Report. This provides further substantiation that the issue was not whether midwifery would be funded but how. It would take several years, however, for this to be made explicit. It was not until December 1992, when NDP Minister of Health, Frances Lankin, formally announced what many has assumed all along: that the government was committed to funding midwifery services in Ontario. No other occupation with newly endowed self regulatory status under the RHPA was given such a promise. Nevertheless, the way the government intended to implement midwifery funding represented a challenge to midwives and the midwifery model of practice in particular.

NEGOTIATING THE FUNDING MECHANISM FOR MIDWIVES

The implementation of a funding mechanism for midwifery services was highlighted early on as a potential threat to the way midwives wanted to practice and to the model developed by the MOPP and IRCM:

When we began to look at funding, we looked to ... some of the people who were critiquing the ... Canadian health care system, and the way that the funding system ... had a major impact on patterns of health delivery and the way that the system of payment creates incentives and disincentives to kinds of care. So we went in with our eyes wide open. The basic principle was that the model must drive the funding system, not the funding system drives the model. We realized that unless we carefully think this through, after all of the hard work, after achieving malpractice insurance regulations, after doing all this, funding could wreck it all, it really could. We were very anxious about that. (Midwife Vicki Van Wagner, personal communication 1995)

In a preliminary report on funding dated January 1992, the AOM stated that it "hopes to work with the government towards a method of funding which will support the philosophy and approach to midwifery care which Ontario consumers have worked for over the past decade and which is reflected in the Interim Regulatory Council on Midwifery (IRCM) *Philosophy of Midwifery Care in Ontario* statement" (AOM Newsletter 8, no. 1, March 1992, Appendix B: 21). It also asserted that the "planning of payment for midwifery care must take into consideration the impact of funding on practice" (AOM Newsletter 8, no. 1, March 1992, Appendix B: 22). The AOM recommended that midwifery funding be channelled through group practices already established to provide continuity of care.

Many of the recommendations made by the AOM in this preliminary report were reiterated by the MOPP Committee. It too addressed the challenge the organization of funding had on the model of midwifery practice by arguing that the model should direct the funding mechanism rather than the reverse: "We recommended that the Ministry of Health ensure that an equitable formula for funding of midwifery be structured to fully support our recommended model of practice" (*The Gazette* 3, no. 2, August 1992: 2). One of the MOPP Committee recommendations highlights how funding should not affect the principle of choice of birthplace: "The ways by which midwives and facilities receive money to provide midwifery care should be designed to eliminate disincentives to choice of birthplace ... [M]idwives should be paid equitably for births regardless of setting" (MOPP Report, June 19, 1992: 9). Various payment options were examined and discussed in the MOPP Committee report, and, as in the AOM document, a fee-for-service model was rejected as it was considered inappropriate for midwifery care. Instead, the MOPP recommended either a "capitation" model, under which payment is made according to a number of clients in a practice, or a salary model (*The Gazette* 3, no. 2, August 1992: 2). Payments, it was suggested, could be channelled to midwives working in group practices or other organizations.

With respect to the level of funding or remuneration, the MOPP committee recommended that "funding must reflect midwives" level of skill and responsibility as primary caregiver, education at a baccalaureate level, the realities of working on call and the time-intensive nature of midwifery care" (MOPP Report, June 19, 1992: 10). It was suggested that a midwife's remuneration should fall somewhere between that of a senior salaried nurse and a family physician. The MOPP Committee, largely reiterating recommendations made by the AOM in its preliminary funding report, additionally recommended that funding for midwifery care accommodate the different costs of providing care for specific client populations (some with greater needs than others), for different geographic locations (e.g., Northern Ontario), and various birth settings. They also suggested that overhead costs, costs of setting up new practices (initially with low volumes), travel time, part-time practice, and professional activities (i.e., continuing education and clinical teaching) also be taken into account when determining remuneration level.

Funding Organization Negotiations

Ministry decision-making regarding the funding mechanism for midwifery, the Ontario Midwifery Program (OMP), began in earnest in the Spring of 1993, less than a year before proclamation was anticipated. It had already been decided that midwifery would be funded through the Community Health Branch (CHB) of the Ministry of Health as this was seen by Ministry officials as most compatible with the community-based practices of midwives. Unsure about whether they would be involved in negotiations involving the establishment of the OMP, given that the Ministry was within its rights to make unilateral decisions regarding funding, midwives in the AOM requested a meeting with CHB representatives to express their concern "that how midwifery is funded is going to have an impact on the model of practice" (Midwife Jane Kilthei, personal communication 1995).

To support their position, AOM representatives were accompanied by MTFO President and former IRCM member Diane Pudas, and Transitional Council Chair Mary Eberts. Pudas and Eberts presented the model of practice developed by the IRCM and urged that the model of funding be established in accordance with that model. AOM representatives also expressed the view that they should be involved in negotiations for midwifery funding: "It took a little while to get recognition from the Ministry of Health that the body that represented the interests of midwives was who they should be talking to ... I think there were certainly enough people internal to the Ministry of Health that this was appropriate just the same way that they would talk to the Ontario Medical Association about what physicians get paid, that they should be talking to the AOM" (Kilthei, personal communication 1995).

The AOM representatives were ultimately successful at securing a seat at the funding decision-making table, attributed by Kilthei to their focus on the model: "We went to them to say, "yes, the level of payment is an issue, but much more important to us is having a mode, a mechanism for funding the midwifery program to protect the model of practice." And I think we got a certain respect from the people within the Ministry of Health that we laid that out as our top priority" (personal communication 1995). Formal negotiations between the AOM and CHB began in May 1993, involving the AOM President, Jane Kilthei, and President Elect, Eileen Hutton, and Sue Davy and Jim Shea from the CHB, both parties with legal council.

At the outset, AOM representatives presented a list of principles which they felt to be critical to the funding negotiations. These were: 1) the funding arrangement must support the Ontario Model of Midwifery Care which includes continuity of care, informed choice, and choice of birthplace; 2) the funding arrangement must acknowledge midwives as autonomous practitioners; 3) current midwifery practices must be "grandmothered" into the funding system; 4) funding must allow for two midwives at all births except in cases of transfer of care to a physician (where one midwife would attend with a physician); 5) funding must permit midwives to work with other health care providers; and 6) funding must allow access to or working relationships with existing health care facilities (AOM Newsletter 8, no. 4, December 1992). In addition, it was argued that there should be one central negotiation process in which the AOM has a direct relationship with the government, and one funding arrangement for all midwives (AOM Newsletter 8, no. 4, December 1992). These latter two recommendations were considered particularly important given that midwives were a small group, and hence were vulnerable in the negotiations process.

The Ministry's initial position was in general agreement with the MOPP/IRCM recommendations that payment for midwives could be channelled through existing organizations such as Community Health Centres (CHCs), already funded by the CHB.[6] CHCs could act as local transfer payment agencies for midwifery funding. The government's proposal followed "the idea of funding midwifery as a community-based health service rather than as a profession" (CHB representative Jim Shea, personal communication 1995). Organizing midwifery funding in this manner would prevent the need to set up a separate bureaucracy to administer the OMP and avoid the "whole situation of setting up the accountability between the profession and Ministry; the accountability would be more directly with the community" (CHB representative Jim Shea, personal communication 1995).

This proposal provoked considerable apprehension among midwives and CHCs alike. CHCs were concerned because they thought they would have to fund midwives from their existing base budget. Midwives were concerned with this arrangement because of the incongruity of their model of practice and the CHC "team" approach. Midwives felt that the CHC approach would result in dividing up a pregnant woman's care among different professionals working in the CHC, which was not compatible with the establishment of the close personal relationship that midwives felt was an important part of their model of care: "Community health centres ... very much have a team approach. A client will see any one of several health professionals – you know nurse, doctor, social worker, etc. – and everyone collaborates on taking care of the client. Midwives had concerns with fitting into the team approach because midwives can't share care with the doctor or nurse. They would be concerned that their model of practice would be eroded that way, and the College very specifically wrote into the regulations the kind of model of practice so that it would not be diluted that way" (Midwifery consumer Betty Dondertman, personal communication 1994). The AOM representatives felt that a great deal of discussion would be needed to orient all CHCs to the model of midwifery practice. Additionally, there was the problem that many communities had no CHC, and those CHCs that did exist did not have adequate facilities available for midwives.

The CHB's task of responding to the concerns of both CHCs and midwives was considered overwhelming in light of the urgent need to set the funding mechanism in place before the official integration of midwifery, expected at the end of 1993. Subsequently, AOM and CHB representatives discussed alternative funding arrangement possibilities. AOM representative Jane Kilthei described the funding alternative that emanated from these discussions: "We actually did some creative brainstorming and problem solving on a variety of ways that that could work before we all sort of mutually came up with this idea of a central agency that's consumer-based that would do the first three or four years and sort of shepherd the process of moving midwifery practices to being connected with local agencies" (personal communication 1995). Thus, in the end, the

government decided that it would have to set up a centralized bureaucracy to manage the first midwifery funding program, at least temporarily. CHB representative Jim Shea described the reasoning behind the
government's decision:

Some of the barriers were that midwifery wasn't well enough understood and
the model, therefore, wasn't well enough supported around the Province by
enough transfer payment agencies – and this was a judgement call that we had
to make very quickly. If we were to force midwives into transfer payment agencies that weren't ready for them, and midwives themselves were anxious enough,
we could have created real problems. I don't think either the midwives or the
transfer payment agencies were really ready for that yet. But we did agree that's
where we wanted to go. So we decided to take an interim step. (personal
communication 1995)

Establishing this interim payment agency therefore "bought them some
time in terms of getting to the ultimate position which is still to somehow
integrate midwives into existing facilities" (midwifery consumer Betty
Dondertman, personal communication 1995).

The next question that needed to be addressed was the form this
bureaucracy would take. Midwifery representatives suggested that a con-
sumer-run organization was well-suited to the philosophies of both midwifery and the CHB: "At the AOM we have always seen midwifery as it's
developed in Ontario as being very consumer driven. That and Community Health Branch is very consumer focused and so it was very much a
meeting of ideas" (Jane Kilthei, personal communication 1995). CHB representatives concurred with this argument: "Part of the model of practice
being very much consumer oriented and the Ministry's interest in maintaining a very consumer oriented service here ... Why not have the
interim managers of the system be the consumers?" (Jim Shea, personal
communication 1995). They were nevertheless still faced with time constraints. Because of this situation, the AOM representatives suggested that
this consumer-based funding organization could be developed as an offshoot of the existing MTFO. Jane Kilthei described the process of coming
up with this suggestion: "[We said,] 'Well, is there an agency anywhere
that could do this provincially? No, there really isn't one. If we're going
to create one, where could it grow out of and because it had to happen
fairly quickly, [because] it needed an existing organization to kind of feed
it, but to not actually be part of that organization'" (personal communication 1995). CHB representatives agreed with this suggestion and it was

decided that the MTFO would become involved in establishing this interim funding bureaucracy.

Executive members of the MTFO were subsequently contacted to help establish a steering committee for this central funding agency, the Lebel Midwifery Care Organization (LMCO).[7] Although membership in the MTFO was not mandatory, the steering committee was made up entirely of MTFO members. Once established, the steering committee began to recruit Board members discreetly through MTFO channels in the fall of 1993. Discretion was necessary as the Minister of Health had not yet formally announced the government decisions about the funding of midwifery.

Concurrent with the efforts to begin establishing the central funding agency, AOM and CHB representatives continued to discuss the manner in which midwives would receive compensation. Kilthei described the argument the AOM made regarding why existing midwifery practice groups should become the fundamental bases for midwifery funding: "We spent ... a lot of sessions just giving the Community Health people information about how midwifery worked now, and part of what we were driving at in that process is to say, 'Let's not throw out the baby with the bath water here. We've got something that works. Let's look at what are the good parts of that.' And part of what's good about the way midwifery evolves with practice groups is that there's a unit there that provides care co-operatively together that also is in place to do peer review, to make sure that there's ongoing quality improvement" (personal communication 1995). This idea satisfied the CHB representatives and it was subsequently agreed that midwives were not to be paid a salary directly by the government, but would receive a salary, or compensation package, through their practice group.

By the time these decisions regarding the channelling of funds had been made, the Board of the LMCO had, with the assistance of the AOM and CHB representatives, drawn up its terms of reference. These were 1) to provide ongoing funding and support to midwifery practice groups in accordance with the OMP guidelines; 2) to develop a network of local transfer payment agencies for midwifery throughout Ontario; and 3) to completely transfer the authority of the LMCO to these local agencies by December 1997, and to monitor this transition period (LMCO 1993/94 Annual Report, p. 2).

The Board of the LMCO had also come to some decisions regarding the staffing of the organization. One of these staff positions was that of the Executive Director, filled by previous MTFO President Betty Dondertman. She described the process of how she was chosen for the position: "They hired me largely because of the midwifery background that I had ... because the board was very concerned about maintaining the model of practice and having somebody coming in who understood that side of things" (Dondertman, personal communication 1995). Thus, MTFO involvement in the LMCO was evident in several stages of the development process.

Because of its temporary nature, the LMCO was required to educate local transfer payment agencies about the midwifery model and divest its responsibilities to these transfer payment agencies. So part of the mandate of the LMCO was essentially to self-destruct. In the interim, however, it would first have to develop contracts with existing midwifery practice groups for midwifery services under the terms developed out of the negotiations between the AOM and CHB. Although LMCO representatives were included at the negotiation table, decisions were still made between the AOM and CHB: "When the LMCO was created, they were brought into the process to bring the consumer perspective into the process. But the negotiation still remained fundamentally between the AOM and the Ministry of Health. And really the way it worked is the AOM and the Ministry negotiated the funding agreement; and the LMCO is the body that implements that agreement. And so they were brought on stream so they would understand the roots of where this agreement that they were going to implement came from" (Midwife Jane Kilthei, personal communication 1995). LMCO representatives felt at times powerless to influence decision-making on the details of the contract that they would ultimately have to implement.

Funding Level Negotiations

Once the decision around the organization of the funding mechanism was in place, the next step in the negotiations process focused on the terms of the agreements between the LMCO and individual practice groups, including midwives' case load and the level of remuneration. Case load was generally regarded by members of the midwifery community to be a significant factor affecting midwives' ability to practice according to the desired model of care. For example, midwifery consumer and MTFO member Susan Meyer highlighted the effect of a large case load on the principle of informed choice:

In considering how to promote informed choice I've always thought the important issues were around how midwives practice and how they get paid. Informed choice takes time, time to convey information, time for the client to digest information. If there isn't the time to teach and to be taught, there can't be informed choice. So beyond what a midwife learns in her education, if a midwife has to process so many clients to earn her living that she hasn't got the time to teach as well as deliver babies, informed choice will be lost. Clients need time and knowledge to have the confidence to make choices. (Meyer as cited in Van Wagner 1991, 125)

In anticipation of the need to set case loads, midwife Vicki Van Wagner conducted background research, based on local and international midwifery practices, to help recommend an appropriate case load given the instituted model of care developed by the MOPP and IRCM. Based on Van Wagner's research, the AOM recommended to the CHB that a full case load be eighty births per year: forty complete courses of care as primary midwife and forty cases as backup midwife.[8] This number was determined using both international standards and current community midwifery practices in Ontario (Van Wagner, personal communication 1995). CHB representatives were persuaded by the evidence collected. A provision for midwives to work part-time with reduced case loads was also recommended by the AOM representatives and agreed to by the CHB.

Decisions regarding remuneration followed those made for the recommended case loads. In order to help determine an appropriate level, the CHB representatives contracted the services of an independent pay equity consultant. AOM representative Jane Kilthei described how this consultant came up with an appropriate figure for midwives' compensation: "The Ministry brought in consultants who did work in pay equity. And so what we did was ... took the midwives' job description and issues of education level at a baccalaureate level, issues of work stress, the on-call [nature of midwifery work] and we took it through a pay equity exercise and used as the comparators a physician in a community health centre and a primary care nurse at a community health centre" (personal communication 1995). As a result of this exercise, a salary range was established with the full-time entry-level salary beginning at $55,000 and extending up to $77,000 for midwives with more than ten years of work experience.[9]

Once the AOM and CHB had determined the compensation range, the LMCO had the task of deciding where individual midwives would be placed on that range. CHB representatives agreed to include a midwife's self-reported years of practice experience prior to official integration in the determination of her appropriate salary level. Thus, for each practice group, the LMCO had to ascertain how many midwives were working in the group, what their work load would be (whether full or part-time), and at what pay level. The LMCO also had to determine each practice groups' operating expenses, including travel, office, and liability insurance premiums, as these were also funded by the government. CHB representative Jim Shea described why midwives' operating expenses were also to be covered by Ministry funding: "What we were doing was in taking the community-based health approach we were going at it from a salary and expenses perspective rather than pay a fee-for-service or capitation where you roll it all into one and just say we'll take care of everything. If we envisioned midwives to be part of community health organizations, everyone in, for example, CHCs, is paid on salary and expenses are part of the budget" (personal communication 1995).

Following all of these negotiations, Health Minister Ruth Grier made the formal announcement in October 1993, that beginning in 1994, midwifery services would be paid for by the Ontario government. As Grier stated: "Now women in Ontario will be able to choose low-risk, high touch, low-tech care ... This profession will be a real partner to women in their childbearing years" (As cited in Sweet, *Toronto Star*, Oct 3, 1993, p. A3). Shortly thereafter, AOM members ratified the agreement worked out by their representatives with the Ministry by a vote of 82.5 per cent in favour (AOM Newsletter 9, no. 3, December 1993: 24). Despite this overwhelming vote of confidence, many midwives expressed concern with the rushed nature of the process. The following excerpt from the AOM newsletter (9, no. 3, December 1993) described the complaints made and the AOM's response: "Concerns were raised about the process. Some felt that the materials were not available soon enough to be read properly, digested and discussed. However, the framework document reflected the past two years of discussions in AOM committees, regional meetings and Annual General Meetings. Time was a major factor as the government had committed to funding by January '94 and the AOM pushed for funding by January 1, 1994. The priority has been to ensure funded midwifery for women and midwives as soon as possible" (24).

With the proclamation of the Midwifery Act, the LMCO established contracts with twenty-one practice groups including fifty-eight midwives. In looking back at the outcome of the funding negotiations, AOM representative Jane Kilthei described that the outcome "felt like a good beginning in acknowledging midwives as primary caregivers" (*The Gazette* 1, no. 2, December 1993: 4). Moreover, the model of midwifery practice was upheld throughout the establishment of the funding arrangement. Determination of case loads was cognizant of the principles of continuity of care and choice of birthplace. Perhaps it was because these standards were already written into the regulations of the Midwifery Act that they had such persuasive power with CHB representatives. Consumers' involvement in the setting up of the LMCO also helped maintain the consumer-oriented midwifery model.

Some physicians felt differently. One physician, for example, in a series of letters to the editor of the *Canadian Medical Association Journal* on the issue of the "cost of midwifery" stated: "In this day of hospital cutbacks and fee rollbacks, paying midwives a salary of $52,580 or more for normal deliveries is shocking and discriminatory toward all physicians. In Ontario family physicians and obstetricians receive $360 ($600 less 40 per cent for office overhead) for a normal delivery, whereas midwives receive about $1314 (40 births at a salary of $52,580). In addition, because two midwives must be present at every birth the cost is raised to $2629 per birth" (Dobkin 1994). Thus, despite the Task Force's intention to organize funding to prevent such comparisons between midwives "pay and physicians" fees, it inevitably ensued. In response to the issues raised in this and other letters, midwife Jane Kilthei (1994) responded:

Dr Dobkin makes the common mistake of dividing a midwife's salary by his or her caseload and comparing the result with a physician's fee-for-service earnings for pregnancy and childbirth, which is like comparing apples and oranges. A midwife carries out not only the primary care functions performed by the physician but also the education, counselling, support and monitoring functions commonly considered part of nursing care ... As for cost-effectiveness we know from studies in jurisdictions other than Ontario that rates of intervention are low in midwife-attended births, with no attendant increase in rates of perinatal mortality or morbidity. In Ontario the use of analgesia, anaesthesia and forceps as well as the rates of episiotomy and cesarean section – procedures that increase costs – have been found to be low in midwife-attended births. As well, midwives tend to order ultrasonography less often, bring women into hospital at a later stage of labour and discharge women sooner than most physicians. Midwife-attended home births provide the least expensive maternity care option. (516)

Mirroring Kilthei's comments, the Toronto Hospital officials were reported to hope to save money with midwifery by cutting the length of hospital stays because "[p]regnant women using midwives often stay at home during early labor and are discharged as early as 12 hours after delivery" (as cited in Brooke, J. Medical Post 30(5), 33).

In addition to the issue of cost effectiveness, there were other outstanding concerns, not the least of which related to the temporary nature of the centralized LMCO. Depending on the success of the LMCO's educational efforts, the challenges to the midwifery model may lie in the negotiated agreements with the new community-based transfer payment agencies. AOM representative Jane Kilthei described some of her concerns with the move of midwifery funding from the centralized LMCO to individual CHCS: "I am concerned about the move to local transfer payment agencies. I think one of the things we're going to face is another round of pressure to have midwives be employees ... A lot of the community health centres ... just have an employee model fixed in their mind and so I think that protecting the model as we move to local transfer payment agencies is going to be a challenge" (personal communication 1995). Kilthei further points out that the concern with the pressure toward an employee model (see also Giacomini and Peters 1996) may also be exacerbated by the lack of a centralized negotiation process: "And I think some of that too is we've got a lot of good clinical midwives out there; but some midwives are more able to negotiate and deal with a funding agency than others. And the nice thing about having a central agency is it's easy for the AOM to advocate around policy development and things like that. It will be much harder when we've got 50 different agencies in the province" (personal communication 1995). Kilthei's comments highlight the potential for the fragmentation of midwives' funding arrangements across several funding agencies. These concerns are exacerbated by the fact that given the level of funding midwives have negotiated, there may be some underlying uncertainties regarding whether midwifery care will in fact prove to be cost-effective. The standard funding agreement hammered out between the AOM and CHB may prove to be instrumental in preventing such fragmentation.

SUMMARY

The achievement of midwives in Ontario to secure public funding for their services was remarkable particularly compared with similar efforts in other jurisdictions. In some cases where direct-entry midwives have secured legislation in the United States, they have been less successful in garnering third party insurance coverage for their services, especially for home births (Hartley and Gasbarro 2001). But one need not look as far as the United States to compare these outcomes. Although midwives in the province of Alberta were successful in achieving legislation, this did not come with the benefit of public funding (James and Bourgeault 2004; McKendry and Langford 2000). Further, the form that funding has taken supports the midwifery model of practice is also a significant achievement. As Giacomini and Peters (1996) argue, "many stakeholders relate the model of payment to the legitimacy and autonomy of the midwifery profession, as well as its status relative to other professions such as medicine and nursing" (9). The level of funding that midwives negotiated and that state officials supported is also a strong indication of their professional status. It was definitely a far cry from the days when midwives barely made $20,000 a year and out of this had to pay their own expenses. Further, being funded through a different branch of the government than nursing and medicine is another source of professional autonomy (Giacomini and Peters 1996).

In those jurisdictions where public funding or coverage of services has been attained, the challenges to the model of care have been much more extensive. Funding for midwifery in Australia and the UK, for example, largely follows a staff as opposed to a primary care provider model. A salaried model – where midwives are paid through the Regional Health Authorities – was also implemented in Manitoba after the passage of its Midwifery Act in 1997 but the impact of this remains to be fully investigated. Further, in an examination of the relationship between payer source (self-pay, Medicaid, commercial insurance, and HMO) and practice of nurse-midwives in a hospital-based maternity service in the United States, Carr (1993) found that source significantly affected services provided. Fetal testing, for example, was higher in commercial and HMO groups than self-pay and Medicaid groups. Midwifery practice patterns and clinical decision-making are clearly influenced by reimbursement policies.

A recurring theme that is also salient in this achievement of midwives is the strong support for public funding on behalf of the state. One of the most salient indications of the strength of the support by government representatives was how various barriers were mediated in order to ensure public funding would concur with official integration. This is consistent with how other challenges to the model of practice and regulation were overcome with internal state support.

Over and above these important achievements, the funding arrangement not only poses future challenges, it represents a significant change from the time when clients paid midwives directly. Although this is definitely a positive change for consumers in that midwifery services are potentially available to more women,[10] the funding arrangement may also bring about some unexpected consequences. One of these is how the payment for midwifery services by a third party, the government, serves as yet another intermediary between a woman and her midwife. This, in addition to College standards and hospital policies, has the potential to diminish the client-centred focus of midwifery care by diffusing midwives' accountability. It is true that consumer representatives from the MTFO were involved in the implementation of public funding through the LMCO, but they were not necessarily part of the decision-making process for how midwives were to be funded. This was considered a professional issue. So too was the issue of how midwives should be best educated. It is this issue, perhaps more than the others, that reveals the greatest degree of professionalization and exclusionary social closure.

CHAPTER NINE

Educating Midwives
for Independence

Decisions regarding entry to practice issues, including the manner in which future midwives would be educated and trained and the grand-mothering in of current practitioners, would prove to be the most polit-ically contentious in the midwifery community throughout the entire integration process. In this chapter I address changes in the manner in which women learned to become midwives and the evolution of the model of midwifery education during the integration process. A shift occurred in the educational model from one in which women and their midwives learned from each other to a bureaucratically administered model producing professional experts. The recruitment of new midwives also changed from an experience-based, apprenticeship model to a more rigidly defined, university-based academic admission process. In the sub-sequent chapter I detail how this increased rigidity in the recruitment of midwives played out in the process of grandmothering currently practis-ing midwives into "legitimate" practice. Although a cadre of carefully selected "ambassadors" of the new midwifery profession would be cre-ated through the grandmothering process, it also would exclude some capable women from legally practising as midwives.

Although midwifery leaders had a significant influence on the state in the implementation of their model of midwifery education and the grand-mothering of midwives, their proposals represented a significant depar-ture from the original form of training and entry to midwifery practice and from the way some within the midwifery community wanted women to become qualified as midwives. These moves toward a more standard-ized and formalized educational model and recruitment process were largely a response to midwives' perception of what physicians and the state, through the HPLR, would deem acceptable. That is, controlling how midwives were trained and who could become midwives became important in achieving legitimacy through the enhancement of the professional image of midwifery. Ultimately, midwifery leaders proved to be accurate in their perception of what constituted an acceptable form of education. In exchange for the reshaping of their educational model, midwives secured significant state support for its implementation. The price paid for legitimacy through the education and integration programs, however, was substantial dissent within the midwifery community.

BECOMING A MIDWIFE PRIOR TO INTEGRATION

As suggested in chapter 4, midwives often entered into the practice of midwifery because of their experience with motherhood and home birth. Midwifery supporter and author Eleanor Barrington (1985) described the career path of early Canadian midwives:

Midwifery is typically a second career, a discovery of "right livelihood" that comes after post-secondary education, some other occupation, and usually parenthood ... An informal survey of a dozen practising midwives reveals a curious array of past lives: one actress, three nurses, two journalists, a teacher, an occupational therapist, a weaver, an x-ray technician, a massage therapist, and a bookkeeper. Clearly there is no prescribed career path into this profession. All that the midwives have in common is motherhood. The only prerequisites are life experience, quick intelligence, a giving personality, and a passion for birth. (41)

Just as midwives came from many different backgrounds, their work as midwives arose from many different circumstances. Many began as assistants to home birth physicians and were self-taught, often drawing on the assistance, expertise, and experience of others in study groups. Barrington (1985) describes how "some women moved gradually from prenatal teaching or women's self-health groups into the midwifery field, responding to the needs of those around them" (42).

The system of midwifery education was also varied. Often midwives learned midwifery from their clients; that is, they learned by doing. This experiential learning was supplemented with self-directed reading in reproductive health care. For example, midwifery supporter Jutta Mason (1990) notes, of a new midwife, that "to find out what she needed to know, she read books, talked to other women doing the same thing, and watched the labouring women." (1). Increasingly these birth attendants and "midwives" sought to improve their skills through apprenticeships with doctors, through correspondence courses, and generally through absorbing any information they could access: "The nature of midwifery training has been almost as variable as the motivations for it. Some simply learn by doing, others go abroad to earn foreign credentials. Apprenticeships to doctors or midwives, self-study and correspondence courses, conferences and workshops all fill some of the skills gaps" (Barrington 1985: 43). A few midwives also took the lay midwifery training available at Shari Daniels' El Paso Maternity Centre mentioned in chapter 4. Although the apprenticeship training here was more formalized, it did not lead to any recognized credential.

As the number of local midwives increased and had "developed a comprehensive base of experience" (Barrington 1985: 44), apprenticeships were sought with more experienced midwives. Barrington (1985) described the inherent flexibility of this apprentice-based approach: "It adapted to the needs of the community and the circumstances of the aspiring midwife. In rural districts an apprenticeship might last several years, because there are relatively few births to attend. In ... Toronto an apprentice might accumulate enough birth experience inside of one year" (44).

With the rise of more midwifery apprenticeships, this model of training became more formalized. Barrington (1985) described how Jane Kilthei's apprenticeship to midwife Theo Dawson in Toronto represented a usual case:

Over the course of a year, Jane accumulated 3,000 hours of clinical experience, including 50 births. For the first while, she followed Theo everywhere. Observing Jane's growing abilities, the senior midwife gradually assigned her tasks like postpartum visits and hospital labour coaching. Jane took Theo's nine-week course "The Art and Practice of Midwifery" and assisted with teaching prenatal classes. She earned her certification in cardiopulmonary resuscitation through the Red Cross. In addition, Theo asked her to begin a three-year "Apprentice Academics" midwifery study programme from the United States, a course which required critical reviews of 50 books on childbirth, and then moved through all the major obstetrical texts currently studied by medical students. ... Her apprenticeship ended at the pre-appointed time because she had seen and helped manage all the common complications of pregnancy and childbirth. Both she and Theo were confident in her abilities. Nevertheless, Theo, or another more experienced midwife, continued to attend all Jane's births for many months. (45)

Thus, although the model of midwifery care had begun in a varied, diverse, and unstandardized way, it was becoming more formalized.

These more "formal" apprenticeships were regarded by some as less accessible for some women over others, as indicated by the following comment in *Issue* (3, no. 2, Spring 1983) by Louise Norman: "Those training options that do exist are generally inaccessible to women outside a few urban centres – training options outside Ontario are generally accessible only to single women, or women who can afford to leave home for an extended period of time – numerous obstacles and difficulties such as finding a supportive doctor, or insufficient interest to fill prenatal classes discourage many potential midwives at an early stage" (7–8). Proponents of the apprenticeship model argued that these problems were not inherent to the model, but were due to the shortage of midwives (a problem they hoped would be ameliorated by integration). The model, they maintained, was fundamentally flexible and accessible. The apprenticeship model also helped to ensure a strong commitment on the part of the would-be midwife to the model of midwifery practice and principle of continuity of care, including being on-call: "Many women set out to become midwives and change their minds. The romantic allure of birthwork is rapidly offset by the exhausting hours and the emotional demands. Vicki Van Wagner began her apprenticeship along with five others. Within three months she was the only student left" (Barrington 1985: 50). Because of the advantages of this model, when contacted by the HPLR, the Midwifery Coalition argued that the apprenticeship model should somehow be integrated into any formal education program envisioned in Ontario.

DECIDING ON HOW TO EDUCATE MIDWIVES

From Apprenticeship to Clinical Internship –
Midwives' Submissions to the HPLR

The trend toward increased formalization of midwifery training proposals continued with the Midwifery Coalition's submission to the HPLR. Initial contact with the HPLR committee made it clear to the members of the Coalition that a standardized, formal education program would be a requirement for integration and self-regulatory status. Although Coalition members conceded that they would need to have a more formal system of educating midwives, they nevertheless strove to maintain the practical component of the apprenticeship model. The elements of such a program were proposed in the Coalition's first submission: "The effective practice of the midwifery profession depends on both specific and/ or advanced education. This education consists of both intensive theory and practical preparation ... The best way midwifery can be taught is by a formal recognized programme of education with ... a period of internship...integrated into the programme" (first submission to HPLR, December 1983: 10). The proposed program was to be three years long. To ensure that "educational standards [were] consistent with the principles of midwifery," the Midwifery Coalition members asserted that the "design of the course work should be the responsibility of the College or University and its faculty and approved by the governing body of the profession" (First Submission to HPLR, December 1983: 23).

In keeping with the spirit of the coalition of lay or practising midwives and nurse midwives, the Coalition also argued for multiple routes of entry to practice including "midwives who learn through formal programmes and through empirical experience" (Lenske 1984, *The Ontario Midwife* 1, no. 2: 6). In making this proposal for multiple routes of entry (direct-entry as well as through nursing), the Coalition had to debunk the contention that prior nursing training was necessary for midwifery training: "Training and practice in either nursing or medicine alone does not prepare one for midwifery practice. Midwifery cannot be adequately learned as a short post-graduate training programme developed for a nurse or doctor. Midwifery cannot be a specialty of nursing or medicine. The basic philosophies and approaches of these professions are too diverse" (first submission to HPLR, December 1983: 6). At the same time, however, Coalition members stated that a formal training program for midwifery would include "a basic nursing component" (first submission to HPLR, December 1983: 22).

Thus, in this initial educational proposal of the Midwifery Coalition to the HPLR, the direction toward increased formalization of midwifery education and training was forged. This direction was further reinforced in the consultations between the Midwifery Coalition and the nursing and medical professions following the submission. Given this strong push for "formal" education by the HPLR, midwives felt it politically necessary to accept it at an early stage in the HPLR discussions. This they hoped would increase their chances of being taken seriously and enhance their case for integration.

This increased formalization of the proposed midwifery training program resulted in considerable concern within the midwifery community. Some midwives and midwifery supporters felt that a pure apprenticeship model should be maintained. They argued that this model would "ensure the art, as well as the science of midwifery is taught, and would enable student or apprentice midwives to remain in their own communities during training" (TFIMO 1987: 124). Midwifery Coalition members agreed with these assertions but felt that such a proposal would not be regarded positively by the HPLR. They felt that a formal program would be a necessity for integration, and that midwives should focus their efforts on formulating a program that integrated the apprenticeship model as much as possible.

By the time of the third submission to the HPLR, the Midwifery Coalition (now the AOM) had formulated an even more detailed proposal for a midwifery education program. First, in response to queries by the HPLR Committee, they argued that there was a strong desire on the part of midwives for a standardized educational program: "Midwives have in these ways attempted to overcome the lack of available midwifery education in Ontario, but since the 1970s with the inception of the Ontario Association of Midwives they have indicated a desire for standardized education" (third submission to the HPLR, October 1985: 36). In line with this desire for standardization, the AOM consulted with local "midwives, apprentices, teachers, a nurse and a doctor" (AOM Newsletter 1, no. 2, September 1985: 33), and additionally reviewed "models of international midwifery programmes" (AOM Newsletter 1, no. 2, September 1985: 15). Based on this research, the AOM's Education Committee "identified aspects of existing programmes which should be integrated into midwifery education in this province" (third submission to the HPLR, October 1985: 37). It recommended: "A four year degree programme, leading to a Bachelor of Science in Midwifery degree (BScM) ... completed in three calendar years; an emphasis on immediate and ongoing clinical experience under supervision; direct entry to midwifery education; and admission policies allowing for a variety of educational backgrounds" (37).

It was through this emphasis on "ongoing clinical experience under supervision" that the AOM intended to build the apprenticeship model into its proposed program. It argued strongly that "the great strength of self-directed midwifery education has been preceptorship," and that "a formal educational programme must include the benefits of preceptorship" (third submission to the HPLR, October 1985: 38). This "apprenticeship" was proposed to take the following form: "Clinical experience will be integrated throughout the three years of the programme ... Each student must work with at least three preceptors approved by the school as clinical instructors, of whom at least two must be practising midwives. During these preceptorships the student will be involved in the documented continuous care of 50 clients throughout the maternity cycle" (third submission to the HPLR, October 1985: 40). In addition to this

clinical component, the AOM's proposed curriculum also included a
theoretical component which would include instruction in midwifery
skills (pregnancy, labour and birth, postpartum, childbirth education, and
detecting obstetric pathology), as well as anatomy and physiology, general physical assessment, embryology and genetics, chemistry, pharma-
cology, gynecology and family planning, pediatrics, nutrition, psychology
and counselling, sexuality, sociology of health care, statistics and epide-
miology, and laboratory techniques.

The admissions requirements proposed for the program were intended
to ensure that all women with the prerequisite education (then grade 13
or OAC) would be eligible for admission. It was further recommended
that the program begin small, working up to full operation within three
years.

Not only did the proposed program include the core components of
the apprenticeship model, it was asserted that "a future midwifery education programme must be based on the application of a midwifery
model" (third submission to the HPLR, October 1985: 37). In order to support the model of practice, the AOM prepared a statement of philosophy
for the proposed midwifery school which endorsed the international definition of a midwife and supported the principles of normal birth, choice
of birth place, continuity of care, accessibility and informed choice:

The School believes that midwives should be responsible for normal deliveries
on her own responsibility ... (and the programme will be oriented to normal
birth) ... She may practice in hospitals, health units, or domiciliary services ...
The School believes that midwives should be primary contact professionals who
will provide continuous care throughout pregnancy, labour, delivery, and the
postpartum period ... The School will accept students from a variety of backgrounds and experience and supports access to health education for people in
isolated communities. ... The School will support the right of parents to actively
participate in their birth experience. A midwife's training will enable her to facilitate the decision-making process and to respond effectively to the individual
choices made. (third submission to the HPLR, October 1985: 40–1)

The AOM's proposal also included a list of "key competencies" that
successful midwifery students must possess. These included the abilities
to "act as a teacher and counsellor to the mother and/or family during
the childbearing year and facilitate client's decision-making, ... demonstrate professional values in all aspects of midwifery, ... [and] function
in a collegial relationship with other members of the professional health

care team" (third submission to the HPLR, October 1985: 41). Thus, although the educational program was intended to foster informed choice, these key competencies suggest a greater degree of professionalization and hierarchy vis-à-vis clients than originally envisaged under the principle of informed choice.

This proposed program was a far cry from the early years of self-motivated and self-directed midwifery training. Again, the formality and standardization of the program was regarded by midwifery leaders as necessary to secure legitimacy as primary practitioners in the eyes of the public and other health care professionals: "In Ontario public trust in midwifery care would be fostered by a consistent standard of university education leading to the BSCM" (third submission to the HPLR, October 1985: 37). Midwife Vicki Van Wagner also highlighted the necessity of adequate training for midwives to be primary caregivers and for compliance with international standards: "As primary care givers and 'integral' members of the health care team, midwives must have adequate training to prepare for this role. In order to meet international standards, it may be necessary to implement midwifery training at a university level" (*Issue* 9, October 1985: 14).

The AOM also argued that a degree-based program would enable midwives to continue on in graduate work in midwifery research. This would prevent a midwifery training programme from becoming a "ghetto" affording graduates little flexibility for further education. Potential continuation into graduate programmes would also foster development of a knowledge base for midwifery through midwifery research, rather than it being based solely on medical (i.e., obstetrical) and nursing research: "The university environment allows the development of graduate programmes in midwifery, with advanced level research. Such research would have practical application to midwifery practice and would raise the standards of care in midwifery" (third submission to the HPLR, October 1985: 3). The midwifery educational programme outlined above formed the basis of the AOM's submission to the HPLR as well as to the Task Force on the Implementation of Midwifery in Ontario struck in early 1986.

Task Force on the Implementation of Midwifery in Ontario

As noted in chapter 6, one of the mandates of the Task Force was to make recommendations to the Minister of Health regarding "how midwives should be educated" (Hansard 1986: 3373). In order to make these recommendations, the Task Force had to gather information from several sources. This included consultations with local stakeholder groups, through formal written submissions and public hearings, and consultation with international experts on midwifery education.

In its submission to the Task Force, the AOM largely reiterated its third submission to the HPLR. It outlined a midwifery educational program with the following elements: "A four year degree programme completed in three calendar years; emphasis on immediate and ongoing clinical experience under supervision; direct entry to midwifery education; and admission programmes allowing for a variety of educational backgrounds; access to education for people in isolated communities; and standards for continuing education" (AOM Submission to Task Force, September 1986: 18). The importance of apprenticeship or preceptorship for midwifery education was again emphasized in this submission.

Anticipating that the Task Force might recommend nursing as a prerequisite for midwifery, the AOM made a strong case for the direct-entry training option: "It must be emphasized that midwifery has its own philosophy, process and scope of practice. According to international experts and midwifery organizations, direct entry training programmes are an important means of preserving distinct qualities of midwifery education and practice" (AOM Submission to Task Force, September 1986: 19). To support the direct-entry option, the AOM argued that, among other positive features, it was cost-effective "because [it prepares] competent practitioners without first requiring training and proficiency in another profession" (AOM Submission to Task Force, September 1986: 21). Prior nursing education, it was argued, would "needlessly extend the cost and duration of midwives' education" given that "much of nursing preparation is not relevant to midwifery" (TFIMO 1987: 121). Both consumer and women's groups strongly endorsed the AOM's education proposals. MTFO chapter groups specifically argued that if nursing training was required as a prerequisite for midwifery, consumers would continue to seek out non-nurse midwives in Ontario.

The AOM also elaborated on the "phasing-in" of the educational program it outlined in its third submission to the HPLR. This involved first assessing the present level of clinical skills and the educational needs of practising and foreign trained midwives; upgrading and standardizing these skills according to international midwifery education standards; employing these upgraded midwives as teachers, clinical instructors, and preceptors for initial midwifery education programs; and concurrently generating curriculum recommendations for future midwifery education programs (AOM Submission to Task Force, September 1986: 22). Proposing that currently practising midwives become part of the educational program was a measure to help ensure the continuation of the model of midwifery care. The AOM also stipulated that "ideally, all midwifery educators would also be in current practice" (AOM Submission to Task Force, September 1986: 19). This was suggested because "currently practising midwives felt that many of their practices and policies had been handed down by other midwives and that no other profession could adequately teach these aspects of midwifery" (TFIMO 1987: 251). To help implement this phasing-in plan, the AOM recommended that the ministers of Health and Education, in conjunction with the provisional governing body, appoint a midwifery educator as program director to oversee the process.

The AOM submission also made provisions for ensuring the accessibility of midwifery education to women from remote areas of the province. These included giving these women "priority access to educational opportunities" and providing "educational equivalencies through alternate educational structures" limiting the amount of time they would need to spend at university centres (AOM Submission to Task Force, September 1986: 21).

The Task Force also received submissions from the medical and nursing professions and hospitals regarding the education of midwives. Submissions from several medical organizations indicated that formal, direct-entry education based at either a college or university was acceptable, as long as it was based on international standards. Following the nursing profession's assertion that midwifery was a specialty of nursing, the CNO, RNAO, and ONA all argued that nursing education should be a prerequisite to midwifery education. They argued that integrating midwifery education programs within existing faculties of nursing would save the costs of establishing a completely separate program. The RNAO also argued that midwifery education should be either at the baccalaureate or the post-graduate level. Most hospitals (97 per cent) surveyed by the OHA also felt that midwives should have prior nursing training. The OHA, however, concluded that since many countries do not require this, it would be open to the possibility of direct-entry education for midwives. The issue for many hospitals was not whether a midwife was a nurse but "whether she was qualified, competent and adequately prepared" (TFIMO 1987: 236). Most hospitals indicated their preference for a university-based education program.

From their international consultations, the Task Force found that in Europe there is little distinction made between midwives who have prior nursing training and those who do not. They concluded that their international survey "indicated that there is no universally held view in the developed world that only nurses should become midwives" and in fact "there is a drive to increase the number of direct entry programs." (TFIMO 1987: 119). From these sources of information, the Task Force identified two potential models of midwifery education: "One model requires every person who wishes to study midwifery to obtain an education in nursing first. The other model permits a person to study midwifery without prior education in nursing" (TFIMO 1987: 119). In deciding between these two models the Task Force argued that the decision was, in fact, about whether or not nursing should have a monopoly over midwifery. TFIMO member Karyn Kaufman – who had both nursing and midwifery training – recalled how the decisions regarding midwifery education were the most difficult for the Task Force to make: "I think on the whole, probably the only areas where there was ever a lot of discussion was around educational programmes. And we struggled and struggled with the whole idea of how to accommodate the variety of backgrounds of women that we knew would probably be interested in a midwifery programme" (personal communication 1995).

In the end, the Task Force recommended that "there be multiple routes of entry to midwifery education in Ontario" (TFIMO 1987: 121). These multiple routes would include: 1) a four-year direct-entry stream leading to a baccalaureate degree in midwifery; and 2) a twelve- to eighteen-month diploma stream for those applicants who have university-level preparation in nursing (TFIMO 1987: 123). Midwives taught in either stream would practise according to the same scope of *practice*. Part of the reason given for deciding on multiple routes of entry was related to accessibility:

A vocation for midwifery sometimes develops when a woman has children of her own, or becomes involved in childbirth education. Immigrant women may have functioned as birth attendants in the countries from which they have come. It is difficult enough for mature women, especially those with children, to qualify for a new profession, without having, in effect to qualify for two. Mandatory nursing education would only deflect them into what many of them might view as an irrelevant educational experience. We think that multiple routes of entry will make midwifery education accessible to a considerably wider group of potential aspirants. (TFIMO 1987: 122)

The Task Force also argued that restricting entry to nurses would not yield "significant cost advantages over the long term" (TFIMO 1987: 123). Its most compelling reasons for not limiting midwifery to nurses was to prevent the development of an unregulated, underground profession of midwives with no enforceable standards of practice: "It is precisely to safeguard the public by ensuring that all midwives are properly prepared and that they practise in accordance with high standards, that the Government of Ontario has decided to recognize and regulate the profession. Its objective could well be defeated if only nurses are permitted to become midwives" (TFIMO 1987: 123).

Given the Task Force recommendation that midwifery education should be at the baccalaureate level, the implication was that the program would be limited to degree-granting institutions. The Task Force argued that apprenticeship alone was not a "realistic option for Ontario given the predominance of university and college-based education for the health disciplines" (TFIMO 1987: 124). It added that "apprentice-educated midwives would not gain acceptance with hospitals or other health professionals" (TFIMO 1987: 124) and that a university-based education was critically important for midwives' legitimacy: "Midwifery, as a new profession in Ontario, must gain the trust of consumers and other health professionals. Physicians and nurses must regard midwives as colleagues and peers, and they must be willing to trust their clinical judgment. We believe both consumers and other health professionals may have a more positive attitude toward midwives whose educational preparation is at the university level" (TFIMO 1987: 125). TFIMO member Karyn Kaufman emphasized that "if we really expected that midwives would have a place in this spectrum of health professions, it was pretty difficult to see how you could confer professional autonomy, hospital privileges ... to people without a university degree, given the North American penchant for educational credentials" (personal communication 1995). In addition, the Task Force argued, as the AOM had previously done, that a baccalaureate program enabled the possibility of graduate studies in midwifery research and the development of midwifery-based knowledge:

The other thing that we wanted to accomplish was we wanted to have a programme that would give people access to further graduate study. Because we always believed that a programme, a profession that wasn't always sort of self-consciously reflecting and researching about its own work would not really be able to go anywhere. We want to be able to provide the basis for generating its own cadre of researchers who had researched the pregnancy and birth experience from a midwifery perspective, so that midwifery was not always having to cope with the research of nurses and doctors, which would be done from their own point of view. (Mary Eberts, personal communication 1995)

Beyond just being university-based, the Task Force also recommended that a midwifery education program should be located at one of Ontario's health science centres. This was recommended in order to encourage "contact among midwifery, medical and nursing students" which would "facilitate the integration of midwifery into the health care system" (TFIMO 1987: 125).

Understanding that its recommendations for the midwifery education program might limit the accessibility of midwifery education to some segments of the population, the Task Force recommended that provisions be made for midwifery students from the north and those with franco-phone backgrounds. In addition, the Task Force made an argument that experience should play a vital role in the program admission process: "The Task Force recommends that selection of students not be based solely on academic achievement and that procedures include assessment of applicants' personal suitability for midwifery, including their maturity, motivation, resourcefulness, service orientation and ability to relate to others. We recommend that admission to the baccalaureate component be considered for students who can demonstrate that their life experience (including work, homemaking, childrearing, and volunteer activities) qualifies them for entry" (TFIMO 1987: 127).

With respect to the curriculum for the new midwifery program, the Task Force recommended that the first two years of the program focus on sub-jects in the humanities, social sciences, basic sciences, and health sciences. The following two years would focus on midwifery practice subjects and clinical education. This organization of courses would more easily enable nurses with advanced standing to upgrade to midwifery by sharing third and fourth year courses with the direct-entry students. Requirements for graduation were to be developed by the governing body for midwifery to address "numbers of clinical experiences, including examinations, super-vision and care of pregnant women, deliveries, postpartum examinations, and newborn examinations" (TFIMO 1987: 130).

The Task Force also recommended that the government provide funding for the development of the midwifery education program and that it "select a centre through a competitive tendering process open to all health sciences centres" (TFIMO 1987: 127). Criteria for selection recommended by the Task Force included accessibility to northern and francophone students, accessibility to clinical education sites in hospital and community settings, and integration of midwifery, nursing, and medical faculties and students.

Given that these recommendations strongly resembled the AOM's proposals, they were viewed quite favourably by midwives. The AOM strongly supported the Task Force's "position that midwifery education should not be limited to nurses only (AOM newsletter 3, no. 4, December 1987: 16). There were, however, some concerns within the AOM that the multiple routes of entry to midwifery practice would create two classes of midwives, that is, that the program for nurses would be significantly different than that for non-nurses.

There were also continuing concerns among a small but growing number of midwives and supporters about the recommendation for a baccalaureate program. Although the AOM had proposed to the HPLR that midwifery education should be standardized and formalized as a baccalaureate degree program, some members of the midwifery community wanted to maintain the local apprenticeship-based programs. One midwife described the intraprofessional dynamics between the AOM executive, largely based in Toronto, and midwives outside Toronto regarding important decisions such as the education program proposals:

The AOM sends out a rep. from Toronto to tell the people in the area that ... they are consulting. Then the people here say what they want and the rep. from Toronto says, "This is why you shouldn't think that way because the government wouldn't like it. This is the way we should think instead." Then they think that they've got everybody in the area convinced that that's the best way to do it, and often the people from Toronto ... leave assuming that they convinced the outer group to think that way, and they go home back to Toronto and say basically to the people in Toronto, "It's okay, we've got them under hand now." And after they've gone back to Toronto, that's when the women up north or back east start to realize that they weren't ever really convinced. (personal communication 1995)

Midwives less active in the AOM continued to believe that apprentice-based programs would be more accessible and more supportive of midwifery philosophy. TFIMO member Karyn Kaufman described the overall view of this group of midwives: "I think there's always been a group who felt that any kind of formal education was a violation of the fundamental precepts of midwifery; that it's the one-to-one, it's the informal basis, that the minute you institutionalize it you lose it" (personal communication

1995). Although the arguments of this group of midwives were not fully developed at this point, they were to become more fully articulated with the continued conceptualization of an increasingly formalized and standardized midwifery education program.

Evolution of AOM Education Program Proposals after the Task Force

Following the Task Force report, the AOM came to realize the importance of education policy in the integration process: "The Education Committee will become increasingly important as legislation and integration into the health care system draws closer. It is crucial that we develop our own ideas about the education of midwives so that we can influence government decisions which will directly affect us and future midwifery practice in the province" (AOM newsletter 4, no. 3, September 1988: 6). The form of midwifery education was highlighted as having an important influence on the philosophy and model of midwifery care. The AOM felt that it was important for midwives to have a strong influence on the process of developing midwifery education in order to protect its ideal midwifery model: "As always, it is probably better for us as midwives to determine what the essentials of education are rather than to have someone else do it for us!" (AOM newsletter 4, no. 3, September 1988: 6, emphasis in original).

One focus of the AOM was the development of core competencies, that is, a "list of midwifery skills, behaviours and fundamental knowledge, which might be expected of a beginning graduate practitioner" (AOM newsletter 4, no. 3, September 1988: 6). This list addressed general components of midwifery care, education and counselling, collaboration with other caregivers, antepartum care, intrapartum care, postpartum care of the newborn and mother, sexuality and gynecology, and professional/ legal aspects of midwifery care. Under general components of midwifery care, for example, core competencies included 1) providing care focused on the woman and her family; 2) promoting normal birth and appropriate use of technology; 3) providing care in a variety of settings, including home, birth centre and hospital; 4) providing care consistent with the philosophy of midwifery care in Ontario; 5) providing continuity of care over the childbearing cycle; and 6) facilitating informed choice (AOM Core Competencies, September 1990: 2). In developing core competencies, the AOM intended to provide a foundation for a midwifery education program that would sustain the midwifery model of practice: "The AOM remains committed to: continuity of care, community care, and choice of birthplace ... Our current struggles over issues of midwifery education all relate back to these essentials" (Kilthei, AOM Newsletter 5, no. 1, April 1989: 26–7). The AOM also began to expand on the curriculum that it had developed in its previous submissions to the HPLR and Task Force to reflect these core competencies and the model of midwifery care.

Concurrent with these conceptual developments, the AOM was becoming increasingly concerned with what they perceived to be a lack of action on the part of the Ministry of Health and the Ministry of Colleges and Universities to embark on the integration process. In response to this concern, the AOM prepared a brief addressing issues in midwifery education and distributed it to representatives of these Ministries. This brief essentially contained all the writings of the AOM on educational issues from the HPLR and Task Force and included the list of core competencies it had developed. The AOM hoped that presenting this brief would spark some activity within the Ministries.

This strategy proved to be successful and subsequently in the fall of 1988 the newly appointed Midwifery Coordinator, Karyn Kaufman, began to discuss the establishment of a midwifery education program with the Michener Institute for Applied Health Sciences. The Michener was a post-secondary educational institution funded entirely by the Ministry of Health to provide health science courses and programs (e.g., for radiation therapists and chiropodists) to meet the needs of the health care system (*The Gazette* 3, no. 1, May 1992: 1). Kaufman stated that the decision to work with the Michener Institute was made by then-Minister Elinor Caplan: "You're looking at Ministers who say, 'Look, we provide that group with money, we like what they do, so get them involved.' ... There are some things Ministers just tell you to do" (personal communication 1995). Caplan viewed the Michener as an appropriate site for midwifery education. She had expressed concerns regarding the recommendation to have midwifery education at the baccalaureate level because she wanted to avoid the rising credentialism that plagued many health care occupations: "My own view was that there tends to be an over-credentialization in the delivery of health services and I was not so much concerned about whether or not it was a university degree granting, I was more concerned with were we going to have people who were properly and well-trained to be able to meet the needs of women in Ontario" (Elinor Caplan, personal communication 1995). Task Force members such as Rachel Edney felt that the Minister and the government were also concerned with the costs of implementing a baccalaureate program, which were much higher than they would be for a community college program: "There was some concern from the government that it would be cheaper to put it into a non-university programme from the government's point of view" (Rachel Edney, personal communication 1995). Whatever the reasons, Kaufman and the executive director of the Michener Institute, Diana Schatz, began to discuss the development of a midwifery curriculum development project.

The decision to situate a midwifery education project at the Michener was initially regarded with apprehension by the AOM and by several key midwifery supporters because of their commitment to a baccalaureate program. They specifically expressed concern that a program at the Michener Institute would not "prepare a midwife who will be accepted as a primary caregiver [and]…would ensure that midwives will have an education that will provide access to graduate education and the ability to participate in research, policy and education" (AOM newsletter 5, no. 1, April 1989: 11). The AOM emphasized these concerns in a meeting with the Minister of Health: "In our meeting with Elinor Caplan, we stressed the importance of education, research and administration as part of a basic midwifery programme. She agreed that this would be desirable and possible through [the Michener Institute]" (AOM newsletter 5, no. 2, October 1989: 5). The Minister's affirmation of the midwives' concerns, in addition to the recognition that the Michener "offered more possibilities for AOM input and community practice" encouraged the AOM to "support the establishment of a midwifery school in this institution" (AOM newsletter 5, no. 2, October 1989: 5). AOM representatives also highlighted the Michener Institute's "emphasis on clinical education, flexible entry requirements, distance learning, and experience in establishing clinical sites for education and practice in community-based hospitals" (AOM annual report, June 1989: 9–10). In May 1989, Minister of Health Elinor Caplan announced the development of the Curriculum Design Committee to be headed by Diana Schatz, Executive Director of the Michener Institute.

The Curriculum Design Committee

The Curriculum Design Committee (CDC) was a multi-disciplinary committee coordinated by midwife Holliday Tyson, including twelve members – from medicine (obstetrician Henry Muggah, family physician Anthony Reid), nursing (professor Ellen Hodnett, Margo Kowalchuk, and nurse-midwife Helen McDonald), consumers (Monique Charron, Robert Couchman, MTFO president Michelle Lahay), and for the first time in an official capacity, midwifery (practising midwives Elizabeth Allemang, Eileen Hutton, Leslie Shear and Vicki Van Wagner). Four representatives from the Ministry of Health and the Ministry of Colleges and Universities also sat on the committee ex officio. Two members of the IRCM, Winifred Hunsburger and Catherine Oliver, acted as liaison between it and the CDC.

The mandate of the CDC was to "describe in detail the essential components of midwifery education in Ontario" (CDC Report 1990: 16) including program length and composition, didactic and clinical content, clinical requirements, academic structure, faculty, and site. The work of the CDC was to take six months and consisted of gathering information about midwifery education in European, British, and American settings, and inviting written submissions and oral presentations from "approximately 100 health profession educators, practitioners, interest groups and consumers about the essential components of midwifery education in Ontario" (CDC Report, May 1990: 5). Tyson recalled that the CDC asked people to direct their submissions so as to answer "what do you think midwifery education should look like; what do you want, and not want; and what should a midwife look like at the end of the day?" (personal communication 1995).

In the submissions, Tyson recalled a sense of convergence from different groups about how midwives should be educated:

There was certainly a convergence toward what people thought a midwife should be and should be able to do. People wanted someone who was well-rounded, able to have admitting privileges, able to work easily with physicians and nurses as well as clients, able to move back and forth between home and hospital setting with some comfort, someone who was able to understand consultation-transfer mechanisms, be safe, and to be an independent practitioner. All those things everyone generally agreed on, ... such as a midwife needs to have some sciences but not a lot of sciences. "Don't keep them too long in the classroom." That's a major problem when you keep them in the classroom and they are not adequately prepared for the reality of the clinical life. There was remarkable convergence. (personal communication 1995)

What proved controversial was *where* midwives should be educated. CDC Coordinator Tyson described this as "the single biggest debate during the life of the CDC ... that people were violently split on" (personal communication 1995). Submissions from medical and nursing groups strongly asserted that midwives should be educated in a university setting: "The vast majority of doctors and nurses said midwives should be educated in university. 'That's the only place to be, there is no question about it. It is the only place you can have a good education, and besides all doctors are trained in universities, and nursing is already going that way. If you don't put them in universities, you will be trying five years later to put them into university. Don't make the mistake nursing made'" (Tyson, personal communication 1995). Other arguments for a university-based education addressed midwives' ability to do research and to secure hospital admitting privileges.

Arguments against implementing a university-based midwifery education program were brought to the CDC by several individual midwives and consumers, as well as organizations that they had developed, including the Coalition of Ontario Midwifery Birth Schools (COMBS), and Students Organizing for Midwifery Education (SOME). As highlighted previously, several midwives and their supporters were concerned with the AOM's proposals for a formal degree program. By the time the CDC had begun, many of their arguments in opposition to university-based midwifery education became crystallized.

The Coalition of Ontario Midwifery Birth Schools (COMBS), which represented a networking group of community-based "schools" for midwifery (in Ottawa, Kingston, Cornwall, North Bay, and Windsor) and who promoted a regional-based, self-directed apprenticeship approach to midwifery education, emphatically stated in its presentation to the CDC that:

We believe that many educational systems have come and gone for midwives but the one that has been tested, over and over again, for centuries, is the system of apprenticeship ... We understand that it has been suggested that a "part" of our curriculum in the future in Ontario be apprenticeship. Yet apprenticeship to some of us is a whole learning style, an entire attitude and approach, not part of a curriculum. It is an entire outlook on one's educational process and the crucial factor is that it is completely self-directed ... It is a self-directed and self-motivated learning process requiring the student to be able to perceive and choose the best way to acquire and retain core competencies. It trains one in useful principles by which decision-making can be carried out. It is by nature a personalized learning process which helps one to teach in a personalized way and respect each person for their unique way of approaching their pregnancy and birth. (3–4)

Thus, making apprenticeship part of a university-based program, as the AOM suggested, would mean that the fundamental component of apprenticeship – individualized, self-directed training – would be lost.

The submission presented by the Students Organizing for Midwifery Education (SOME) also supported apprenticeship training for midwifery based on its philosophical compatibility with the midwifery model of care. They argued "how can we be advocates for women's choices in childbirth if we haven't the courage to exercise choice around where, how and by whom we will be taught?" (Monk 1989, Submission to the CDC, Midwifery Education: An Alternative Approach: 9). They emphasized the importance of the emotional aspects of midwifery which might be suppressed in a didactic academic program: "Classroom learning is notorious ... for depressing the feeling and spiritual dimension, making it suitable only for the passing on of "cold" information – anatomy ... and so on. Feelings must not be depressed in the educational environment of student midwives. Lack of feeling and emotional support is what drives many local women to midwives in the first place. If we simply repeat this medical training pattern we replicate all the problems associated with allopathic practitioners, creating "medical midwives" (Monk 1989: 3).

Both COMBS and SOME attempted to debunk the thesis that a formal training program produced more competent midwives: "The idea that an intensive three-year period of institutional technical training based primarily upon the medical student/internship model guarantees superior maternal health care is an unwarranted assumption ... What does seem to be the case is that traditional apprenticeship, in most instances coupled with conscientious, ongoing, self-directed study, yields community midwives with skills and statistics at the very least on par with their 'professionally' trained peers" (Monk 1989: 1). The COMBS submission asserted that "credentialling ... improves credibility not competency" (3).

These groups also argued that a university-based education was inaccessible to many women, especially those interested in midwifery (older, often with children, etc). As an alternative, COMBS proposed having midwifery education in existing regional schools as opposed to establishing it in a large university: "We were trying to get them to recognize schools that already existed ... and that they make use of the schools that were scattered around the province ... If you are going to start a profession from the grass roots up you start at where these midwives in these various communities are starting; you use their workshops and their spaces rather than start an institution and not make use of any of this incredible community workup that's happened" (Midwife Betty-Anne Davis, personal communication 1995). Ultimately COMBS and SOME realized that "a lot of the decisions had already been made" and that "the whole notion of apprenticeship was sinking at the time" but they nevertheless felt it important to point out that they "didn't necessarily like the decisions they were making" (Midwife Betty-Anne Davis, personal communication 1995).

The AOM's submission largely reiterated its earlier position statements to the HPLR and Task Force. Although the midwifery leaders in the AOM had previously recommended a baccalaureate program for midwifery education, they too expressed concerns with accessibility. These midwives ultimately came to the position that "although a degree was desirable for several reasons, including accessibility to graduate education and credibility with the public and other health professionals, it was not absolutely necessary; the philosophy, design and content of the program were seen as paramount" (AOM Newsletter 6, no. 2, August 1990: 14).

The CDC produced its report to the Minister of Health and Minister of Colleges and Universities on May 30, 1990.[1] It recommended a "baccalaureate degree as the appropriate credential for midwifery education in Ontario" (CDC Report 1990: 14). CDC midwife representative Vicki Van Wagner described how a university degree program was regarded as necessary to earn respect, a fact that was a major factor behind the recommendation:

We didn't think you achieved power simply from having a university degree; the situation is more complex than that. We did not agree with the argument that we had to have a baccalaureate degree to be a good midwife ... But in the end it was the physicians and nurses on the CDC who said, "The bottom line is without a degree it is going to be a struggle for midwives; you will not get the day-to-day respect, not get into graduate school, you will not get acceptance within the system given the big push for baccalaureate nurses. The whole myth about midwives is that you are uneducated, and given that you're looking to be the colleagues of medicine and nursing, you need a degree. Without a degree you are not going to get the autonomy that you're asking for." In the end, we became convinced that in terms of the way we think about professions in our society, the degree of power in the health care system that midwives were asking for in order to support women's choices, we needed university education. (personal communication 1995)

An important corollary to this argument addressed the necessity that midwives secure hospital admitting privileges to practise according to the principle of choice of birth place: "The input we got from people in hospitals was, 'Don't try to get admitting privileges if you don't have a university-prepared person'" (Holliday Tyson, personal communication 1995). Maintaining the model of care, especially choice of birth place, was considered "more important than haggling over university/non-university" (Vicki Van Wagner, personal communication 1995) and the AOM in the end "expressed [its] support for the CDC recommendation of a degree-granting programme in order to give midwives access to graduate level education, and to enhance midwives' interprofessional relationships and their opportunity to gain hospital privileges" (AOM Newsletter 6, no. 3, November 1990: 11).

Although it was decided to situate the midwifery education program in a university, the CDC wanted to integrate as much of the apprenticeship approach as possible. It recommended that a clinical as well as a theoretical component be integrated into a four-year program (which could be completed in three calendar years). Topics for the theoretical component included basic sciences, health sciences, health education and promotion, professional studies of midwifery, social sciences, education and research, and alternative health care practices. At least half the program would include clinical practice experience with a practising midwife at home births and hospital births. During this clinical experience, the student would be required to attend sixty births, forty of these as primary caregiver and thirty within a program of continuity of care.

To guide the development of the curriculum for the midwifery education program, the CDC developed a list of "guiding principles" which formed the philosophical framework of midwifery education. These largely reflected the core principles of the model of midwifery practice, which included primary care, informed choice, normal birth, woman-centred care, continuity of care, and choice of birth place. The CDC was also guided by the list of core competencies, originally developed by the AOM and later revised by the IRCM.

The midwifery education program designed by the CDC was to meet the needs of aspiring midwives with no previous health profession training as well as those with training in related health care backgrounds (who might qualify for advanced standing). Although part of the CDC's mandate was to also address the needs of applicants with prior midwifery experience, it felt that this was too large a task to be able to address in its six-month term. It did, however, create parameters around which such an integration program should be designed and recommended that "immediate attention be given to more detailed planning of the integration program" (see discussion in the following chapter on the integration of midwives).

The CDC thus decided that a middle ground for a midwifery education program would be sought – a baccalaureate program with a large apprentice-based component including a flexible format, immediate hands-on experience, and mentorship. But the CDC was only an advisory committee. Its recommendations continued to be challenged by the government over concerns that a university-based program would be too expensive:

Within the Ministry we ran into opposition from fairly senior level people who said "It's too expensive. We don't want to do that. Put it in the Community College. This just isn't worth it." And we actually argued from the perspective of the profession, and I think the consumer group at that point as well, that that was really going to disadvantage midwives; that you would be, I think, putting them into a non-credible position vis à vis other health professions ... And it was a long uphill climb, but we finally through Health, through the Ministry of Colleges and Universities as a joint Cabinet submission got it approved. (Karyn Kaufman, personal communication 1995)

The CDC ultimately managed to convince government representatives that in order to have midwifery implemented in the manner the government wanted, midwives would have to have a university-based education. On October 15, 1991, it was officially announced jointly by the new NDP Minister of Colleges and Universities, Richard Allen, and the Minister of Health, Frances Lankin, that Ontario would establish the first university degree program in Canada for midwives. Ontario universities were subsequently invited to develop proposals to include a bachelor's degree program in midwifery in their curricula.

Establishing the Baccalaureate Program[2]

Once government approval of the CDC recommendations was given, the selection of the university or universities to house the baccalaureate program proved yet another challenge to the model. To help maintain the education model, the CDC had developed a list of criteria from which a university's proposal for a midwifery education program could be assessed. These criteria addressed the need for flexibility of access to the program, a separate, autonomous academic structure open to input from practising midwives, flexible arrangements in the appointment of academic staff so that instructors could continue to practise, and access to graduate studies and research initiatives. AOM representative on the site selection process Michelle Kryzanauskas described the reasoning behind these criteria:

The request for proposals included things like the expectation around the model of practice, what we thought was necessary for the clinical component, access in relation to the French bilingual commitment and also aboriginal issues ... We also needed to know that whatever sites were going to have the programme were going to find a way to mount a very large portion of the programme in a clinical aspect because the apprenticeship model is very much the model we felt was important to continue to educate midwives in ... Those were all very major components of the selection process. (personal communication 1995)

These selection criteria were disseminated to the universities competing for the midwifery education program. Realizing that it would be difficult for one institution to meet all criteria, the CDC recommended that universities collaborate on proposals. The government also encouraged competing universities to draw from existing courses and structures in their proposals to ensure cost-effectiveness.

The AOM also endorsed a collaborative proposal, specifically between a degree and non-degree granting institution due to its "concerns that many degree granting institutions will not have the ability to be sufficiently flexible to create a midwifery programme" (AOM Newsletter 7, no. 3, October 1991: 30). Additionally, the AOM directly contacted those sites that had expressed initial interest in developing a midwifery education program, to offer its technical assistance in helping develop a program proposal that was in keeping with their model of practice and philosophy of midwifery. Several of the sites did invite AOM representatives to brainstorming sessions and also requested that the AOM review drafts of their proposals.

Proposals were subsequently submitted on June 15, 1992, by two university consortiums: 1) Laurentian University in Sudbury, McMaster University in Hamilton, and Ryerson Polytechnical Institute in Toronto; and 2) University of Ottawa (with La Cité Collegiale), Lakehead University in Thunder Bay, the University of Windsor, and the Michener Institute in Toronto. To evaluate these proposals and negotiate the budget to establish the program, a midwifery education program site selection panel was set up shortly following the submissions. This panel was chaired by Joy Cohnstaedt, Chair of the Ontario Council on University Affairs, and Mary Eberts, IRCM Chair (*The Gazette* 3, no. 1, January, 1993: 1–2). Panel members also included representatives from the Ministry of Colleges and Universities and from the AOM (Bobbi Soderstrom and Michelle Kryzanauskas). AOM representatives were included to provide technical advice on the establishment of the program. From the midwives' point of view, their inclusion would help sustain their desired model of education.

The site selection panel met with the deans of the departments involved at each university to assess their commitment to the midwifery model of practice and adherence to the criteria developed by the CDC. On December 21, 1992, the Minister of Colleges and Universities, Richard Allen, announced that the Laurentian/McMaster/Ryerson proposal was successful and that the midwifery baccalaureate program would begin at those universities in September, 1993. This consortium's proposal offered both the credibility of a health science centre, and the flexibility and accessibility of a community college. Vicki Van Wagner highlighted some of the strengths of the Laurentian/McMaster/Ryerson proposal: "The consortium that was chosen had a non-university famous for access, Ryerson,[3] and a health science centre, McMaster, which sort of was the compromise between those two positions" (personal communication 1995). It also accommodated francophone students and distance learning at the Laurentian location, and included a part-time program at Ryerson: "There is flexibility. People can choose to go from anywhere [between] three [and] seven years and the important thing that Ryerson offered the consortium of universities was the possibility of part-time" (Vicki Van Wagner, personal communication 1995).

Following the success of the proposal, the Consortium appointed programme directors: Karyn Kaufman, as overall director at McMaster, Vicki Van Wagner at Ryerson, and Holliday Tyson at Laurentian. Faculty were chosen during the Spring of 1993 from currently practising midwives with advanced standing from the Michener program (discussed in chapter 10) and who had advanced university degrees. As highlighted above, recruiting faculty from the group of current practitioners was intended to help sustain the philosophy of midwifery and the midwifery model of care.

Following the announcement of the establishment of the program, course development began in earnest with ongoing AOM input. The AOM wanted to ensure that the core components of the apprenticeship model were appropriately integrated into the clinical component of the program, and that the principles of the midwifery model of practice (e.g., choice of birth place through educating student midwives in all settings, and teaching continuity of care from the beginning of the program) were also promoted. A common curriculum for all three institutions included basic sciences, social sciences, health sciences and women's studies, in addition to clinical courses and electives (*The Gazette* 3, no. 1, January 1993: 1–2). As Vicki Van Wagner noted, "it's one programme, administered through three institutions" (as cited in *The Gazette* 1, no. 2, December 1993: 5).

As recommended, the program was designed to be a four-year program which would run year-round, and could be completed in three calendar years. Half of this time would be devoted to the theoretical component and the other half to the clinical component. Each student would be assigned to a midwifery practice group for an extended period of practice for the clinical component (*The Gazette* 3, no. 1, January 1993: 1–2). To ensure students' compatibility with the midwifery lifestyle, all students were required to be on call from the inception of the program and throughout their studies. Due to the complexity of launching the mid-wifery program in its entirety, the curriculum was developed as needed, one year at a time. The total enrolment in all three years of the program was projected to be 122 students by 1996 and was estimated to cost approximately $2 million annually.

Beginning in March 1993, more than 1800 information packages were mailed out and 400 applications for the approximately thirty positions in this new educational program were subsequently received (*The Gazette* 1, no. 1, July 1993: 3). The three-step admissions process included first, assessing academic eligibility; second, evaluating a written autobiograph-ical submission; finally, undergoing in-person interview scheduled in June. Approximately 100 individuals were interviewed and thirty-three students were accepted to fill a total of twenty-six-full-time equivalent places in the first year of the four-year program. McMaster accepted seven full-time students, Ryerson, fourteen part-time students, and Laurentian twelve full-time students (six English-speaking and six francophone) (*The Gazette* 1, no. 1, July 1993: 3). Vicki Van Wagner emphasized that "even though sixty-two percent of students already have previous degrees, the basic requirement is high school, which is very important to us in terms of the principle of access" (personal communication 1995).

The successful establishment of the baccalaureate program is yet another indication of both the significant influence of midwives in the AOM on the state regarding the integration of midwifery and the strong support the state gave to the midwifery initiative. Midwifery leaders were involved and influential at every stage in the development of the mid-wifery education program, and were thus able to help implement a pro-gram they believed would help sustain what they felt were the core aspects of midwifery.

Nonetheless, concerns continued to be expressed over the de-emphasis of the traditional apprenticeship components and restriction of accessi-bility because of the centralized locations, lack of distance education, and rigid academic admission process. Even Task Force, IRCM and Transi-tional Council Chair Mary Eberts, who so strongly recommended a bac-calaureate program, conceded that the admissions process of the education program as implemented did indeed limit accessibility:

Well, I think in retrospect we were somewhat more naive about how accessible that programme could or would be made, than it turned out to be ... Universities do guard and preserve their independence very jealously, and their own admission standards just automatically clicked in once a programme had been established. And I think a lot of the hopes of accessibility of the Task Force and also of the committee that chose the site, the Site Selection Committee, were confounded when the universities got at it because they do a lot of things reflexively like put everybody through the university admissions programme ... and that made it very difficult to maintain as open a programme as we had wanted. (personal communication 1995)

Long-time midwifery supporter Jutta Mason (1990) also expressed her concern with the establishment of the midwifery education program: "In the plans laid down for midwifery education, the midwives have repudiated much of their own non-medical birth culture and have constructed a curriculum that is at times indistinguishable from any other progressive medical curriculum" (4). It would be curious to note whether Mason's opinion expressed prior to the creation of the program, would differ once the actual program was examined.

SUMMARY

Clearly, the importance of achieving legitimacy is one of the main themes that emerged from this examination of the changes in midwifery education and entry-to-practice policy. A formalized, standardized, baccalaureate educational program for midwifery professionals was seen as necessary for midwives to be acknowledged as professionals within the mainstream maternity care system. Legitimacy of midwives' educational preparation was especially important to secure hospital admitting privileges and by extension, the maintenance of the midwifery model of practice. As two of the architects of midwifery education in Ontario later reflected, "The development of the educational program has contributed to greater visibility of the profession, strengthened the autonomy of the profession, and also furthered its integration into the overall health care system" (Kaufman and Soderstrom 2004: 201). Garnering legitimation via entry-to-practice requirements is not unique to the midwifery professional project. It is a typical strategy used by aspiring health professions, such as chiropractic (Biggs 1989; Willis 1989), nursing (Heap and Stuart 1995; Saks 1994; Witz 1990, 1992), and naturopathy (Boon 1998, Gort and Coburn 1988). Nurses' push for a baccalaureate degree as an entry to practice requirement in particular informed midwives' evolution of their educational model.

In contrast to the other elements of midwifery integration, state support for legitimation through changes in midwifery education was mixed. The government ultimately did fund a new university-based program but it did so rather reluctantly. In fact, there was a strong push particularly by the Minister of Health at the time to base the program at the community college level so as to avoid what was considered to be unnecessary credentialism. If this initial decision had been implemented, it may have responded to some of the concerns about accessibility that were raised by some advocates both prior to and following integration.

Consumer support for the shift in midwifery education was also mixed. How midwives were trained was not as salient an issue as were the funding and the model of practice. This was much more of a professional issue. If midwifery entry-to-practice requirements had to change to ensure the model, this was largely viewed as a necessary compromise. Perhaps the government's mixed feelings reflected the lack of a strong consumer voice on the issue. The relative cost of a university versus college-based program quite likely was also another critical criterion in the government's decision. Curiously, it was the insistence of members of the other professions – nursing and medicine – that led to the Ministry supporting the baccalaureate initiative. Midwifery integration was like a house of cards and the aspect that consumers and in turn the state most strongly supported – the model of practice – needed a baccalaureate preparation to serve as its basis in order to be sustained in the mainstream system. If this element of midwifery integration was removed, the house of cards would likely have collapsed. The state supported midwifery enough to see the whole house through even though it may have supported some elements less than others.

It is important to emphasize that the changes to the orientation of the midwifery education program originated from within the midwifery community. Midwifery leaders did, however, make these changes in response to their perception of what other professions within the health care system, especially medicine, would deem acceptable. In seeking legitimacy through these means, it could be argued that midwifery leaders compromised what some within the community regarded as an essential component of Ontario midwifery.

Throughout the integration process, several significant changes occurred in how women became midwives and how they learned their craft. Before integration, a midwife's learning came directly from her own birth experience and her direct experience with clients, augmented by ad hoc courses, lectures, and reading; academic modes of learning supplemented experience. With the establishment of a baccalaureate educational program, it could be argued that the emphasis went in the opposite direction; that is, clinical experience supplemented academic learning. Moreover, it could also be argued that standardization has become emphasized over individualized, hands-on experience with birth. That is, throughout the integration process, texts and formalized professional knowledge have been prioritized over the experiential client-based knowledge. The implications of this shift in daily practice and client-midwife relations remain to be seen. This reorientation of midwives' knowledge base may serve as yet another means of distancing midwives from their clients consistent with professionalization. Will it be as Jutta Mason (1990) predicts, that the midwife will now be the teacher and not the taught, and the woman her pupil rather than a partner in the birthing process?

The recruitment of midwives and entry-to-practice midwifery has also changed from a system in which midwives became interested in midwifery through their own life experiences and through seeking mentorship with a more experienced midwife, into a bureaucratically administered admissions process for a university-based educational program. This may serve to limit the accessibility to becoming a midwife for many women and, in turn, limit the accessibility of women to midwives, which was one of the main objectives to the midwifery integration process. At the same time, because the government considers the midwifery education program to be a legitimate educational program, accessibility may be increased through the availability of student loans to pay for midwifery education. This was not possible in the earlier apprenticeship models.

Although these changes to entry to midwifery practice were regarded as compromises which were necessary to maintain the house of cards through the integration process, the potential for these changes to continue to affect midwifery are significant. The effect of these changes in educational and entry-to-practice policy are also not only limited to this domain. They have some potential wide-ranging effects on other domains of midwifery, most notably on the maintenance of the midwifery model of practice. Having said this, the evolution of midwifery education in Ontario is not out of sync with what has been happening elsewhere. Benoit and Davis-Floyd (2004), for example, identify the move toward direct-entry and higher level of education as a key international trend in midwifery education (see also Benoit et al 2000). Perhaps it is because there were no pre-existing programs that midwifery leaders were able to work with a clean slate and develop something that midwives the world over have envisioned. Indeed, the Ontario model of midwifery education has become recognized internationally as a unique program and one that is or should be emulated (Kaufman and Soderstrom 2004).

Nevertheless, it is important to acknowledge the differing opinions on the changes that occurred. As noted above, these concerns over midwifery education and entry-to-practice criteria created perhaps the greatest dissent within the midwifery community of any integration issue. This feeling was exacerbated significantly when the issue of how currently practising midwives could legitimately enter the new profession of midwifery was addressed. Here again we will see the issue of seeking legitimacy through restricting access to the official practice of midwifery raised.

CHAPTER TEN

Acknowledging Expertise through "Grandmothering," but Not for All

Related to the issue of establishing a training program for the new generation of midwives was the issue of how to integrate midwives who were currently practising in the province and those who had previous midwifery training. It is here where Witz' (1992) dual closure model of female professional projects seem most apropos. This is because the result of this grandmothering process was the exclusion of several potential midwives. Their exclusion became a critical issue because the newly drafted legislation would make their continued practice not just illegitimate but also illegal. As was the case for the evolution of the model of midwifery education, the issue of legitimacy was also apparent in this decision-making process. Legitimacy would be fostered by credentialling a carefully selected, highly competent and "safe" cadre of midwives to act as ambassadors of the new midwifery and promoters of its professional image. But what may have garnered external legitimacy resulted in extensive divisiveness within the midwifery community.

DECIDING ON WHO WILL BE "AMBASSADORS" OF THE NEW MIDWIFERY

Midwives' Proposals to the HPLR and Task Force

The issue of acknowledging existing midwifery expertise was identified by midwives early on in the integration process. In its first submission to the HPLR, the Midwifery Coalition stipulated the need to make provisions to include those women in the province with foreign midwifery training, and those currently in practise: "Midwives trained in other countries through programmes approved by the College of Midwives of Ontario may apply for a licence after sitting a challenge examination. Midwives who have practised for at least two years prior to this act and attended a specified number of births may also qualify for the challenge examination" (first submission to HPLR 1983: 22). This "challenge examination" was proposed to "test the applicant's ability, competency and knowledge of the theory and practice of midwifery," the results of which "would identify areas in which further study would be necessary before a licence is granted" (first submission to HPLR 1983: 22).

The 1985 Toronto Island Inquest jury also addressed this issue when it made the following recommendation: "Foreign trained midwives would need to pass [an] exam before being licensed in Ontario. Midwives without formal training but with five or more years of experience as practising midwives could make submissions for advanced standing, then requiring only the final year of midwifery training before sitting board exams" (*Issue* 8, July 1985: 7).

The AOM readdressed the issue of integrating currently practising midwives and foreign-trained midwives in the "Phasing-In" plan it presented in its third submission to the HPLR. Instead of an exam, it proposed an integration program: "In order to integrate both currently practising and foreign trained midwives, a skills assessment programme is necessary to determine what areas of training are most important for upgrading. This would be accessible to "lay" midwives with a minimum level of experience, for a limited period of time [and] ... a refresher programme for foreign trained midwives who wish to sit exams" (third submission to HPLR, October 1985: 26). The goal of this integration program was mainly to "standardize academic and clinical knowledge of midwives in Ontario" (third submission to HPLR, October 1985: 27).

Like the jury from the 1985 Inquest, the AOM felt that it was important to establish eligibility criteria for an integration program. It was not comfortable with the jury's recommendation of five years of experience given "the diversity in training and experience of Ontario midwives" (AOM third submission to HPLR, October 1985: 29). In accordance with international educational standards, the AOM recommended that practising midwives who had attended at least fifty births, thirty as primary caregiver, within the last five years should be eligible for a "granny clause." Foreign-trained midwives would have to provide evidence of graduation from an accredited midwifery school as well as evidence of practice within the last five years. It was then proposed that eligible midwives would have their clinical practices evaluated, highlighting the clinical skills that required upgrading.

The need for an integration program was also noted by the AOM in its submission to the Task Force on the Implementation of Midwifery. The AOM's position was succinctly put by one midwife in her submission to the Task Force:

The currently practising midwives have responded to the demands and needs of people and have relearned the art of supporting natural childbirth and confidence in women's ability to give birth. Years of preparation have gone into this and the 30–35 midwives now working in Ontario possess experience, skills, knowledge and intuition that cannot be mass produced in midwifery education and institutions. It is for this reason that these women be allowed to continue to practise under a "granny clause" in legislation for to lose what we have learned and have to offer would be a retrogressive step of the worst kind. Perhaps these women could be best used in individual centres of the province to offer learning experience for aspiring midwives and training. It is the only way to preserve what we now have and know. While most of us will be very willing to be examined individually and to meet certain criteria to assure equal standards of competence and skill, it must be remembered that we have spent years offering prenatal care, managing on our own childbirths in and out of hospital settings, and providing care and counselling, and we have a very high level of satisfaction among the families we serve. (TFIMO 1987: 251–2)

The AOM also submitted to the Task Force its proposals for the HPLR. They argued that the number of applicants for an integration program should reflect a balance between "the phasing-in of a high quality midwifery system, and the need for appropriate numbers of midwives to meet the demands of self-regulation and the demands of the health care system" (AOM Submission to Task Force, September 1986: 24). They also elaborated on the importance of developing a unity of philosophy, practice, and standard of care through the integration program in creating for the public and other health professions a "distinct profession with a clearly defined role" (AOM Submission to Task Force, September 1986: 24). The standards for this program would be the same as those expected in the recommended midwifery educational program.

The Task Force Recommendations

In addressing the issue of currently practising midwives, the Task Force identified three options: 1) make all currently practising midwives go through the newly developed school of midwifery; 2) "rubber stamp" all current practitioners with approval to practice; and 3) grandparent a cadre of qualified practising midwives after assessing their knowledge and clinical competency. The Task Force recommended the third (middle-ground) option and justified this choice in terms of not losing the valuable resources and expertise these midwives represented: "There are indeed people in Ontario whose knowledge, clinical skills, and experience in midwifery should not be wasted. The province needs these people to develop the profession: to be the first cadre of qualified practising midwives, to serve in the College of Midwives, and to participate in the education of the second generation of midwives" (TFIMO 1987: 147).

In order to make recommendations regarding the content and feasibility of an integration program, the Task Force attempted to identify groups likely to seek integration. Data were gathered via two province-wide surveys which investigated the extent of midwifery education and experience among RNs and RNAs, and among practising and non-practising direct-entry midwives (TFIMO 1987: 11). The survey of nurses was conducted by the CNO. Based on the survey population of 5,400, the Task Force estimated that approximately 1,000 CNO registrants would have a definite interest in practising midwifery. More than 80 per cent of CNO survey respondents, however, had acquired their midwifery training prior to 1970. Because of this, the CNO emphasized to the Task Force that: "Clearly, the midwifery knowledge and skill of these registrants is, for the most part, outdated and there is an obvious need for refresher courses as well as basic midwifery education programmes. It could be argued that the midwifery training of many registrants is so out of date that a refresher programme would be insufficient and completion of a basic programme should be required for them to resume practice as qualified midwives" (CNO 1987: 23, as cited in TFIMO 1987: 148). The Task Force concluded that relatively few of these nurses and assistants would be eligible for an advanced standing integration program.

The second survey of currently practising and non-practising direct-entry midwives revealed that there were fifty midwives currently practising in Ontario, forty of whom intended to continue practising upon legalization.[1] The survey also highlighted, as the AOM had previously asserted, that there was "tremendous variability in the educational preparation and practice experience of these practitioners" (TFIMO: 148). This would prove challenging in creating a standardized integration program. This survey also investigated fifty-nine non-practising midwives. The surveyors realized, however, that it was next to impossible to estimate the total number of non-practising midwives in Ontario and concluded that "the information obtained for this group is therefore of limited usefulness" (TFIMO 1987: 148).

Based on the data collected in these surveys, the Task Force emphasized that "the integration process must enable a potentially large number of people to be comprehensively and intensively assessed with respect to their knowledge and clinical competency in midwifery" (TFIMO 1987: 149). They also recommended that "the process should ideally take place in a short time, and its cost, both to the individual and to the government of Ontario, should not be excessive" (TFIMO 1987: 149).

Following this recommendation, the Task Force outlined the admission requirements, selection procedures, content, and assessment of midwives' competency through a "Midwifery Integration Programme" (TFIMO 1987: 152). It recommended that applicants be current residents of Ontario with "educational preparation or significant experience in midwifery, maternal/infant nursing, or medicine" and proficiency in written and spoken English (TFIMO 1987: 152).[2] All applicants who met these admission requirements would then go through a two-step selection process. The first step was "a written multiple choice examination covering the appropriate subject areas in the basic sciences and midwifery" (TFIMO 1987: 152). Having passed this step, the applicant would then take "an Objective Structured Clinical Examination (OSCE) covering all areas of midwifery practice" (TFIMO 1987: 152). Applicants passing these two steps would then be granted admission depending on "the number of hospital sites and preceptors available to provide clinical placements and supervision" (TFIMO 1987: 152).

The Midwifery Integration Programme was to be "structured to permit students to proceed at their own pace" (TFIMO 1987: 153). It included clinical preceptorships and provisions for students to "provide care in all areas of midwifery, including the management of women throughout pregnancy, labour, birth and the post-partum period" (TFIMO 1987: 153). The Task Force recommended continuous assessment of students' performance during this clinical component (prenatal and postpartum visits, births, and newborn assessments) by their preceptors. Successful completion of the program would be indicated in a final clinical exam. Graduates would then be able to apply to the College of Midwives for registration. In addition to the one-time only program, the Task Force recommended the development of another ongoing program to assess the qualifications of foreign-trained midwives seeking registration in the future.

Again, these recommendations of the Task Force were viewed favourably by the AOM. It formally stated in its newsletter following the presentation of the Task Force report: "In order to fully integrate midwives into the health care system the Task Force has recognized the importance of currently practising midwives, and the AOM supports the provisions that they have made for their integration and licensing" (AOM Newsletter 3, no. 4, December 1987: 16). Following the Task Force report, the Curriculum Design Committee became the next government-appointed committee to address the issue of the integration of currently practising midwives.

The Curriculum Design Committee Recommendations

One of the tasks of the CDC was to make recommendations regarding the integration of persons in the province with prior midwifery experience. Although the CDC felt that this task was beyond its six-month mandate, and it ultimately proposed the immediate establishment of a Midwifery Integration Planning Project (MIPP) to address the details of integration, it did draft some overall parameters that an integration program should follow. First, an integration program should give priority to currently practising midwives in Ontario, and such a program should not simply "grandmother" these practitioners without some sort of assessment and standardization of skill:

The CDC did set out the clinical requirements for a midwifery graduate. And then we said people who have that much experience already and have been previously practising, people who are currently doing that should have an opportunity to prove that they do know what they're doing. But there should be a process for it. There shouldn't be a rubber stamp, and the reason it needs to be an assessment process is because it is still controversial, to establish credibility with the other professions, and this is something the AOM believed should happen all along. (Vicki Van Wagner, personal communication 1995)

The need to ensure that the first registered midwives in Ontario are seen as credible and competent may not be compatible with an automatic "grandmothering" of existing practitioners. (CDC Report 1990: 35)

The CDC identified the purpose of this programme as being to "provide public protection through a credible process which balances the recognition of experience and existing skills with the need to provide a structured opportunity to achieve uniform standards" (CDC Report 1990: 35). The CDC also recommended that this integration program should not exceed one year, that it be available for a limited time, and that it be individually tailored to meet the needs of each entrant.

The Midwifery Integration Planning Project

The Midwifery Integration Planning Project (MIPP) was initiated in October 1990 following the recommendation of the CDC. It had a six-month mandate (which was extended to eight months) to develop, refine, and agree upon the structure and process for assessment of current practitioners including admission criteria, length of program, assessment methods, and educational review process (MIPP Report 1991: 1). Like the CDC, this project was provided administrative support by the Michener Institute, was headed by Diana Schatz and coordinated by Holliday Tyson. MIPP members included Dr Anthony Reid, a family physician; Ina Caissey, a registered nurse; Dr Murray Enkin, an obstetrician; Vicki Van Wagner and Jane Kilthei, both members of the IRCM's Liaison Committee with the AOM. MIPP members had sat on either or both the CDC and IRCM. The committee was also advised by Midwifery Coordinator Karyn Kaufman.

Like the CDC before it, the MIPP received input from consumer and stakeholder groups (medicine, nursing, hospitals), and also gathered information about "grandmothering" and credentialling programs for other professions in Ontario (MIPP Report 1991: 16). The purpose of the integration program (now called the pre-registration program) was to "prepare currently practising midwives for registration with the College of Midwives through a process which [had] sufficient rigour to ensure competency of practitioners and credibility to the public and health profession" (MIPP Report 1991: 17). These midwives would then become "founding practitioners of regulated midwifery in the Province of Ontario" (MIPP Report 1991: 17), and essentially ambassadors to the new midwifery profession. The guiding principles for the MIPP included the international definition of the midwife, statement of philosophy of midwifery care (developed by the IRCM), core competencies (developed by the AOM and IRCM), and principles for midwifery education (defined by the CDC).

In its report made in June 1991, the MIPP addressed the areas of notification and assessment of applicants to the pre-registration program, and the structure, content, and operation of the program. Following the recommendation of the AOM, the MIPP committee recommended that in order to give candidates sufficient time to prepare, public notification of the program should be made twelve months prior to its onset.[3]

Criteria for admission into the pre-registration program were developed based on the CDC recommendations regarding the skills and experience required of a graduate of the baccalaureate program and from the European Economic Community Requirements for Midwives. These stipulated that 1) the candidate must have actively practised midwifery for at least two years in Ontario (immediately preceding the onset of the pre-registration program), one of which must have been as primary caregiver without supervision; 2) the candidate must have attended sixty births; forty of these attended as primary caregiver; thirty must have included provision of continuity of care; thirty must have been attended in Ontario; and at least twenty must have been home births (MIPP Report 1991: 33). These criteria were to reflect the principles of the Ontario midwifery model of practice which were written into regulations, including primary care (only truly available at home prior to integration) and continuity of care. MIPP member Murray Enkin asserted that "Ontario experience was a must" (personal communication 1995).

Like the CDC, the MIPP recommended that the pre-registration program be no longer than one year. All midwives would be required to attend an educational review session at a central location which was short and intensive so as to minimize the disruption to midwives' practices. Individualized, needs-based assessment would be structured around those review sessions. Midwives would be continually assessed throughout the program with a combination of a review of written records, chart-stimulated recall, observation in clinical settings, structured oral exams, and written exams.

The MIPP committee also made recommendations regarding the faculty for the program. MIPP Coordinator Holliday Tyson described how there were essentially three choices regarding the recruitment of faculty: "Do we have midwives from Ontario assess other midwives, or do we have Canadian people or North American people assess us (and should these people not be midwives but nurses who are nurse-midwives)? The third option was to find international midwives who might be sympathetic to the way we practice but have the necessary distance to have some respect from our Minister of Health and our health care providers, and have them assess us. We decided on the third option" (personal communication 1995). It was decided that midwifery assessments would be accomplished by three full-time faculty recruited from other countries who were practising midwifery, had teaching experience in a wide range of settings, and had some familiarity with the Ontario midwifery community. It was recommended that recruitment be undertaken immediately.

Following the final report of the MIPP, the site for the midwifery pre-registration program was chosen. Given its involvement in both the CDC and MIPP, the Michener Institute was chosen to administer the program and it began working with the MIPP to develop the midwifery assessment program in late 1991. In October 1991, the Ministers of Health and of Colleges and Universities announced that a special, one-time program organized by the Michener Institute would be established commencing October 1992 to approve existing midwives for practice (*The Gazette* 2, no. 2, December 1991: 1). The Michener was then faced with the task of implementing the recommendations made by the MIPP into a workable assessment program.

The Michener Pre-Registration Programme

The main objectives of the Michener Pre-Registration Programme were to ensure that the midwife had the necessary professional competencies and personal qualities to work *safely* as a midwife by practising according to the standards and philosophy of midwifery care in Ontario, and to ensure that the midwife had the knowledge necessary to participate in the integration of the midwifery profession into the health care system (Michener Introductory Document: 1, emphasis in original). Essentially, the Michener was to create a cadre of safe, standardized ambassadors of the midwifery profession.

One of the first items on the Michener's agenda was to recruit international midwifery faculty. Midwifery Coordinator Karyn Kaufman described the recruitment process: "It's a combination of things. One, you want somebody who's credible within their own setting; somebody who's willing to pack up their life and move to Toronto for a year. And so because we had some international contacts, either through the Task Force travel, through the International Confederation of Midwives, people who had gone to various European countries, we said here are some names, call them up, see if somebody might want to come over here" (personal communication 1995). Midwives in the AOM who had been involved in several international midwifery conferences and had made international contacts submitted names of midwives whom they felt would be appropriate assessors. Midwife Holliday Tyson described how the AOM put together a list of midwives they recommended as faculty:

We pulled a couple of people from Education and from the Midwives' Association and said, "Let's get together a list of names." It happened that a number of us had, since the early 80s, gone to the International Confederation of Midwives Conference every three years, and we had representation there. In addition, some of the midwives from other countries had visited Ontario over the years so we did have a pool of names. It wasn't too difficult to put together [a list] of people who had current clinical experience, had home birth experience, knew something about Ontario, and had educational experience. (personal communication 1995)

Midwives' recommendations for faculty were seriously considered by Michener director Diana Schatz. Early in 1992, she announced the appointment of Susanne Houd as program director of the pre-registration program. Houd was a practising midwife from Denmark, active in both teaching and research with the World Health Organization. She was known by the members of the Task Force, as she had arranged a "midwifery study tour" for them in Denmark back in 1986 (Houd, personal communication 1993). Following this introduction, Houd was invited on occasion to speak at midwifery related conferences in Ontario. She described how through this initial contact, she became "fascinated with what was going on in Ontario" and kept in contact (personal communication 1993). In Schatz' announcement of Houd's appointment, she described Houd as "a midwife of international stature who understands community care, has research expertise and a broad understanding of midwifery across the world" (*The Gazette* 3, no. 1, May 1992: 1). The AOM commented on how Houd was "strongly committed to continuity of care, choice of birthplace, informed choice and integrating research evidence into practice" (AOM newsletter 8, no. 3, July 1992: 16), that is, all of the principles of midwifery the AOM promoted.

As program director, Houd was required to contribute to and oversee the development of the pre-registration program and its implementation including faculty recruitment (*The Gazette* 3, no. 1, May 1992: 1). Houd noted that the "criteria were that people had a teaching background, that they had tried to work in a community-based practice: they should be comfortable with home births, but also have some hospital experience" (personal communication 1995). Subsequently, Dutch midwife Annamiek Cuppen, British midwife Jilly Rosser, and New Zealand midwife Joan Donley were recruited. All had extensive backgrounds in practise, research, and teaching.

Concurrent with the recruitment of faculty, the Michener began the admissions process and an admissions committee was struck in March, 1992. Following the MIPP recommendations, the Committee included a member of the IRCM; a physician experienced in working with Ontario

midwives; a registered nurse with maternity care experience and familiarity with the practice of midwifery in Ontario; one consumer from the
MTFO; and a midwife credentialled in another jurisdiction, a position filled
by program director Houd (MIPP Report 1991: 31). Currently practising
midwives were formally excluded from the admissions committee. The
criteria for admission followed the MIPP recommendations. Also following the recommendations of the MIPP committee, applicants were required
to provide the following: 1) a statement and documentation to show that
they have fulfilled eligibility criteria; 2) a detailed biographical letter; and
3) three letters of reference – one from a midwife colleague, one from a
physician working in obstetrics, and one from a client. Applicants were
also required to provide evidence of past adherence to practice standards
and express their future commitment to the IRCM Standards of Practice.

Although the CDC had estimated that "there may be up to seventy-five
individuals who could meet the definition of current practitioner and
who may apply of the integration programme" (36), and the MIPP had
estimated that there would be fewer than 100 eligible applicants to the
pre-registration program (32), over 120 applications to the program were
received. IRCM Chair Mary Eberts explained that not only was the Admissions Committee inundated with many more applications than expected,
the documentation on applications was also problematic:

People were desperate to get into that programme. It was the beginning of the
end if they didn't get into it. And so the emotional energy that went into the
search for a place was just unbelievable ... There were all kinds of what I would
call "evidentiary" problems. People were double-counting births, people were
arguing about whose birth was whose, they were saying that they had done
certain things and they were contesting versions of whether they had done them,
so that the combinations of all the exercise of discretion in administering the
criteria at the margin ... just made a mess all around ... And so what happened
was because of the absence of experience and the absence of the uniform criteria
beforehand, all of this stuff was a battleground open to interpretation. (personal
communication 1995)

In addition to these problems, the Admissions Committee was strongly
encouraged by the IRCM to be flexible in its decision-making, and to use
an "exceptional category" in certain circumstances to include midwives
who might otherwise be excluded from the program. IRCM chair Mary
Eberts described the reasoning behind the IRCM's insistence to include

"exceptional" cases: "We wanted there to be room in the Michener admissions process for accommodation where there was a clear case that a duty could arise because of some family circumstance or health circumstance, or ... the rural midwife, because of the demands imposed upon her by any single pregnancy or birth, all the driving and this and that, would have fewer numbers ... If they were reasonably satisfied that the person would still be a good candidate but for these kinds of reasons she couldn't meet the technical requirements" (personal communication 1995). This "exceptional" category was "applied on an individual basis for applicants who, although short some entry criteria ... had other strengths in education and experience such that ... [they] did meet the objective of the Pre-Registration Programme and would be able to meet all programme requirements" (Michener Institute's Report on the Admission Process, Pre-Registration Program, Midwifery, August 24, 1992: 2). Thus, although there was to be flexibility, the IRCM maintained that the purpose of the program was to integrate *currently* practising midwives:

The Executive came to the conclusion that while some flexibility would be desirable, it should be borne in mind that the purpose of the Pre-Registration program is to integrate currently practising midwives. The central question, even in the exercise of discretion inherent in "flexibility" should therefore be, "is the person a currently practising midwife?" The "flexible" approach should be used to benefit those of whom it could be said that they are currently practising midwives, but who are slightly outside the formal requirements [(eg.,] because of pregnancy or educational leave). It should not be used to broaden access to the program, so that, for example, apprentice midwives, those trained in other jurisdictions but not now actively practising in Ontario, or others well outside the criteria, could gain admission. (MIPP Report 1991: 34)

Although many agreed with the need to be flexible, the use of an "exceptional" category for the inclusion of midwives "led to the accusation of subjectivity" (Vicki Van Wagner, personal communication 1995). Ultimately the success of a candidate rested on his or her ability to convince the Admissions committee that he or she was indeed exceptional:

"You had to show somehow exceptional status and for some people they didn't really have anything to demonstrate as exceptional ... It meant that people were trying to prove that they were more exceptional than the next." (Michelle Kryzanauskas, personal communication 1995)

"The admissions committee made judgements about which applicants had a set of strengths that made them exceptional. Those not deemed exceptional found the decision hard to accept." (Vicki Van Wagner, personal communication 1995)

In the end, seventy-two practising midwives (including one man) gained entrance to the program. Those not accepted into this "grandmothering" program were excluded mainly because of their low number of births recently attended (particularly in Ontario), and lack of home birth experience. Successful applicants were not charged a fee for the program, as the AOM successfully argued that midwives would already be experiencing financial burdens as a result of a reduction in their practice during the education programme. The Michener also provided accommodation for out-of-Toronto midwives as well as some expense funds.

Once successful applicants were notified of their admission, they were required to fill out a needs assessment form to help faculty identify areas in which midwives wanted and needed more knowledge (*The Gazette* 3, no. 2, August 1992: 7). These generally followed those identified by the AOM Education Committee, which included: 1) working in the role of primary caregiver in the hospital setting; 2) using pharmacological agents as specified by regulations; 3) making a physical assessment; 4) obtaining specimens; 5) administering venipuncture and intravenous; and 6) interpreting results of screening and diagnostic tests (as specified by regulations) and electronic fetal heart monitors (MIPP Report 1991: 56). These areas were focused on ensuring that midwives could work competently in hospitals.

The content and framework of the program were largely based on these needs assessments, and were designed by an Advisory Council which included consumer representatives, members of the IRCM, interdisciplinary representatives of relevant health professions, and AOM representatives. Through this Advisory Council it was decided that the program would consist of three parts: 1) educational review – a four-week intensive review of theory using a mixture of lectures, group work, and problem solving; 2) clinical assessment – faculty observation of midwives' ante-, intra- and postpartum care, chart review, and case studies; and 3) health care system orientation – observation of practitioners in community and hospital settings, and participation in consumer organizations (AOM newsletter 8, no. 2, July 1992: 17).

Although the program was intended to be flexible, many midwives felt that it ended up being overly structured. Much of the program was also criticized for being too focused on the medical aspects of midwifery, such as prescribing drugs, taking blood, and conducting a physical exam, and working within the hospital environment: "They were training people to not embarrass midwifery when they first came into the hospital. That was a terribly important thing; once you've decided to join that monopoly you've got to be able to deal there" (Jutta Mason, personal communication 1995). Moreover, many midwives felt that the important issue became safe, standardized practice rather than connectedness with clients: "The most important thing here was to produce *safe* practitioners. ... There was also rigid ordering and labelling so the more rigid and stricter you could appear the safer you appeared the better but for years we as midwives played the opposite role – now there were new mores and new norms ... Anecdotal material was discouraged and the very way midwives learn to appreciate and be in tune with the woman by just being there and use that experience later with other clients was discouraged" (Midwife, personal communication 1995; emphasis in original). To be fair, the content of the program was not to be a reflection of the overall emphasis of midwifery. It was not a midwifery education program but an assessment and upgrading program. Being that the "pre-registrants" were midwives who were practising or had practised in the province, they would have been well versed in the provisions of women – centred midwifery care. These skills did not necessarily need to be upgraded. What was needed to meet the challenges of an expanded model of practice – particularly in the hospital setting – was to have complementary skills in some of the more high-tech requirements that midwives had less of an opportunity to develop because of their previous lack of status.

Over and above this issue, some felt that the program was important in creating a stronger sense of sisterhood among midwives: "Participating in the programme was an experience I would not have missed for anything! As hard and intense as the whole evaluation process was, it was also wonderful to get to know other midwives and to add to midwifery lore in the time-honoured tradition of swapping birth stories" (midwife Heather Keffer as cited in *The Gazette* 1, no. 2, December 1993: 2).

One year later, on October 2, 1993, sixty-three midwives graduated from the program. These midwives were now prepared for registration with the College of Midwives. The nine midwives who did not graduate with the others in the fall of 1993 had received an "incomplete" assessment on some portion of their program. Some of these cases were due to a legitimate need to upgrade in a certain area. Other cases were more controversial and highlighted serious concerns some had with the perceived biases of the faculty towards the elite group of midwives and the "professional" aspects of midwifery, and the lack of an appeals process to express these concerns. Although it was meant to only run for one year, the Michener extended the pre-registration program, largely in response to vociferous lobbying on the part of midwives who received an "incomplete" and their consumer supporters, to ensure that all midwives admitted to the program were allowed to finish it.

The process of deciding how to integrate currently practising midwives through the CDC, MIPP, and Michener program was heavily influenced by the AOM, specifically the Education Committee. Thus, the AOM had little criticism of the process. They did not, however, view it as perfect. Concerns were particularly noted of the admissions process. The exclusion of midwives resulting from their admission process became quite controversial and produced considerable criticism. It also served to spark the organization of the protest group, the "Committee for More Midwives."

The Excluded Midwives

As mentioned above, the exclusion of midwives from the Michener program was due mainly to the criteria regarding numbers and home-birth attendance. Although these criteria were not chosen to explicitly exclude people from the profession but rather because they best represented the skill set considered necessary for the practice of midwifery, exclusion was indeed an outcome. Excluded were the occasionally practising midwives who did not meet the criteria regarding numbers of births; maternity care nurses (including those who worked in the newly developed in-hospital birthing centres) who did not meet the primary care, continuity of care, and home birth criteria; and foreign-trained midwives who did not meet the "practised recently in Ontario" criteria.

Reflecting upon these specific criteria, Nestel (2004) reveals the dilemma faced in particular by immigrant midwives: "Immigrant midwives of colour, while anxious to work in their profession, feared legal prosecution and deportation if they were to practise in the legal limbo that characterized the period prior to legalization" (295). Compounding this dilemma was the paradoxical situation whereby "immigrant midwives of colour were unable to use their professional expertise in Ontario, [but] practice experience acquired in the "Third World" enabled white Ontario midwives to qualify for registration in the province" (295).

Although some of these excluded midwives tried, they were unsuccessful in convincing the Michener's admissions committee that they were "exceptional" candidates. Indeed, the major criticism some of these women had of the admission process was not with the criteria specifically, but with the use of the "exceptional" category: "The purpose of the Admission Review was to ensure equitable application of criteria. This objective was not met. In light of the many exceptions to the Michener's own admission policy, the reasons for excluding our member midwives do not hold water (fax from Committee for More Midwives to Minister of Health Ruth Grier, May 13, 1993, 3).

In response to their exclusion, some of these "midwives," numbering approximately nine community midwives and seven birth centre nurses, established the Committee for More Midwives. This group engaged in a fierce lobbying campaign directed toward the AOM, IRCM, Transitional Council, Midwifery Coordinator, Minister of Health, Minister of College and Universities, the Baccalaureate program, the Michener program, their MPPs and the provincial Ombudsman. They argued that the level of experience of the individuals in their group did not warrant them going through the entire three years of the recently established baccalaureate program. They also argued that the delay and interruption to their services would result in fewer women having access to midwifery services: "*Accessibility* is guaranteed only in part by financial subsidy. Midwifery care is not truly *accessible* if there are insufficient numbers of midwives to accommodate the demand for their services" (fax from Committee for More Midwives to Minister of Health Ruth Grier, April 5, 1993, emphasis in original).

Access to midwifery services was especially important to consumers in eastern Ontario who organized the Eastern Ontario Midwifery Support Group to protest the exclusion of eleven of the midwives in Eastern Ontario. They argued that "only three of the fourteen midwives who have worked in that capacity in Eastern Ontario [would] be allowed to continue to practice" and that ironically midwifery care in their area would actually be reduced by legislation rather than increased (Eastern Ontario Midwifery Support Group, Press Release, December 30, 1993: 1). It is noteworthy that this group formed separately from the MTFO Eastern Ontario Chapter group. Many of its members felt that their concerns were falling on deaf ears by the executive of the MTFO, who like the AOM, was largely based out of Toronto. These eastern Ontario consumers felt that the MTFO was simply "rubberstamping" policies proposed by the AOM.

To ameliorate this situation of exclusion and inaccessibility, the Committee for More Midwives proposed the establishment of "a supplementary short term programme that would allow [them] to resume providing midwifery services to [their] communities as soon as possible" (letter from the Committee for More Midwives to the Transitional Council, February 8, 1993). Following this proposition, the Committee drafted an integration plan outlining eligibility criteria and updating requirements needed by the members of the committee, such as supervised home birth practice.

When contacted about this request for an additional program, the AOM expressed opposition and referred the committee members to the baccalaureate program: "The AOM does not support the establishment of a second pre-registration program. We believe that there should be early development of advanced standing opportunities in the baccalaureate program and that community midwives should be given priority in completing their education" (AOM newsletter 9, no. 2, August 1993: 8). The reasons the AOM cited for their lack of support for another pre-registration program included 1) that it would foster a two-tier system of midwifery preparation (baccalaureate and otherwise); 2) that it would be impossible to accommodate the substantial diversity in the experience, education, and model of midwifery practised by those excluded from the Michener; and 3) that mounting such a program would take substantially more time than seeking advanced standing in the baccalaureate program. The Committee for More Midwives counterargued that there was already a two-tiered system of midwifery preparation (the Michener and the baccalaureate program) and that the diversity of their group was not any greater than that of those who originally entered the Michener program.

The Transitional Council of the College of Midwives also opposed this request from the Committee for More Midwives. It argued that the Michener pre-registration program "was not intended as a 'privilege' for midwives but as a requirement to ensure the protection of the public." (Letter from the Transitional Council to the Committee for More Midwives, May 21, 1993: 2). They also argued that the creation of a second Michener program "would be a complex task, rather than the simple one which [the Committee] seems to envision" (3). Moreover, they felt that creating another pre-registration program to meet the needs of the committee's members, some of whom were nurses, would doubtless raise "the same cries of injustice" from other nurses that the committee was levelling against the Michener program. For these reasons, the Council stated quite emphatically: "We will not be available to assist you in designing any such program, we will not support any requests to the Minister for such a program, and we will offer no assurances whatever that if any such program is to be established by you as an independent venture the College will consider its completion as equivalent to its registration requirements" (3).

Thus, the members of the Committee for More Midwives were left only with the possibility of waiting for advanced standing in the baccalaureate program. But securing advanced standing was problematic: it was not immediately available, as the program was being developed year by year: "It certainly didn't occur to me early on, although it became clear to me that there was no way the university programme could offer advanced standing until they had at least three regular years of the programme ... I think people really didn't think all of that through. They didn't really think well these people who are left out will be able to get advanced standing in the university programme but ... they are stopped from practising for at least three years because they can't get advanced standing which may then prohibit them from getting advanced standing" (Midwifery Coordinator, Margaret Ann McHugh, personal communication 1995). During this delay, these "midwives" would not be able to practise: "We fear that our abilities and expertise will be wasted. Our time in exile from community practice will effectively eradicate our livelihoods as well as half the midwifery services available to Ontario, at a time when the government's highly publicized intention is to provide employment and bring accessible midwifery to the women of our province" (fax from Committee for More Midwives to Minister of Health Ruth Grier, May 13, 1993, 3). Not only was there the problem of a delay, there were also limited spots for candidates with advanced standing. Directors of the baccalaureate program felt that their ability to accommodate students with advanced standing was limited by available clinical and financial resources. In fact there have been no advanced standing spots made available.

Realizing these problems with the advanced standing option, the excluded midwives were subsequently referred to the Prior Learning Assessment (PLA) program which was being developed by the Transitional Council.[4] The PLA program was aimed at assessing the readiness for registration of those midwives who did not complete the Michener program or have the Ontario baccalaureate degree but who nevertheless had midwifery qualifications in other countries. Because these midwives would have a variety of credentials (formal, informal, and from various countries), the Transitional Council assigned the task of designing a fair and equitable PLA process to consultants. These consultants recommended a five-step process, including an orientation session, taking a profession-specific language proficiency exam, developing an education portfolio, assessing this portfolio, and undergoing a multifaceted intensive assessment. Throughout this process, applicants' knowledge and clinical skills would be assessed with respect to the core competencies regulated by the College. All applicants would be required to go through all of these stages in order to be determined equivalent. The cost of this assessment would be borne by the applicant for a fee comparable to the financial commitment of a baccalaureate applicant.

Although this consultancy regarding the PLA was considered essential to ensure that the process was equitable for all applicants, it nevertheless resulted in further delays in the start-up of the program. Commenting on the "success" of the PLA, Nestel (2004) summarizes: "[T]he CMO had received close to 1,000 inquiries about registration from trained midwives. While 337 women attended the 1995 PLA orientation, only 165 applications were received and eventually only 126 took the first language exam. Half that number (63) sat the second language exam, 56 submitted portfolios to the College and 51 took the Multifaceted Assessment I exam. By March 1998, the [PLA] program had produced only seventeen registrants" (297). Without trying to diminish the complexity of making a fair assessment of credentials from other jurisdictions, particularly in light of the unique baccalaureate entry to practice requirements in Ontario and the lack of internationally agreed-upon standards of midwifery training, these have been the outcomes. To be sure, the success of the program was also limited by financial constraints and the lack of a budget to properly and inexpensively assess the number interested in practising midwifery in the province.

In the final analysis, the pursuit of standardization resulted in several women who had a strong commitment to midwifery being excluded. Midwifery Coordinator Margaret Ann McHugh aptly described how this outcome was the unfortunate consequence of the system of midwifery in Ontario: "I don't think that there was any actual attempt to discriminate against them. I don't think there was any attempt to stop them from becoming practising midwives in Ontario, but the system as it fell out did in fact squeeze them out and it was just an accident. There are sort of personal tragedies but they weren't systematically intentional" (personal communication 1995). Whether it was intentional or not, with the proclamation of the Midwifery Act on December 31, 1993, these excluded "midwives" were no longer able to practise midwifery legally in Ontario. Despite the Transitional Council's assertion, midwives who were allowed to take the pre-registration program were privileged in that they could continue to practise.

Proclamation and the New "Illegal Midwives"

With the proclamation of the Midwifery Act, midwifery as defined and regulated by the College of Midwives was officially legitimized. At the same time, however, midwifery outside this regulated system became illegal.[5] For the first time in Ontario, practising midwifery without a license was a criminal act punishable by law. Midwife Betty-Anne Davis stated emphatically that the criminalization of midwifery was objectionable: "Women will always rise up in their communities to serve other women, calling themselves midwives. We consider it an affront to history and to our own philosophy that they should be considered criminals in the future if they cannot access a license or their communities prefer that they obtain their learning outside of an institution. The title 'licensed midwife' can be owned by the government. But the title 'midwife' is governed by birthing women. They name their midwives" (letter to Minister of Health Evelyn Gigantes, April 15, 1991: 3). In direct response to this criminalization of midwifery, another midwifery consumer support group, the Friends of Midwifery, formed. This group boldly asked: "Why does midwifery need friends? We need to decriminalize midwifery. Bill 56 (The Midwifery Act) and Bill 43 (The Regulated Health Professions Act) make practising midwifery without a licence a criminal offense. Women must be able to choose whoever they wish to attend them in pregnancy and delivery without risk of prosecution and conviction" (Lorna Irwin, Friends of Midwifery Brochure, 1993: 2).

When she addressed the IRCM earlier about her concerns with the restrictive proposals for legislation, aspiring midwife Hilary Monk (1989) noted the options that excluded midwives would face: "More than one practising midwife and more than one aspiring midwife are resignedly considering that, if legislation in its proposed restrictive form becomes law, they will have only a few options open to them. They can give up midwifery, give up midwifery here and go outside their communities to practise, or be driven back underground in order to practise as they see fit" (4). Even obstetrician and midwifery advocate Murray Enkin who strove to help make midwifery a legitimate health profession, admitted that lay midwifery might persist: "I guess the whole question of lay midwifery is going to remain with us I think as midwifery becomes a licensed, regulated organization. There are going to be pregnant women and would-be midwives who are not going to want to work within the constraints and then you will get a new lay midwifery movement growing up. When, where, how, I don't know but I think it is just as certain as we've got alternative practitioners in medicine. It is bound to come. I think lay midwifery is not lost … That's a crystal ball based on what's happened to every other profession" (personal communication 1995). But Ontario has not witnessed a backlash to regulated midwifery in terms of the development of another lay midwifery movement. Indeed, some of the excluded midwives have been integrated either through the PLA program or the baccalaureate program. Legitimacy was the way that some chose – others simply quit midwifery or quit aspiring to midwifery entirely. This has not been entirely the case for the integration of midwives in British Columbia where a vocal midwife – Celine Lemay – has opted to practice outside the system, much to the dismay of the regulated midwives in that province. This persistence of lay midwifery despite legislation has also proved to be the case in other jurisdictions, such as the United States (DeVries 1986).

Proclamation of the Midwifery Act also created an instantaneous shortage of midwives. With many communities without a registered midwife, more consumers were seeking the services of fewer midwives. Also, with fewer registered midwives, there were fewer left to keep the College, the Association, and the baccalaureate program functioning: "It's overwhelming. Trying to get the College to function, trying to keep the AOM functioning, getting the education programme to where it is, increasing the numbers that are enrolled. In many ways it's too much and it leaves a fairly fragile environment for a lot of practices, and it doesn't take much to turn people into feeling pretty miserable some days" (Karyn Kaufman, personal communication 1995). Given the problem of so few practitioners, the exclusion of midwives seems not only unfortunate for those excluded but also for those who are overwhelmed by providing care to all the consumers wanting midwives, and keeping a self-regulating profession operating. It is also equally distressing in light of the current human resources crisis in maternity care (discussed more fully in the conclusion).

SUMMARY

As noted throughout this discussion, the legitimacy of midwifery in Ontario was seen to be dependent not just on the form with which it was integrated but also in large part on the midwives who would be the ambassadors of the profession. They would become the human face of the various policies that so many had worked so hard to develop and have implemented. This was particularly the case for those policies created to ensure the sustainability of the model of midwifery practice. Choice of birth place and home birth in particular was critical to the practice of midwifery in the province so if a potential midwife was not supportive of that aspect of the model she was excluded as a result. This helps to explain why nurses, including those working in hospital-based birth centres, were not considered part of the ambassadorial cadre. It is less clear why some potential midwives who were affiliated with the home birth community were not.[6]

The Ontario midwifery professional project is not unique among professional projects in its exercise of exclusionary social closure strategies. Biggs (1989; Coburn and Biggs 1986) describes how the "straights" in the chiropractic profession (i.e., those who focused primarily on disorders of the spine) came to exclude a more mixed practice through control of their educational program. Legislative efforts undertaken by chiropractors also reflect this closure pattern. Larkin (1983) and Willis (1989) describe similar tensions and takeovers by different factions of the optometry professions in Britain and Australia respectively. Exclusion was also evident in other midwifery professional projects. Heagerty (1990), for example, details the extensive efforts midwifery leaders went to in Britain to exclude lower class "untrained handywoman." Class issues may not have been the criteria for exclusion as they had been in Britain, but Sheryl Nestel's (1996/97; 2000) analysis posits that nationality and by extension race played a part in the exclusionary social closure strategies evoked in Ontario.[7] As she argues: "[T]he struggle for the legalization of midwifery and its subsequent implementation in Ontario represent racist processes inasmuch as they have enacted exclusions which impact systematically and dramatically on racialized groups of women. Structural inequalities and symbolic processes in which racism plays a central role have not just gone unchallenged by the midwifery movement they have, in fact, been essential to the formulation of politically efficacious strategies" (Nestel 2004: 301). Was this too an unfortunate consequence of the integration process or could it be seen as consistent with the need to create a professional and socially acceptable group of midwifery ambassadors? One would hope that, given the contemporary midwifery profession's roots in feminism, it was the former.

Advancing Conceptualizations of Women, Professions, and the State

Since its revival in the mid-to late 1970s, midwifery in Ontario has undergone dramatic changes. Midwifery originated as an amorphous alternative childbirth movement made up of birth attendants, consumers, and supporters who organized to bring about changes to mainstream maternity care. Throughout the late 1970s and early 1980s, this community evolved into an effective lobby force that drew upon national and international support to confront numerous local challenges from other professional groups. They garnered strong state support for their efforts to achieve integration into the provincial maternity care system and took on the role of creating a unique form of midwifery renowned throughout the world. This included not only state recognition through self-regulatory status, but also public funding for an expanded scope of practice and an independent educational program.

To achieve these ends, some changes occurred in the alternative birth community from which midwives evolved. First, midwifery became more bureaucratically organized into a professional project with overlapping but nevertheless separate institutionalized interests of professionals and consumers. With professional legitimacy at stake, midwives had to take on the tasks of developing standards of practice and a standardized educational program within the confines of a recognized university setting. Professional standards, the policies of the hospitals midwives have privileges at, and the funding agencies that pay midwives together can serve to constrain midwives' ability to be as responsive to birthing women in the spirit of women-centred care as they were previously. These changes, while significant, are far fewer than those experienced by most other professional projects.

In this concluding chapter, I address the questions, "How did midwives and their supporters realize such dramatic achievements?" and "Why do

System of Professions

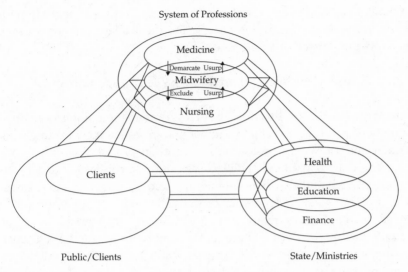

Figure 4
Conceptual map of the interrelations between midwives, consumers, professions, and the state

these outcomes differ from integration projects for midwives in other jurisdictions and from those of other aspiring health professions?" In answering these questions, I revisit the conceptual framework presented in chapter 1. I first discuss the dynamics of the relations within the midwifery community – specifically between midwives and consumer supporters – detailing how the midwifery integration project came to be defined by its proponents and the strategies undertaken to propel it forward. Following this, I contextualize this integration project within the "system of health professions," highlighting the interprofessional relations between midwifery, medicine, and nursing. I then examine the dynamic between midwives, consumers, and the state, expanding upon Larson's and Witz' conceptualization of profession–state relations within patriarchal, capitalist society. A more complete framework reflecting the elements of this case study is depicted in figure 4 above. A common theme across all three levels of analysis is the importance of the combination of the agency of midwives and their supporters and the structural context of the system in which they were attempting to become integrated.

Many of the conclusions reached in this three-level discussion parallel those of other studies of professionalization. But given the uniqueness of midwifery and the contemporary Canadian socio-political context, an expanded conceptualization of the impact of gender on the role that the state and consumers play in professionalization projects becomes possible.

In the final section of this conclusion, I comment on the changes to midwifery through the integration process and the challenges it continues to face revealing areas for future research.

One of the key themes that arose from this examination of the integration of midwifery is how an "elite" group of midwives emerged, leading what became the midwifery profession's integration project. As Jutta Mason (1990) described, in all the "political campaigns, a core group of activists has done much of the work of submission-writing, lobbying, and organizing" (2). These leaders tended to be the same group of approximately a dozen or so midwives, many of whom at some point worked out of the Toronto-based Midwives' Collective. These midwifery leaders also formed the majority of the executive of the AOM. Though formally excluded from some of the key state-appointed committees, these midwifery leaders came to have a profound influence on the integration process across all four domains – organization, regulation, practice, and education.

Larson's (1977, 1979) and Witz's (1990, 1992) works are helpful in illuminating the strategic importance of the emergence of an elite group in directing an integration project. First, as noted in chapter 1, Larson (1977, 1979) introduced the concept of a *professional project* which involves, among other things, the control over a market for expertise. According to Larson, control over a market involves both the creation of a distinctive professional product, as through a unique cognitive base, and the concurrent control over who becomes a member of the profession. In leading this integration project, midwifery leaders created a distinct yet marketable professional product – the Ontario midwifery model of care.

As noted previously, members of the alternative childbirth community came from many different backgrounds and perspectives, and their reasons for being involved in this community varied greatly. The one common thread holding this diverse community together was their support for a women-centred model of maternity care. Midwifery was originally regarded by many within this community as a means to the end of greater consumer choice and control of childbirth. Those within this community who later came to head the midwifery movement essentially took this consumer-responsive form of childbirth care and packaged it into a midwifery professional project palatable to what they regarded as the "powers that be" – the HPLR, other professions (notably medicine) and the state. In this sense, it could be argued that midwifery leaders co-opted this aspect of the alternative childbirth movement, making it into a professional project.

But the decision to develop this project did not only come from within the profession. It is in explaining the reasoning behind the development of this professional movement and the strategies used to promote it that Witz's (1990, 1992) work is particularly relevant. Following Witz, one could describe female professional projects as developing in response to exclusion. This is true of the Ontario midwifery case. It was largely in response to midwives' exclusion from the publicly funded and administered health care system that this professional project was undertaken. Midwifery leaders hoped that with integration, their services would be more accessible to a wider group of clientele, and in addition, that they would secure protection from legal harassment. To achieve this end, midwifery leaders employed strategies similar to the "gendered occupation closure strategies" Witz (1990, 1992) described. These strategies involved both the intraoccupational strategy of "exclusion" as a means of controlling midwifery, and the interoccupational strategy of "usurpation" as a means to distinguish midwifery from medicine and nursing (discussed more fully in the subsequent section on the system of professions level).

The professional product being "marketed" by the leaders of the integration project – the model of midwifery care – became the priority of the movement. To maintain the model, these leaders realized that other elements of midwifery considered to be less critical might have to be compromised. The existence of a somewhat accommodating elite group within an aspiring professional group (or within an established professional group for that matter (Tuohy 1988) willing to make compromises is by no means a rare occurrence. Several other studies (e.g., Biggs 1989; Cant and Sharma 1996; Coburn 1988; Willis 1989; Witz 1992) highlight similar intraprofessional dynamics in other professionalization projects as discussed in chapters 1 and 10.

One of the compromises made by midwifery leaders throughout the integration process was in the shift of the educational model away from an apprentice-based approach towards a university-based, baccalaureate degree. Establishing the program within a university at the baccalaureate level was not necessarily regarded as the best way to educate midwives and indeed, some felt that this could create barriers for some women to become midwives. It was, however, viewed as necessary by some of the professional supporters of midwifery in order to gain legitimacy within the health care system. Midwifery leaders came to agree.

Compromising for the sake of legitimacy, however, may not have been the only reason behind the reformulation of the midwifery educational model. The standardization of the entry to midwifery practice into a baccalaureate program could also be construed as a method whereby the professionalizing elite could control who became a member of the profession (akin to Larson's (1977, 1979) "control of the production of the producers"). That is, it could be regarded as a means of controlling the supply of entrants to midwifery which in turn was a way to control the professional product (Parkin 1979). This control over entry into the profession could have been possible through an apprenticeship program but it would not have garnered the kind of legitimacy that a baccalaureate program would. Thus, the changes in education were both a compromise to gain legitimacy as well as a mechanism for controlling the profession and the professional "product" in the future. Limiting midwifery entrants to those who were committed to the philosophy and model of midwifery practice in Ontario and excluding those who did not fit the model (e.g., those who were not comfortable attending at home births), along the lines of Witz's model of intraoccupational exclusion, was a means of ensuring the promotion of that model, or the professional product.[1]

But midwifery leaders' willingness to accommodate should not be overstated. They actively attempted to minimize compromises through several strategies. One of their strategies was to draw on research and on the sponsorship of the broader national and international midwifery community to provide justification for the midwifery model of care. This proved to have a great deal of currency with some of the key decision-makers. Another strategy was to shape and control the "midwifery product" through such means as controlling midwifery input to key policy-making committees, developing standards of practice, and controlling the image of midwifery – generally promoting a "professional" appearance through a variety of means (e.g., media presentation protocols). Controlling what midwifery was or was seen to be is similar to what Witz (1990, 1992) and Donnison (1977) described of British midwives' attempts to raise the status of midwifery. Ontario midwifery leaders promoted midwifery as both an educated, upper-middle-class movement (which to a large extent it was prior to integration) by emphasizing its professional aspects and at the same time downplaying its counterculture fringe roots.

These legitimizing yet controlling strategies resulted in general feelings of exclusion among some rank-and-file midwives that were exacerbated by the hurried nature of the integration process. For example, Jutta Mason (1990) explained how the creation of a sense of urgency also created an environment of exclusion: "Right from the beginning of the campaign there was also a sense that *there just wasn't time* to debate issues that didn't relate strategically to the goal of legalization" (2, emphasis in original). The often hasty nature of responses and actions resulted in AOM meetings being less and less open, and less likely to be held outside Toronto. Even when meetings were attended by midwives outside the elite group, many felt that a lot of the decisions had already been made prior to the meetings by the midwives driving the integration project.

At the same time, however, the "excluded" midwives felt the work accomplished by those leading their profession was impressive, as one midwife described: "I don't feel bitter because I feel that there was a lot of great work that happened, but it was very hard to feel inclusive about it. There wasn't the sense that people felt welcome" (personal communication 1995).

Although these controlling strategies of midwifery leaders created dissension, they proved to be successful in establishing a professional image that achieved respect from key policy decision-makers. This is exemplified in the following comment by Task Force, IRCM, and Transitional Council chair Mary Eberts:

I've heard some of the doctors describe them as "talented outside agitators." They really did appear to be larger than life and when you think of it that only a handful of people were doing all of this ... They are very high energy, they are very highly organized and the ones that I met, mostly the AOM and large practice midwives were amazing professionals. They really had struggled to create a profession and find the essence of professionalism in a totally unregulated situation. The leadership in that community is just outstanding, really magnificent leadership. They are women who drive themselves hard ... They're such negotiators and they're such leaders and they're really amazing people ... I have an enormous amount of respect for them. (personal communication 1995)

Another policy decision maker, IRCM member Wendy Sutton, also commented that she had "never seen a group of people that was able to function and direct their circumstances so effectively" (personal communication 1994). Internationally renowned midwife and director of the Michener integration program Susanne Houd also commented on the importance of the impact of the leaders of Ontario midwifery:

I think it's no secret that the Midwives' Collective, and Vicki and Holliday and so on are the ones that are the leaders of midwives and I think they should have all the credit in the world for what they've done ... I know that sometimes they can be intimidating and all that because they are so strong and they have a vision and they went for it no matter what, but I think the other side of that is because of the persistence and the incredible I mean, they had no private life, it was to do this, 24 hours a day they worked for this cause and they've been doing this for years ... Of course, it wouldn't have happened without the elite. They had to be extremely clever, extremely political, smart. It has been really fascinating to follow that. (personal communication 1993)

The "internal" control over midwifery and the respect for midwifery leaders by key policy decision makers would prove to be important for the midwifery integration project. When the strategic actions of midwifery leaders faced the structural constraints of the system of health professions, the credibility of the midwifery elite proved crucial. Nevertheless, the hierarchy inherent in the increased elite control over midwives and midwifery represented a shift from the egalitarian social movement from which it originated.

MIDWIFERY AND THE SYSTEM OF HEALTH PROFESSIONS

As noted above, Witz (1992) described female professional projects as involving the dual closure strategies of exclusion within the profession and usurpation between professions. Usurpation as initially conceptualized by Parkin (1979) and defined by Witz, entails "the mobilization of power by one group or collectivity against another that stands in a relationship of dominance to it" (Witz 1992: 74). In the case of midwifery, the "dominant" profession midwifery leaders had to face was medicine but they also faced the more established (albeit not dominant) profession of nursing. It was vis-à-vis these two professions that midwifery leaders had to mark the distinctiveness of the midwifery model, their professional product. This is in fact what they did right from the beginning, as clearly exemplified in their first submission to the HPLR: "Midwifery is a separate entity *distinct from nursing and medicine*. Its specific focus on normal pregnancy and childbirth contrasts sharply with both the broad scope of nursing and general practice medicine, and the focus on the abnormal of the obstetrician" (Lenske 1984: 9, emphasis added). It is clear that given this particular model of practice, those in medicine and especially nursing would be excluded from the midwifery professional project unless they became part of it.

But the midwifery model of care was not developed in a vacuum. The women who became midwives responded to the need of an increasing number of women who were looking for care that differed significantly from that which was available in the mainstream maternity care system. It was in this way a response to the "lack" of a certain kind of service by the established professions that midwifery developed. In Abbott's terms, this new model of midwifery was made possible either by the "external system disturbance" of the counterculture movement or women's desire for more control during childbirth; either way it was a new take on the existing jurisdiction of the provision of maternity care.

The success of midwifery leaders' usurpationary efforts was due to several factors at the "system of professions" level. As previously noted, both medicine and nursing were preoccupied with other issues emanating largely from the HPLR process. That is, because of the HPLR, nursing and medicine were faced with several other occupational struggles over and above that of midwifery (e.g., medicine with chiropractic and naturopathy, nursing with nursing assistants, etc.). Former Minister of Health Elinor Caplan noted the importance of the diffusion of interest of these "traditional naysayers": "Perhaps the timing was right [in that] ... the traditional naysayers who oppose this kind of change were busy with other issues. Because of the Health Professions Legislation coming in, I would say the other providers who normally would be threatened by the entry of midwives were more concerned about their scope of practice and their issues under the Health Professions Legislation rather than focusing their time and attention [on midwifery]" (personal communication 1995). This is not to say that nursing and medicine were uninterested in midwifery, it is just that the resources each profession had available to address the midwifery issue were limited and diffused across many other issues.

This diffusion of resources largely resulting from the HPLR was also exacerbated by other factors. Within nursing, for example, many of those most interested in the implementation of midwifery and who would have been most active in lobbying for nurse-midwifery had for the most part already been essentially co-opted into the midwifery integration project. The medical profession was also preoccupied with its confrontation with the government over the extra billing issue. This had culminated in the physician strike in the summer of 1986 (serendipitously the same year that the government announced its intentions to integrate midwifery), and continued into a sort of "cold war" between the state and medicine throughout the late 1980s (Coburn, Rappolt and Bourgeault 1997). During this period, it could be argued that the state was continually chipping away at the mantle of medical dominance in an effort to rationalize the health care system (Coburn 1993). Thus medical opposition to midwifery leaders' integration efforts was substantially muted.

In addition, many physicians (obstretrician/gynecologists and family physicians alike) were abandoning the practice of obstetrics: "If you look at the people going into family practice ... some family practitioners are not doing obstetrics, and the age at which obstetricians want to get out of doing general obstetrics seems to be getting younger and younger. So there's a kind of shortage of manpower/health human resources to do normal obstetrics" (Karyn Kaufman, personal communication 1995). This exodus from obstetrics has several causes, including lifestyle factors and significantly larger malpractice insurance fees for obstetrics, a result of the 1984 Canadian Medical Protective Association review (Lofsky 1995). Borrowing again from Abbott's (1988) terminology, physicians were beginning to vacate the jurisdiction of childbirth attendance, leaving an opening for midwives. In this way, it could be argued that midwives were partly filling a void rather than usurping turf from physicians – but they were filling it in a different way. Furthermore, the effect of this jurisdictional vacancy was to leave fewer advocates within medicine deeply interested in the midwifery issue; the majority were engaged in other issues considered more salient. Some physicians within the maternity care community also either were or became key advocates of the midwifery professional project. The development of strategic medical alliances is similar to what has been found of other professional projects including other midwifery professional projects (Donnison 1977; Witz 1992; Kornelsen and Carty 2004).

Following this lack or diffusion of interest, medicine and nursing were somewhat invisible at the midwifery integration decision-making table. Despite this invisibility at the policy level, however, it could be argued that medicine was nevertheless indirectly influential at the implementation level due to its ideologically and structurally embedded dominance within the health care system (Alford 1975; Kazanjian 1993). Medicine was influential at the ideological level in terms of the model of midwifery education and regulation. That is, many of the integration decisions were made by midwives themselves, but were formulated in terms of how they would be viewed by the medical profession. This was especially true of the decision to have a formal baccalaureate educational program housed within a university-based health science centre. Midwife Robin Kilpatrick noted how throughout the integration process, midwifery leaders continually asked themselves: "What are the politics of articulating this to the medical establishment in moving midwifery into a legitimate kind of profession within the health care community? How do we present this and represent this without losing credibility for the profession?" (personal communication 1995). This conscious attempt to monitor its appearance in the "medical mirror" corroborates what midwives pursuing integration in other jurisdictions have done (Sullivan and Weitz 1984). In this way, midwifery paradoxically came to be partly co-opted by the very system in opposition to which it originally developed.

Medicine's impact on the midwifery integration process was also due to its structurally embedded dominance in existing legislation (Kazanjian 1993). This was most evident in the Public Hospital's Act which structured physicians' privileged position within the hospital. Medicine had an influence, therefore, albeit *in absentia*. Perhaps it is because of a recognition of this embeddedness of medical dominance in concert with its diffusion of interests that organized medicine did not make such an overtly public and concerted effort at the policy level to thwart the midwifery integration project.

Thus, although physicians partly vacated a "jurisdiction" they nevertheless maintained control over it through structurally and ideologically embedded means. Was this demarcation in action? Because of these residuals of medical dominance (as yet relatively untouched by the power of the state), midwifery leaders had to make compromises in their integration project. This shaping of the presentation of midwifery in order to make it palatable to medicine in turn pushed midwifery in particular directions. In attempting to become included in a system, one must play by rules and regulations defined by the dominant group, which in midwifery's case was medicine. This dynamic is a well-documented facet of the integration efforts of many aspiring health professions (e.g., Biggs 1989; Larkin 1983; Wardwell 1981; Willis 1989).

But medicine is not the ultimately determinative force in the Ontario health care system. More and more, the state as regulator and funder has begun to exercise its power within the system of health professions (Coburn 1993). With the rising attention paid to the fiscal crisis, the state has increasingly taken on the task of managing the system, attempting to rationalize the health care division of labour. For a variety of reasons, not the least of which is the open-ended nature of physician remuneration, medicine is often regarded as an obstacle to these efforts. Sponsorship by the state, achieved in part through the consumer support group, helped push midwifery past the structurally and ideologically embedded "leftovers" of medical dominance.

THE NEXUS BETWEEN MIDWIVES,
CONSUMERS AND THE STATE

Although factors within the emerging profession of midwifery (and in the related professions of medicine and nursing) were influential in the integration project, as noted throughout, the nexus between midwives, consumers and the state was particularly important. State support for the midwifery integration project was evident at several levels. One of the first was the establishment of committees to examine the arguments for and against midwifery integration, and the appointment to these committees of people generally in favour of midwifery. This was readily apparent to many involved: "Obviously people in government were supportive of midwifery because of the people they chose to head committees" (midwife Chris Sternberg, personal communication 1995). Over and above this, the government acted on the recommendations of these committees. Although the Task Force was an advisory committee, most of its recommendations were implemented, as were the recommendations from the HPLR and IRCM committees. Former Task Force and HPLR staff member Linda Bohnen stressed the significance of government support through the implementation of reports, not just in one piece of legislation but in several: "Things could have fallen by the wayside because the government had to implement. I mean how many reports do you know of that never saw legislation – *millions*. The government had to have the political will, and then not just one government, but two governments had to have the political will to pull this off in Bills. So that was quite important, because it's very easy to lose the will" (personal communication 1995, emphasis in original). The state also supported the midwifery integration project by funding these advisory committees, as well as the midwifery regulatory body, the new educational program, and midwifery services. These funds were not just given on a one-time basis but represent a continuing funding commitment. All of this came at a time when government funding in health care (and elsewhere) was increasingly being cut back.

The achievement of professional legitimacy via the state is not unique to midwifery in Ontario. As highlighted in chapter 1, Freidson (1970a) has argued that occupations become professions through the granting of legitimate organized autonomy by the state. Johnson (1982) also emphasized the importance of the state historically in the professionalization process. In the professionalization of chiropractic in Ontario, Biggs (1989) specifically emphasizes the importance of sponsorship by state elites for chiropractic. Regarding female professional projects, Witz (1990, 1992) described how "legalistic" tactics via the state were the way British midwives ultimately became successful in securing legislation at the turn of the twentieth century. She asserts that these legalistic tactics at the state level were more successful than were credentialist tactics at the level of civil society. Witz does not, however, address the issue of why the state route to professionalization for midwifery integration was generally more effective than were other strategies.

In trying to understand why there was such strong state support for midwifery and, more generally, why seeking state support can be an effective route for female professional projects, it is important to revisit the earlier discussion of the dual roles of a democratic state – capital accumulation and legitimacy (Simmons and Keohane 1992). Regarding the state's role in capital accumulation, governments have become more interested in better managing their budgets and in curbing deficit in particular. Rising health care costs, which in Ontario contribute to over one third of the provincial budget, are a prime target. Consequently, the state has become more interested in the rationalization of health care resources, which often gets translated into the rationalization of the health care division of labour. Given the argument – or some might claim assumption – that midwifery is a cost-effective form of care (Cherry and Foster 1982; Fooks and Gardiner 1986; Reid and Morris 1979; Rooks 1986), integrating midwifery into the provincial health care system suited the state's efforts in this direction. Although at the time there were few data to support this argument – or for that matter refute it – there was at least the appearance that the government might end up saving money in the long run due in part to midwives' "low-tech" approach to birth.

But although cost-effectiveness initially may have been part of the argument for integrating midwifery, it was not the sole reason (Evans 1981). If the state was simply concerned with cost-effectiveness, it would have most likely implemented a nurse-midwifery model. Such a model would have probably entailed few added costs in establishing a regulatory body, and potentially smaller start up and support costs for an add-on midwifery educational program than for a direct-entry program. At the same time it may have produced similar cost saving outcomes to the direct-entry midwifery strategy, such as lower rates of intervention and lower educational costs per practitioner. But time and again, key decision-makers stated that this was not what they heard was desired by the community. Instead, the state implemented a direct-entry model for reasons beyond cost-effectiveness. Thus, the congruency thesis of the relationship between midwifery and the broader interests of capital (Larson 1977, 1979), or the state on behalf of capital, although accurate, is only part of the equation. More was at issue than cost effectiveness in the state's support of the midwifery integration project.

It is in examining the state's interest in maintaining its own legitimacy vis-à-vis its electorate – and the female portion of that electorate in particular – that a more complete picture of state support for midwifery emerges. Politics do matter and it is because of the political role of the state that consumers and the broad base of active women's groups supporting midwifery (including both left-wing feminist activists and more conservative women's groups) take on such great importance. It is through the support of these groups, especially politically astute, predominantly upper-middle-class feminist supporters, that midwifery leaders and their counterparts in the consumer support group were able to convince the state that there was significant constituency support for the midwifery integration project. Barrington (1985) noted the importance of this alliance between feminists and midwives early on: "Feminism lent the midwifery movement complex new networks, political savvy, and imposing numerical strength. This alliance catapulted the midwifery issue into the mainstream political forums" (153).

But as mentioned before, midwifery was not viewed simply as a left-wing feminist issue; it was a unique issue that had support from women across the political spectrum. Moreover, this support was not just for midwifery generally, but for a specific kind of midwifery that leaders of the midwifery movement advocated. A nurse-midwifery model did not garner the kind of enthusiasm from women that community midwifery had. Barrington (1985) foreshadowed the importance midwifery advocates in Canada would play in the political sphere: "After a decade of public education and media attention on the midwifery cause, it is now understood and advocated by a significant block of parents, feminists and health care professionals. As they translate their opinion into petitions, demonstrations and votes, even the most conservative legislators take note" (155). She was correct. Midwives and their supporters together became, as Mary Eberts described, "a change seeking organism":

The midwifery community, the whole community was an organism that had organized itself to accomplish this work, right, so that these women who were so dedicated and so accomplished were doing it within the context of these practices that had been set up to accommodate on-call work and back-up and to provide substitutes for meetings and to incorporate a method of payment for the professional work that the women did. I mean the whole – the whole community had mobilized to do this … They structured their working environment, including the relations of consumers and professionals so as itself to be the engine driving the change … It was really more than the sum of its parts. It was a change-seeking organism … It's quite remarkable. (personal communication 1995)

The leaders of the professional project not only garnered community support, they endeavoured to attain media support as well. This was a particular focus of the community around the Toronto Island Inquest and the role consumer representatives played was clearly of critical importance to the success of this strategy. Although some media have definitely had a negative impact on the midwifery community in sensationalizing the "disastrous outcomes" of home births, some also helped to promote midwifery as a feminist issue. Garnering media support may not necessarily be a social closure strategy, but it was nevertheless an important strategy for the professional project, perhaps related to the need to create a marketable professional product in line with Larson's (1979) thinking. That is, the media was used to help market midwifery and, in addition to the community support, brought pressure upon the state to respond to the midwifery issue.

Pressure notwithstanding, this broadly supported, politically articulate largely female lobby met with a particularly receptive audience within the state, both within the bureaucracy and more visibly at the level of the ministers of Health:

Midwives were very fortunate in that the last four Ministers were all female and all pro-midwifery across parties so the initiative did not get lost with change in government; and also very fortunate to have the opportunity to have so much input into the implementation process. (IRCM member Ina Caissey, personal communication 1995)

We have been lucky that beginning with Murray Elston, we have had Ministers of Health who had an understanding of the importance of midwifery as a popular issue; but also personally all of the female Ministers have told stories about their own births and related to midwifery in a very personal way. (midwife Vicki Van Wagner, personal communication 1995)

Van Wagner also stressed the importance of timing and the socio-political climate which enabled these women in the state to be more open about taking a women's stance to the midwifery issue: "The women's movement had advanced enough that [these women] had gotten into the kinds of positions where they didn't have to apologize about clearly looking at issues from a women's perspective ... You know ten years earlier – even five years earlier that might not have been able to happen" (Van Wagner 1993, as quoted in Fynes 1994). This was particularly striking in the Liberal government's decision to have an outspoken feminist lawyer head the Task Force. So instead of being confronted with a state which has been described as "institutionalized masculinity" (Connell 1990), they were met with at least a sliver of institutionalized femininity with the temporarily feminized Ministry of Health.

Further, the ideological compatibility Larson (1979) highlights as being critical for professional projects is not only with respect to capital (the dominant ideology) but could also be with respect to the increasingly important ideology of feminism (Adams and Bourgeault 2003; Rushing 1993). Like Barrington (1985) comments above, Rushing (1993) argues that feminism provides an ideology that has both shaped the nature of midwifery practice, and helped midwifery to popularize and legitimate itself with many members of the public. Feminism as an ideology has currency for midwives' professional project because of the contemporary context. The currency of feminism is not just with feminist activists but also within certain segments of the state in part because of its legitimacy function. The consequence of this ideological compatibility is that the midwifery lobby was able to penetrate particular segments of the state and become political "insiders" to the policy process which was to impact upon them, rather than being relegated to the margins. This was most clearly evident in the unofficial status of the midwifery liaison committee of the IRCM. This is quite a remarkable achievement which, in the realm of health policy, is usually only obtained by leaders of the medical profession. It is the feminization of the state – or at least of key segments of the state – and its ideological compatibility with the midwifery project that enabled this strategic "opportunity space" (Waylen 1998) to be created.

That the integration-seeking efforts of midwives went as far as they did in Ontario is due in large part to this confluence of "female" factors around the legitimacy role of the state (see figure 5). The achievement of integration via the state with the help of consumer support may not be unique to midwifery. Biggs (1989) also detailed how the integration efforts of chiropractors in Ontario benefited from the support of organized labour and their lobbying efforts on the government to include chiropractic under the provincial health insurance plan. But it is the

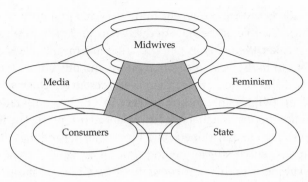

Figure 5
The nexus between midwives, consumer supporters, and the state

gendered perspective on this consumer–profession–state dynamic that represents a unique contribution to the professions and policy literatures.

Melding this historically specific, gender-based consumer–profession–state dynamic with the also historically specific facts that the state in Ontario has an increasingly powerful position within the health care system, and that nursing and medicine were otherwise preoccupied, enables one to better understand why the Ontario midwifery integration project was more successful than other similar professional projects. For example, in comparison with the integration project of British midwives, which occurred roughly one hundred years earlier, both the state's role in the health care system and women's influence on the state were much less pronounced. Because of this context that differed greatly from earlier efforts, the kinds of legalistic social closure strategies undertaken by midwives differ greatly from those described by Witz (1992). In her case, midwifery leaders had to secure proxy state support from men largely because women did not yet have the vote. Midwives at that time – turn of the twentieth-century Britain – were clearly confronted with institutionalized masculinity in the state as well as in civil society. In Ontario, consumers were an integral part of the midwives' legalistic strategies because of the influence they would have on the state. Moreover, midwives were able to draw upon the success they garnered from their legalistic strategies vis-à-vis the state to gain support for their credentialist strategies of securing hospital admitting privileges and establishing a baccalaureate educational program. So this analysis of the midwifery project in the contemporary Canadian context enables a greatly expanded analysis of professionalization strategies possible for female professional projects.

In comparison with more recent midwifery integration projects in the United States, the role of the state in the American health care "system" is markedly weaker than it is in Ontario. This has meant a less conducive environment to midwives' integration efforts in both Britain (at least historically) and the United States, than was present in Ontario. Closer to home, the midwifery integration project in Quebec suffered from far greater medical opposition than was experienced in Ontario (Vadeboncœur 2000, 2004; Vadeboncœur, Maheux and Blais 1996/97) and the Alberta midwives were less successful in gaining state recognition through appointments on key decision-making committees than were Ontario midwives (James and Bourgeault 2004). Both cases also suffered from greater intraprofessional conflict between midwives with and without a nursing background (McKendry and Langford 2000).

Thus, it is not just timing that is important, but timing in concert with the structural context and the interest and relative influence of various actors within the health care system. This not only emphasizes the importance of examining professionalization projects from various levels of analysis, it also highlights the need to regard the interests of the professions and the state as both dynamic and as partly situation-specific. As Biggs (1989) noted of the professionalization of chiropractic in Ontario, there was a "historically specific constellation of interests" (422), which, in the case of midwifery in Ontario, came together to provide a window of opportunity conducive to its professional project. It is because of the dynamic nature of these interests that studies done in different settings at different times have come to different conclusions. This highlights the importance of examining professionalization projects from a comparative perspective (van Teijlinden et al. 2003). It is in doing so that a more complete picture of the process and outcomes of integration is made possible.

The integration of midwifery into the Ontario health care system was a process influenced by structure, agency, and timing. Midwives and their consumer supporters, as exemplified by their representatives, took charge of the fate of midwifery. At the same time, many of their actions were sparked and enabled by broader structural factors, including those emanating from within the state and system of health professions, beyond the control of midwives. The midwifery integration process, however, was not only promoted by the state, it was also bounded and constrained by it. As Briskin (1999) alluded to earlier, "state responsiveness is not without contradiction: issues raised by women are often taken over by the state and solutions reshaped and managed in ways that might not have been foreseen and are not always in women's best interests" (12). That is, although midwifery gained legitimacy and autonomy through the state, this autonomy is ultimately limited and constrained by the state. Midwifery was also constrained by the embedded power of the still-dominant medical profession particularly within the hospital setting. Thus, with integration, midwives may not only feel pressure to come under medical control, as DeVries (1982, 1985, 1986, 1996) and others have argued (see discussion in chapter 1), because of the influential role of the state in the health care system in Ontario, midwives may also feel the pressure of direct or indirect state control. This external control over midwifery ultimately had and will continue to have an effect on midwives and their clients, and on the relationship between these parties.

REFLECTIONS ON THE EFFECTS OF
PROFESSIONALIZATION ON MIDWIFERY

As noted above, there have been some important "side effects" of the professionalization process for midwifery. The strategic reorganization of the community includes a more bureaucratic representation of professional and consumer interests which marks a significant shift in the originally undifferentiated, nonhierarchical organization of midwives and clients. This organizational separation creates the potential for distancing between midwives and their clients (see also Kirkham 1989; Nelson 1983).

The regulation of midwifery has also changed.[2] When midwifery first arose, midwives were "regulated" to a certain extent directly by their clients, but also more crudely by the criminal justice system. Given midwives' negative experiences with inquests, this latter form of regulation came to be regarded not only as inadequate but threatening to the continuation of midwifery. In securing self-regulatory status, midwives garnered protection from harassing courts, but it also marked another step in the distancing of midwives from their clients. The regulation of midwives was no longer in the hands of a few clients but was mediated through a professional self-regulatory body.

The midwifery model of practice, which centred around the consumer-oriented principles of continuity of care, informed choice, and choice of birth place, was a crucial feature of midwifery that midwives and their supporters struggled to maintain. In large part they have succeeded. But due in part to the desire to expand their scope of practice and secure public funding for their services, midwives face continued challenges to their practice model from hospitals and funding agencies. Midwives must not only practise according to what their clients need and want, they must also adhere to professional standards and hospital policies (see more extensive discussion below).

The process through which women become midwives has also shifted from one in which women and their midwives learn from each other in the community to a university-based, bureaucratically administered professional education program.[3] In shifting midwifery education from the community to a university-based program, it has been argued that the accessibility of midwifery practice may be limited.[4] Although these changes to the entry to midwifery practice were regarded as compromises that were necessary to ensure the success of the integration process, the potential for these changes to continue to affect midwifery are significant. Midwifery has not only been changed at the community and organization level, the "new" profession contains many further implications for the future of the profession.

By examining the changes to midwifery separately within each of these domains, one could come to the conclusion that integration has had varying degrees of effect on midwifery. For example, if one were simply to examine the fate of the midwifery model of practice, one could conclude that midwives and their supporters were largely successful in maintaining their model throughout the integration process. An investigation of the changes to education, however, would suggest that midwifery was changed more substantially through the integration process. But, as noted previously, these domains are neither separate nor discrete but rather are interconnected aspects of the profession of midwifery. To truly understand the effects of the integration process, one must step back and examine the totality of changes across all these domains of midwifery and their potential to influence future midwifery practice.

It is in taking a step back to examine the overall effect of integration on midwifery in Ontario, that I have experienced the most difficulty as an "involved" researcher (MacDonald and Bourgeault 2000). Throughout this study my opinion regarding the outcome of the integration process has vacillated from being supportive of integration to being somewhat ambivalent, depending often on who I last interviewed or what document I last read. I can see that in each domain of midwifery I have examined, the changes I have observed had both positive and negative effects on midwives and birthing women. This is especially true of the organization and regulation of midwifery and the education of midwives. The changes in the organization of midwifery in the early stages of the integration process set the stage for the possibility of increased hierarchy between midwives and women. The position of midwifery consumers moved from significant involvement in the regulation and training of midwives to a more marginalized position. The evolution of midwifery training into a university-based, baccalaureate program also serves to distance midwives from their clients. I am not certain, however, that I would agree completely with Benoit's (1987) assertions that midwifery professionalism and client partnership are necessarily contradictory, but I would agree with Barrington's (1985) supposition that with integration midwives may have constrained their ability to fully practise according to their philosophy.

While documenting the process of midwifery integration, I continually asked myself, "Were these changes avoidable? Could midwifery have survived intact without integrating into the Ontario health care system?" I came to the conclusion that midwifery had to change. The same forces that helped propel midwifery forward as a professional project – namely the HPLR – could have quashed community midwifery in favour of another form or the status quo – no midwifery. Indeed, it was very likely that the HPLR would have regulated midwifery in some form. Midwives felt, and I believe rightly so, that the outcomes would be less negative if they participated in the process. Moreover, although I understand fundamentally many of the central tenets of the anti-integration argument, I came to agree with Karyn Kaufman's more pragmatic assertion that the form in which midwifery originally existed was not a sustainable system:

What troubles me with someone like DeVries is that while I accept his argument, he's not a consumer, and he's not a midwife ... It may be fine from an academic point of view to say, "This is the cutting edge. This is how you get social change. This is the grass-roots stuff." Being out there on that cutting edge, being exposed to legal liability, and taking the risks ... from a midwife's point of view, is not a comfortable place to be ... I think you are asking people to be in a very tough place ... Moreover, burning out midwives leaves no one left to be cutting edge. ... I think that there are prospects for erosion ... [But] by having your own regulatory body ... with some very strong principles ... and espousing more feminist methods of how to run a profession ... I think much, if not most, of the original ideas will be retained. (personal communication 1995)

The most important achievement of the integration process, I (and many others in the midwifery community) believe, is public funding for midwives to practice within their preferred model. First, with respect to the model of practice, although the consumer orientation has increasingly been diffused to address professional standards and hospital policies, at the level of policy (and likely at the level of practice) consumers are still the focus of the midwifery model of practice. It is in this way that Ontario midwifery can remain true to its philosophical roots. This maintenance of the midwifery model of practice and the consequent lessening of the severity of the split between professional and client that occurs with professionalization may be due not just to the agency of midwives, but to the structural context of the state–profession–consumer dynamic described above. It could be argued that since consumers were so important in securing state support, a client focus on care would be the least changed element of midwifery. That is, because of the intricate interconnectedness of the content of the midwifery integration project (i.e., its consumer-oriented ideology and practice) and the political strategies of the project (i.e., supportive consumer lobbying), there was a strong motive to maintain this aspect of midwifery. The role of consumers helps explain, in part, why the effects of integration usually experienced by midwifery professional projects elsewhere were minimized in Ontario. Specifically, midwifery consumers were a more active and necessary part of the professional project and the state was a more "friendly" controlling body than medicine likely would have been, because of its legitimacy role vis-à-vis a female electorate.

Midwifery care is also, at least in principle, more widely accessible through public funding. The services midwives provide are still quite different from those available in the traditional system. Given their strength in changing the system from the outside to include midwifery, midwives may also be able to change the system from within, or at least resist undesirable external pressures to conform.

POSTSCRIPT TO INTEGRATION

Looking back at the ten years that have elapsed since the official integration of midwifery into the provincial health care system, there have continued to be changes and challenges. Some have been expected whereas others have not. One of the first changes following the official integration of midwifery into the health care system occurred to the consumer arm of the midwifery professional project – the MTFO. The proclamation of the Midwifery Act meant that the official mandate of the MTFO – the official integration of midwifery into the health care system – was achieved. Therefore the members of the MTFO decided that it would focus on the role of representing the interests of consumers in the ongoing midwifery integration process. In the fall of 1994, the MTFO officially became the Ontario Midwifery Consumer Network (OMCN). Its mandate was to

---

preserve and promote the Ontario model of midwifery care through active participation in the regulation of the profession, its educational programmes, and ongoing public education (OMCN Vision Statement, September 1994). Its underlying goal was to keep Ontario midwifery responsive to consumers.

As an organized provincial entity, the OMCN did not last very long; it dissolved officially in the spring of 2001. Many of the consumer members of the MTFO and later the OMCN who were most interested in midwifery went on to become midwives later, entering the ranks of the profession. Others drifted away from the organization as their children grew up. Although the OMCN had for a short period of time membership on some policy-making committees with the Ministry of Health, there was no formal role for OMCN representatives on the AOM or the CMO. Despite there no longer being a provincial organization, several local community groups continue to exist and two advocates have compiled a popular guide to midwifery (Hawkins and Knox 2003). The role of continuing local groups varies from organized social support for midwifery clients to lobbying for midwifery particularly in underserved areas. These latter efforts have been helpful in securing funding from the provincial Ontario Midwifery Program for placements of new registrants in their communities.

Another change to midwifery following integration alluded to in chapter 8 was the devolution of the funding for midwifery services from the centralized LMCO to local transfer payment agencies. This was cause for much concern within the midwifery community and when the sunset clause of the LMCO was approaching in 1999 tension was high. The hope was that the duration of the LMCO would be extended, perhaps indefinitely. The same concerns that were raised initially with a decentralized model – that it might alter the way midwifery is practised – were again salient. There were sympathies with these concerns within the LMCO perhaps because some of its members were former MTFO officials. Nevertheless, the Ministry forged ahead with the devolution process. To convey its conviction in this regard, it replaced the Executive Director of the LMCO with someone without previous ties to the midwifery community. In the end, several local transfer payment agencies (TPAs) were established to flow funds to midwifery practice groups across the province. To date, there are nineteen TPAs for the forty-seven existing practice groups. Most of these TPAs are community health centres, but where this option is not available, the local hospital or social service agency have taken up the task. Some of the concerns midwives had with devolution have not (or have not yet) come to pass. It would be interesting to see how this evolving situation compares with that in Manitoba where midwives have been integrated as staff of Regional Health Authorities (Kaufert and Robinson 2004).

This status quo situation in midwifery funding is also notable in the case of midwives' salaries which have not changed in the ten years since integration. This is an issue the AOM is presently attempting to negotiate with the Ministry. The only increases in funding that the Ministry has committed to are increases in pay relating to progress through the ranks (as per the years of experience scale), increases in related expenses, and to funding new midwifery registrants (i.e., graduates from the baccalaureate or PLEA programs). But even in this latter issue of funding new midwives, there have been some significant delays causing midwives and their supporters to rally at Queen's Park in 2002.

In terms of regulation, the College continues to be funded by the Ministry of Health in light of there still being less than 300 midwives in the province (College of Midwives statistics as of July 2005. One of the more salient regulatory issues has to do with the necessity of malpractice insurance in the face of rapidly rising premiums. Malpractice insurance premiums for midwives in Ontario have increased from approximately $6,000 in 1997 to approximately $35,000 per midwife in 2003. Luckily, the Ontario Ministry of Health covers the full cost of liability insurance for midwives and has done so ever since integration. In provinces where midwives do not have public funding, such as Alberta, to offset the rising malpractice insurance premiums this has resulted in many a midwife either leaving the province or discontinuing to practice (James and Bourgeault 2004).

Another highly publicized regulatory issue was the 2001 inquest into the May 2000 death of a baby born at Guelph General Hospital. The mother, Kathryn Kelly-Stalker, was under the care of four midwives with the Guelph Midwives practice. At nine days past her due date she went to Guelph General to undergo two routine tests which indicated she needed to have an immediate Caesarean section. Midwife Kelly Dobbin was paged by the hospital with the results and she in turn telephoned the obstetrician on-call – Dr Nabil Namis – to turn over care to him. Dobbin reported that Namis refused to take on the care of the woman claiming that the unit was too busy.[5] Dobbin began to drive the parents to McMaster Hospital in Hamilton, but before leaving Guelph was called by the obstetrician on call at McMaster and told to return to the General and that she would convince Dr Namis to take the case. Namis ultimately performed the Cesarean section later that day. The baby, Eoin Kelly-

Stalker, was born with complications and transferred to McMaster Hospital where he later died from lung complications on May 20, 2000.

The inquest was called to investigate whether the alleged refusal of care by Namis was a unique incident or a sign of "systemic" conflict between doctors and midwives (*Guelph Mercury*, Wed. October 31, 2001). When the Coroner's report was issued, it did not show that the death of Eoin Stalker was linked to the problems between the midwife and obstetrician on call. The jury, however, did call for improved communication amongst obstetrical caregivers, the need for better integration of midwives into the hospital setting and the removal of barriers to effective care (*Guelph Mercury*, Thurs. Dec 6, 2001). Some had wanted the inquest to delve into the issue of funding and how it can impact on relationships between midwives and specialists. As noted by Remi Ejiwunmi, then president of the AOM, in the *Guelph Mercury* (Sat November 10, 2001), "a major funding issue affecting integration of midwives in the health care system is that obstetricians get a lower fee if they provide consulting services to midwives than they can bill OHIP for consultations with physicians ... The impact varies from hospital to hospital, but in non-emergency cases midwives have been refused consultations, and their patients forced to go through family doctors to get obstetrical assistance." The coroner, however, had ruled that funding would not be considered in the inquest because it was not considered to be related to the death of Eoin Stalker. It is, nonetheless, most relevant for the day-to-day working relationship between midwives and physicians.

Albeit an extreme case, the inquest also revealed that although midwifery was officially integrated into the Ontario health care system, the integration into various health care communities and the relations between midwives and physicians across the province as well as across the country varies greatly. In a follow up study of physicians', nurses', and midwives' views of working with each other in the hospital setting, a range of experiences and perspectives from very antagonistic to very supportive was revealed (Bourgeault, Luce and MacDonald 1998). Some physicians vetoed midwives' applications for hospital admitting privileges, whereas other hospitals held wine and cheese celebrations officially welcoming midwives to their hospitals and various decision-making committees. In other cases, midwives and the medical and nursing staff operate under a system which could be called "peaceful coexistence" where midwives come into the hospital and generally oversee a woman's labour and delivery without much interaction with other provider groups. This range of experiences is comparable across Canadian settings where midwifery has been integrated (Blais et al. 1999; Kornelsen and Carty 2004).

The Ontario Midwifery Education Program has also undergone some shifts since its inception in September 1993. It was initially conceived as a four-year baccalaureate program which would be completed in three calendar years. In response to concerns expressed by students about the pace and lack of any real break, the program has been changed to a standard four-year completion time. Extended options to complete the degree in five, six, or seven years are still available at the Ryerson site. In terms of numbers, OMEP Director Karyn Kaufman and faculty member Bobbi Soderstrom (2004) report, "By the autumn of 2002, 153 students had completed programme requirements and were eligible to apply for registration with the College of Midwives ... The graduates of the programme now constitute nearly two-thirds of the number of registered midwives in Ontario" (200). As a result, the profession of midwifery in Ontario is quickly becoming an overwhelmingly young profession. Follow-up surveys of midwifery graduates from 1996 to 1998 (Stewart and Pong 1999a, 1999b) revealed that most were practising within Ontario and felt satisfied with their decision to become midwives. A few opted not to become registered midwives citing the life-style concerns whereas others planned to reduce their workload because of childbearing plans (Kaufman and Soderstrom 2004). New educational programs have also been established in Quebec at the Université du Québec à Trois-Rivières (Vadeboncœur 2004) and at the University of British Columbia (Kornelsen and Carty 2004).

Workload is a salient issue not just for new registrants but for all midwives. In the follow-up research conducted with midwives, a notable theme was the ongoing concern that midwives have with managing the work that is midwifery. Many expressed being particularly stressed by work that is not directly involved in caring for women, such as committee work to maintain hospital admitting privileges, preceptor work to mentor new midwives, and the paperwork involved in being financially accountable to the Provincial Ministry of Health for public funding (Bourgeault, Luce and MacDonald, forthcoming). Several midwives also detail how their work as a midwife, particularly being on-call twenty-four hours a day can result in personal and familial role conflict, but this latter issue has more to do with the model of practice than with integration per se. These are critical issues which must be addressed to maintain the sustainability of the profession.

While discussing midwives' views of hospital integration, the changes to their funding arrangements, and workload issues I also took the opportunity to ask those midwives who practised prior to regulation to reflect on the integration process. The most common response from these pioneer midwives was that many of the changes that ensued from integration were welcome. First and foremost, midwives were pleased with how funding has enabled the expansion of accessibility to midwifery for a greater number of childbearing women. As one midwife noted, "The impact of [funding] on changes in the clientele we are getting is phenomenal. More often we're working much more with women in the working class, and that's good ... This is why we pushed to get midwifery legislated." Others reflected on their new-found increase in professional autonomy. As one midwife noted, "What I really like is if I have a concern I can order the lab, I can order the ultra sound. I don't have to convince some doctor about my concern." This is not to negate how stressful it was getting to that point: "If you look at when we were registered at the end of 1993, first of all, we had never worked in hospital as professionals really. We had never run offices. We were never expected to have huge budgets of money that we had to deal with. We never were employers before. I mean there was so much to learn with so little experience and so little guidance and no preparation to speak of ... I think back now, I have to laugh." A great deal of work was accomplished in a relatively short period of time. Midwives, consumer activists, and supporters within the state together helped build a model of midwifery care that has attracted international recognition. The work of integration is not yet fully accomplished. The sustainability of the model of midwifery care and those who deliver it are at stake.

THE FUTURE OF MIDWIFERY AND OF MIDWIFERY RESEARCH

Since the official integration of midwifery in Ontario in 1994, there has been an explosion of research and writing on midwifery in Canada. This includes three edited collections (Biggs, Burtch and Shroff 1996/97; Bourgeault, Benoit and Davis-Floyd 2004; Shroff 1997), a new journal, *The Canadian Journal of Midwifery Research and Practice*, as well as numerous journal articles/theses examining midwifery integration both within Ontario (e.g., MacDonald 1999; Nestel 2000; Sharpe 2001) and across the country (e.g., Blais 2000; Blais et al. 1999; Collin et al. 2000; Kornelsen and Carty 1999; Lyons and Carty 1999; McKendry and Langford 2000; Reinharz et al. 2000; Vadeboncœur 2000).[6] These have addressed a wide variety of issues from the practice of home birth; midwifery as a cultural phenomenon; the relations between midwives, nurses, and physicians; and the struggles to integrate midwifery into different provincial health care systems. These issues have drawn interest from midwives, social scientists, and health services researchers with significant cross-fertilization of ideas, methods, and concepts (Bourgeault 2002; Bourgeault, Benoit and Davis-Floyd 2004). Indeed, we are at a point where a review of the literature on midwifery in Canada may be warranted.

Despite this new concentration of research, there remain important questions to address, particularly from a comparative interprovincial perspective. Those I highlight here evolve primarily out of the research I have detailed herein but they are informed by this growing literature on midwifery in Canada. Although the emphasis of my investigation has been at a more macro level of analysis, the implication of changes at this level for everyday practice are significant. It is perhaps at this level that some of the more intriguing dynamics of co-optation and resistance may be most evident. As Annandale (1989) found for nurse-midwives in the United States, it is at the "everyday" micro level that midwives were confronted with the greatest challenges to their alternative focus. Midwives must now directly face the "stronger" mainstream maternity care system every day. The pressures to conform to existing practices and preferences may be overwhelming. The conformity of the content and location of the midwifery educational program with that of other health care professional programs in turn may also serve to steer the practices of future midwives toward the mainstream. But perhaps at this everyday level, midwives may be able to bring about change from within the system. These are important issues to investigate across time and across settings.

The focus of this examination has not been of the challenges facing the everyday practice of midwifery. This more "macro," policy-level investigation, however, does identify areas where tensions exist, and in so doing reveals areas for future research on the continuing effects of integration on midwifery. In particular, how midwives practise within the structural constraints that now exist (as a result of the integration process), how these differ across provincial contexts, and how the new educational program will influence midwifery practices, are some fruitful research issues to pursue. It will also be important to examine what happens to the consumer responsiveness of midwifery policies in the absence of an organized consumer voice. Has the dissolution of the OMCN left a vacuum? This question in particular will be important to ask in light of the importance that the nexus between women, professions, and the state has had on midwifery. As these challenges to midwifery in Ontario and across Canada continue so will the need to investigate the outcomes. The struggles of midwifery have not ended; but they continue to take place within a very different context than has previously existed.

The point of departure for this study, however, should not just rest with the future of midwifery research. The purpose of creating a model of the interrelations between consumers, midwives, and state officials is to help advance our thinking on the relations between women, professions, and the state more broadly. Comparative research is critical to expand and test some of the assumptions that lie within this model. I, along with colleagues, have begun to compare the impact consumers have had on maternity care policy where they have been organized – in Canada and the UK – and where they have been less organized – in the United States (Bourgeault, Declercq and Sandall 2001). Susan James and I (James and Bourgeault 2004) have also compared the context of the state-and-midwifery relations between Alberta and Ontario which can help explain in part the different outcomes of midwifery legislation in these two provinces. I have also begun to examine the model comparatively across professions, drawing upon the case of recent initiatives to integrate primary care nurse practitioners into the Ontario health care system, where consumer supporters have played less of a role than was the case for midwifery (Bourgeault, 2005). The possibilities seem endless. I hope that this detailed case study will encourage others to critique, revise, and expand upon the model I propose here as a way to re-ignite the fields of the sociology of the professions, women and the state, and health policy.

An Expanded Discussion of Theory and Methods

MORE ON THEORY ...

This study is situated in the sociology of the professions literature that has evolved from its functionalist roots – where the distinctiveness of the professions is linked to higher education and a service ethic – to a more critical approach that focuses on power (the neo-Weberian approach) or class (the neo-Marxist approach) (Brante 1988; Saks 1983). Contrary to the early professions theorists, neo-Weberian scholars focus less on the positive function of professions within society and more on how they should be viewed as monopoly-seeking, self-interested groups (Abbott 1988; Freidson 1970a, 1970b; Johnson 1972; MacDonald 1985, MacDonald and Ritzer 1988; Parry and Parry 1976). Neo-Marxist theorists go one analytical step further by situating professions within the class structure and within the context of capitalist relations of production (Boreham 1983; Esland 1980; Johnson 1977, 1980). Although there has been as much debate between these two critical perspectives as there was with earlier theories, some scholars stress that the neo-Weberian and neo-Marxist approaches need not be mutually exclusive (Abercrombie and Urry 1983, MacDonald and Ritzer 1988). Indeed, a noteworthy meshing of these two critical perspectives is Larson's (1977, 1979) conceptualization of *professional projects*. Together these critical perspectives and Larson's conceptualization in particular sparked a flurry of studies of the professionalization of medicine and several aspiring occupations.

I began to frame the theoretical context of the study of midwives' professional project with a description of Larson's work followed by an overview of the key studies of various professional projects within the health care division of labour (discussed in chapter 1). In this note on theory, I offer an expanded discussion of Larson's work for those interested in a fuller description.

Larson's Theory of Professional Projects

Larson (1977, 1979) introduces the concept of a *professional project* in an attempt to respond to criticisms neo-Weberian and neo-Marxist scholars of the professions had of each other. Briefly, the neo-Weberian school of thought as applied to the issue of professions in society stressed the importance of power in the professionalization process (cf. Johnson 1972). In light of the fact that power is an essential attribute of closure, many of these theorists either explicitly or implicitly drew on Weber's theory of *social closure* (Brante 1988; Saks 1983). Parkin (1979), for example, identified two generic types of closure action: *exclusion*, power directed downwards through the subordination of socially defined inferiors; and *usurpation*, power directed upwards oriented at improving the position of a subordinate group at the expense of a dominant group. Professionalism, he argued, was a particular type of exclusionary closure based on credentials "designed ... to limit and control the supply of entrants to an occupation in order to safeguard or enhance its market value" (1979: 54).

Neo-Marxist scholars criticize those from the neo-Weberian school of thought for not analyzing the wider sources of power underpinning professionalism. Johnson (1977, 1980), for example, argues that putting the relations of production and the division of labour at the centre of the analysis helps indicate what knowledge is more valuable, and in turn which positions in the social formation possess the potential for the exercise of power on the basis of knowledge. Boreham (1983) also argues that many of the conclusions drawn about the autonomy, legitimacy, and power of professionals overlook the fact that it is only by "identification with appropriate recognized norms and values in the context of the capitalist organisation of the labour process" (713) that professionals achieve and maintain their position.

Larson's (1977, 1979) work draws upon the case of the development of the medical profession in Britain and the United States as a means to reconcile the differences between these two schools of thought. The professional project undertaken by medicine, she claims, involved two interrelated processes of 1) controlling a market of expertise; and 2) embarking on a collective process of upward social mobility. An upwardly mobile occupation must create a need for its services and at the same time create a scarcity of resources – its own members. This is accomplished by controlling the "production of producers" through a standardized, mandatory system of professional training and through professional licensing and certification. Through the process of professionalization, a monopoly of expertise in the market and a monopoly of status in a system of stratification are sought.

Market conditions, however, are insufficient to guarantee professional power. Larson attempts to address this issue by highlighting the relationship that exists between professions and capital. She argues that as a profession attempts to rise upward, it "must form 'organic' ties with significant factions of the ruling class (or of a rising class); persuasion and justification depend on ideological resources, the import and legitimacy of which are ultimately defined by the context of hegemonic power in a ruling class society" (1977: xv). In the case of medicine, for example, she asserts that its collective rise was facilitated by the fit between its emerging doctrines and the ideology that was being used to justify the increasing power of the corporate capitalist class (see also Coburn, Torrance and Kaufert 1983).[1]

Thus, according to Larson, professionalization results when an occupational group seeks upward mobility by controlling its knowledge base, within a sociopolitical context defined by capitalist relations of production. What remains unclear from Larson's analysis, however, is whether it is mainly the *efforts* of an upwardly mobile occupational group organized around a certain knowledge base to form ties with the ruling class that leads to professional power, or whether it is simply the *logic* of capitalism that enables an occupation with a knowledge base congruent with capitalist ideology to become powerful.

In spite of some lack of clarity regarding these origins of the power of professional knowledge, Larson's approach represented a profound reconceptualization of the process of professionalization, and one that has been followed by countless analyses of health occupations in a variety of system contexts. Gender has played an important role in these projects, but it remained relatively underconceptualized until the work of Witz in *Professions and Patriarchy* (1992). Like Larson, Witz attempts to reconcile neo-Weberian and neo-Marxist theories of the professions by drawing on a neo-Weberian closure model and on a neo-Marxist model as a structural and historical framework. Perhaps now considered a problem sufficiently addressed, very little theoretical attention has been focused on expanding upon Witz' work on gender and the professionalization process. But her model is not complete. One of the key points of departure from Witz' work I pursue is with respect to the relations between the professions and the state and women and the state in particular. In so doing, I intend to expand upon the relatively underconceptualized role of the state in female professional projects.

DETAILS ON METHODS ...

The data this case study is based upon is derived from multiple sources including in part participant observation, but more formally and systematically, historical documents and key informant interviews. First, the collection of documentary data involved several primary and secondary sources. Both substantive and theoretical secondary literature was drawn on to help situate the recent professionalization of midwifery historically, to further conceptualize the key characteristics of midwifery and to analyse changes resulting from the integration process. Documents from primary sources included articles in consumer, midwifery, medical, and nursing newsletters and journals; reports; proceedings of, submissions to, and minutes from important midwifery policy-making committees; minutes from other consumer and midwifery committees and organizations; and speeches and legislative proceedings from state officials. From the documents, I began to create a historical chronology of important events and committees.

The second systematic method of data collection included conducting in-depth interviews with key informants knowledgeable of or influential in various aspects of the midwifery integration process. Key informants were identified through my involvement in the midwifery community, from the documentary data collected, and from other key informants. Through interviews with these informants, I sought to obtain information about the integration process that had not been preserved in documents, as well as to clarify what had been written. Several key informants were specifically selected to respond to these "gaps" in the documentary data. Attention was also paid to ensuring that a variety of informants with differing perspectives on the integration process would be interviewed. An initial list of forty-three consumers, midwives, would-be midwives, nurses, physicians, midwifery policy makers, and state officials was compiled.

Each key informant on this list was first sent a personalized introductory letter explaining how her/his current or past position made her/him a significant observer of the matter under study, and requesting a meeting at a time convenient to the interviewee. Interviews were secured with thirty-nine key informants from this list during an intensive six-week process (from late December 1994 to early February 1995) either by phone (n = 17) or in person (n = 22). The four informants that I did not interview were not available because they were too busy, were out of the province, were simply not interested in taking part in the research, or were deemed not necessary once I secured interviews with other informants. My success in securing interviews with most of the informants on my list is due in large part to my initial involvement in the midwifery community (see Foreword).

Interviews were semi-structured, included many open-ended questions, and largely followed the historical chronology of the integration process. Some structure was necessary to ensure that I addressed the key events and committees I had previously identified as important. Open-ended questions allowed me to delve into areas that I had not anticipated, but which were nevertheless important to the research issue at hand. To help orient the questions asked in the interview and situate their involvement along the time line of events in the integration process, informants were first asked when and how they became involved in the midwifery movement in Ontario. Subsequent questions asked each informant to address specific areas of knowledge and expertise. Interviews lasted from thirty minutes (for those involved in only a few aspects of midwifery integration) to almost three hours (for those with greater involvement in the overall process). All interviews, save one, were taped and later transcribed verbatim.[2]

The content of the interview questions evolved not only within each interview but also throughout the interviewing process. For example, questions regarding a particular event or committee were asked of informants until such time that responses across informants became repetitive. Efforts were made, however, to secure more than one perspective on events and committees. These differences were important data indicating disagreement or dissent. Key influences on the midwifery integration process and key events and committees that I originally had not focused on but which were identified as important by informants, were subsequently investigated and became part of the interview schedule for later informants. When necessary, I followed up on some topics by recontacting informants I had interviewed earlier.

Concurrent with this research, I was involved on a project examining recent health policy changes in Ontario focusing on nursing, medicine, and the state (cf., Coburn et al., 1999). Although I do not directly cite this data herein, my experience on the project enabled me to better contextualize the midwifery integration process within the recent dynamics of the broader health care system. Additionally, I was also granted access to data on the early development of midwifery in Ontario that Mary Fynes had collected for her thesis in 1993 on the legitimation of midwifery in Ontario

(1960–1986). This included many documents she had collected and interview excerpts she had received permission to make public domain.

Following the collection of the bulk of the data, more formal analysis began. I found myself confronted with a mass of data which I originally organized in a simple historical chronology. There were, however, so many different events and committees occurring at the same time that I felt presenting the data in this fashion would be confusing. From an initial analysis of the documents and key informant interviews, I realized that key events and committees during the integration process largely revolved around four central aspects of midwifery. These included the organization of midwives, the regulation of midwifery, the model and scope of midwifery practice, and the entry to practice and education of midwives. Data were subsequently sorted, coded, and categorized according to these four areas.

For each area of midwifery – organization, regulation, practice, and education – I began with a description of midwifery as it emerged. I then described the chronological sequence of events highlighting significant events in the change process and factors and forces influencing change. Documenting the process of change was a constant re-iterative process of moving back and forth between documents and interviews, contextualizing this with my personal experience in the midwifery community and my experience from the Ontario health policy project. Key quotes from informants and passages from documents which described significant factors and forces in the change process were identified and drawn upon to help better document the integration process and the changes it produced. These are cited in text as "personal communications." It should be noted that these quotes are taken verbatim and in many cases the language tends to be informal with many colloquialisms.

The presentation of the data in this book is largely from the viewpoint of midwifery itself. This perspective is due in part to my intimate involvement in the midwifery community, but it is justifiable considering the research questions at hand. Taking an "internalist" perspective is logical if the intention is to describe changes to an occupation and how it has been transformed. Therefore, the perspective of those within the midwifery community, midwives and consumers alike, has been emphasized. The perspectives of other actors, such as those within medicine and nursing, are noted but analysed in less detail.

Notes

1 I have often received confused looks at international conferences or lectures, particularly in the UK, when I would suggest that midwifery in North America was similar in many respects to an alternative health profession; but this is indeed how midwifery was regarded by many professionals and lay persons, even as late as the 1990s.

2 The four who did not participate included two midwives and one consumer who did not return my phone calls or correspondence, and one member of a midwifery policy committee who was out of the country during this phase of data collection.

CHAPTER ONE

1 For those interested in a more thorough discussion of the theoretical influences, please refer to the Appendix on "Notes on Theory and Methods."

2 Navarro (1976, 1986) also describes a similar "congruence thesis."

3 Johnson's, Haug's, and Freidson's work is all on established professions.

4 When I refer to "female-dominated professions," I am referring to the numerical domination of women rather than to the control women have over the profession.

5 Randall (1998) notes, "in analyzing the opportunities presented by the political system or the state for women, adequate account must be taken of the variation in the overall form or type of the state, for instance whether authoritarian or liberal-democratic, whether capitalist or state socialist, whether "developed" or "post-colonial" (196).

CHAPTER TWO

1 In fact, the conflict between the elite leaders in medicine and the rank-and-file general practitioners on the midwifery issue led to a challenge by the British Medical Association leadership and its reconstitution in 1902.

2 It was not until 1920 that midwifery won the right to representation on their licensing board, but they were still precluded from comprising a majority (Robinson 1990).

3 Sandall (1996) argues that "the establishment of the NHS also destroyed the economic basis of independent midwifery as it was now cheaper for women to go to hospital than stay home" (218).

4 Although midwifery in Britain existed as a profession independent from nursing, elite midwives (most of whom had prior nursing training) were struggling to make nursing training a prerequisite to registration, thus excluding "untrained" midwives from licensure (see Heagerty 1990). It is likely American reformers wanted to make a fresh start by lobbying for nurse-midwifery from the beginning.

5 Originally the American College of Nurse-Midwifery was a special section of the National Organization for Public Health Nurses – NOPHN – and later developed into a separate professional organization in 1954 (Hogan 1975).

6 The term *lay midwifery* will be used in this paper for simplicity's sake to refer to independent, direct-entry, non-nurse midwives. As DeVries (1996) notes, the term *lay midwife* "was seen as an act of resistance against the overly technical and cold approach of medical "professionals" ... [but more recently] many lay midwives decided the term *lay* created an image of incompetence [and] within a few years ... was abandoned, replaced by a collection of new names: practical midwife, empirical midwife, traditional midwife, community midwife, direct-entry midwife, or sometimes, simply, midwife" (xx).

7 Lay midwives may not think of themselves as in the same category as other "alternative" practitioners, but many have come to realize that this is exactly how much of the public regards them.

8 Some also argue that there are significant differences in their practice patterns (Rothman 1982).

9 Lay or direct-entry midwifery is also not prohibited but not legally regulated in another six States (Midwifery Alliance of North America website, www.mana.org/statechart.html).

10 MANA is actually a transnational organization encompassing not only the United States but Canada and Mexico as well.

11 The lay midwifery group adopted the name "direct-entry" to reflect their desire for a professional credential that would better validate their knowledge and help them interface with the medical system (Davis-Floyd 1999).

12 Caution must be taken when comparing these statistics, as there is likely to be an under-reporting of the number of lay midwives and lay midwifery-attended births due in large part to the precarious legal status of lay midwifery practice in many states.

13 The original legislation stated ten days; currently it is eight days postpartum.

14 State health insurance in the Netherlands covers approximately 70 per cent of the population; the remainder (almost 30 per cent) have private insurance and a few remain uninsured (<2 per cent).

15 DeVries (2001) for example notes that the home birth rate declined from nearly 60 per cent in 1970 to just over 35 per cent in 1980.

CHAPTER THREE

1 There were only thirty to forty physicians in all of Upper Canada (Caniff, 1894 in Rushing, 1991).

2 Mason (1987) argues that based on various mortality surveys medical birth in a hospital was statistically more dangerous than birth accomplished at home in the traditional manner. Other authors also comment on how many obstetrical practices are based more on social custom than on scientific research (Arms 1975; Biggs 1983; Haire 1972).

3 In fact, midwives often practised in areas considered "unprofitable" to many physicians.

4 For an excellent account of the remnants of midwifery across Canada, please refer to the chapter "Midwives Did Not Disappear" in Wendy Mitchinson's Giving Birth in Canada (2002) University of Toronto Press.

5 Nestel's argument will be readdressed in the conclusion.

CHAPTER FOUR

1 This was especially true in major urban centres such as Toronto where there were a number of sympathetic physicians available.

2 Other forms of support from health care professionals came from the Medical Reform Group in Ontario (a group of left-wing physicians), who passed a resolution in May 1980 calling for the recognition and training of midwives, and the Toronto Public Health Department Task Force on High Risk Pregnancy, who recommended in a May 1980 report that midwives be trained and legally recognized.

3 The number of physicians attending home births in Toronto averaged six or seven between 1979 and 1981 but at one time was as high as eleven (Eberts et al. 1987).

4 The term "lay midwife" will be used for ease of presentation to refer to direct-entry midwives and community midwives who entered practice directly usually through an apprenticeship or self-study.

5 Some source documents date the establishment of the OAM to 1979, but this likely refers to the establishment of the Midwives Support and Study which officially became the OAM in 1981.

6 In fact, in Toronto only one physician continued to attend and back up home birth.

7 According to OAM documents, only one birth attendant/midwife discontinued practising when faced with a lack of physician backup.

8 The ICM is an international organization of midwifery associations which began after World War I. Its aim is to promote midwifery through research, study and information. It began holding world wide triennial conferences in 1954.

9 In late 1979, the RNAO formed a task force to develop a plan of action directed toward preparing the groundwork for nurse midwifery in Ontario. Newspaper reports confirm that a proposal was made to the government calling for midwifery to be a specialty of nursing and for nurse-midwifery services to the reimbursed by the government. This proposal was likely relegated to the HPLR.

10 Indeed, as Sheryl Nestel (1996/97) explains, many women with precarious immigration status were particularly concerned not to partake in any activity that could jeopardize their official integration into Canada.

11 As mentioned previously, a group called Choices in Childbirth had formed to protest the constraints the CPSO placed on physicians who assist at home births.

12 It was at the one-day meeting in Toronto in June 1983 that the decision to become integrated was so hotly debated that Mayr put forth the motion to create the MTFO.

13 A full discussion of the third and fourth points of this submission are addressed in chapter 9.

14 Many, however, envisioned that it would be through this project that other changes to maternity care would follow.

CHAPTER FIVE

1 It should also be noted that organized medicine had been focusing much of its attention on the banning of extra-billing, which subsequently resulted

in the breakdown of profession–government relations culminating in the strike held by physicians in the summer of 1986.

2 Over 85 per cent of physicians in Canada belong to the Canadian Medical Protective Association (CMPA), a nonprofit professional association run by physicians. The CMPA charges physicians differential fees dependent upon the kind of work performed for unlimited malpractice coverage. Originally, one standard fee was charged, but this changed with a 1984 review by the CMPA. The differences in membership fee are supposed to reflect the medical–legal costs of coverage. For example, in 1986 the rate for family physicians not doing obstetrics was $650, for a family physician doing obstetrics $1,200, and for an obstetrician $4,900. These higher fees for practising obstetrics purportedly reflected the fact that the largest court settlements in Canada have been made to the parents of damaged babies and women who suffered an injury from anaesthesia during labour (AOM Submission to TFIMO, Sept. 1986).

3 The founder of the ONMA, May Toth, voted against the merger at this meeting arguing the importance of nursing for midwifery. Subsequently, she and a few other ONMA members decided against joining the newly merged organization.

4 The Ontario Institute for Studies in Education – the location of the MANA conference.

5 This included support from Liberal MPP Murray Elston who would later become the Minister of Health.

6 Other committees were later added including a Liaison Committee that liaised with other midwifery related groups and the MTFO; a Membership Committee, which, like a statutory college committee, kept track of the membership of the AOM; and a Research and Statistics Committee.

7 Some questioned the "normality" of the delivery as the mother was in transition for three and a half hours and in second stage for two and a half hours.

8 The 1982 inquest in Kitchener-Waterloo also examined some of the broader issues of midwifery.

9 It should be noted that Dr Wagner wanted to do both – argue the specific case for the care the midwives under investigation provided as well as the case for midwifery in general.

10 One of the original jury members was dismissed because she was a registered nurse and the parents' lawyer argued that she might have been biased.

11 Vicki Van Wagner, the backup midwife who was at the birth for only the last two and a half hours, underwent two full days of cross examination which she felt was a strategy used to increase the saliency of her lack of

formal training in contrast to the primary midwife, Sue Rose, who had previous nursing training in England.

12 The Coroner also made several sexist comments including saying to the parents' lawyer, "Nag, nag, nag; you're just like my wife – never lets me get the last word." Also, his comment about the notes that the mother, Alix McLaughlin, was referring to in her testimony was "You must make a good grocery list" (*Issue* 9, October 1985: 4, 20).

13 Some of those interviewed for this study even contended that the continuation of the whole HPLR, a decision that the new government was faced with, was due to the media spectacle the inquest had created.

14 It could be argued that all forms of self-regulation are inherently biased toward the provider. The problem with having small numbers is ensuring that a provider is not involved in both the professional association (acting in the profession's interest) and the self-regulatory body (acting in the public's interest) in too short an interval.

15 It is noteworthy that the announcement to integrate midwifery was made three months prior to the formal announcement of the HPLR on April 3, 1986, regarding the final list of twenty-four health professions to be included in new legislation.

CHAPTER SIX

1 See chapters 7 and 9 for detailed discussion of practice and education recommendations.

2 It should be noted that although REAL Women supported midwifery, they were not supportive of midwives being involved in conducting abortions.

3 Instead of implementing midwifery, the OMA submission outlined how nurses' role in obstetrical care should be enhanced.

4 Midwife Vicki Van Wagner (1995) added that, "we have to be grateful that [the Task Force] was before the recession, that it was in the 80s. Because it did cost a lot of money and time. But I think in terms of introducing such a big change to the system, it was very very helpful that so much time and careful thought was put into the issue, and that all the players were involved in discussions about it."

5 Its official placement in the Ministry of Health was in the newly created Women's Health Bureau. In fact, midwifery was one of the first items on the agenda of the Women's Health Bureau.

6 None of the three physician members belonged to the OMA. They were members of the more midwifery-friendly Medical Reform Group.

7 With the exception of Dianne Pudas, no MTFO members were officially chosen to be on the IRCM. Pudas recalled that the MTFO was disappointed that more MTFO members weren't chosen to sit on Council (personal communication 1995). The MTFO nevertheless maintained involvement by sending representatives to all IRCM committee meetings and having special monthly liaison meetings with the IRCM.

8 The AOM put out an official statement criticizing their exclusion from the IRCM based on the principle that they had voluntarily, without support, been working as a self-regulatory body. They also felt that they had a good record of representing the public interest (Midwife Robin Kilpatrick, personal communication 1995).

9 Midwife Vicki Van Wagner described the IRCM members as "guardians" or "shepherds" of midwifery.

10 Liaison Committee members also ended up being paid a per diem compensation as were other IRCM members. Funding was for six midwives which was shared amongst nine Liaison committee members.

11 The AOM also needed to develop standards as it continued to act as a self-regulatory body for midwifery.

12 Under the NDP government, the RHPA was modified slightly, stipulating that the College councils be made up of now less than 50 per cent professionals and no less than 40 per cent public representation.

13 Midwifery representation on the Transitional Council was less than for other Transitional Councils where professionals had at least 50 per cent representation.

14 As it stands, with this government subsidy, midwives' College fees are approximately $1,000; this is in sharp contrast to the fees nurses pay to their college which is under $100. Midwives also pay a $2,500 fee to their professional association, the AOM.

CHAPTER SEVEN

1 The "choice" model paralleled the philosophy of the pro-choice movement that midwives increasingly looked to for guidance.

2 In Toronto this began in 1979. It should be noted that in other jurisdictions, midwives had already begun to do this.

3 Women choosing hospital births would often request early discharge whereupon the midwife would resume primary care during the postpartum period (Tate 1988).

4 This document described three categories of responses to risk factors for the ante-, intra- and postpartum periods including: 1) discuss with partner

or back-up midwife the risk factor in question; 2) consult with family physician or general practitioner or obstetrician; and 3) consult with obstetrician or specialist either directly or ensure consultation via family physicians or general practitioner (in situations 2 and 3 the midwife is obliged to follow advice given by the consulting physician).

5 This recommendation was also intended to ensure that midwives' clients would establish an ongoing relationship with a family physician.

6 There were three categories of acts: 1) licensed acts; 2) ordered/delegated acts; and 3) uncontrolled (public domain) acts.

7 Except in those exceptional circumstances when it is not possible to have two midwives – particularly during the first years of regulated midwifery due to small numbers.

8 This was based on the AOM Document "Contraindications for Home Birth."

9 A client was defined as a woman with whom the midwife has a contractual relationship. Clause 12 of the IRCM Code of Ethics largely follows clause 17 from the AOM Code of Ethics: "a midwife may not refuse to attend a client in the course of labour."

10 McHugh became Midwifery Coordinator following Karyn Kaufman (who held the position from July 1988 to October 1991) and Helen McDonald (who held the position from October 1991 to August 1992).

11 Nurses specifically wanted nurse-midwives to be practising in hospitals.

12 Some dentists also have admitting privileges to hospitals under the direction of a physician.

13 In its international consultations, the Task Force found this to be true in the United States much to the detriment of independent domiciliary midwifery.

14 The amount of premiums was never disclosed either in documents or in interviews but were described as affordable.

15 Statutes are the more permanent aspects of a government Act requiring a legislative amendment process; regulatory amendments are more easily made since they do not require legislative approval.

16 A midwife could file a civil suit for undue limitations to her practice if refused privileges but it is difficult to say if this would be successful as hospitals are not really breaking any law by refusing privileges to a midwife.

CHAPTER EIGHT

1 By way of contrast, nurse midwives in the US made between $20,000 and $35,000 US in 1983/84. (Kraus 1984)

2 Chiropractic in Ontario, for example, achieved self-regulatory status along with midwifery in 1993 but did not attain full public funding for its

services. Some argued that midwifery care and particularly attendance at birth was a more essential health care service than chiropractic care.

3 The only mention of finances is with respect to the costs of operating a self-regulatory college and with respect to the cost-effectiveness of a direct-entry education program.

4 This was a problem the government was facing with the funding for medical services – a problem they intended to avoid with midwifery.

5 It is an interesting aside that the second author of this report – Bob Gardiner – also authored two research papers for NDP MPP Dave Cooke who had earlier proposed the Private Member's Bill. The first was on the safety of home versus hospital births. The second was a review of the medical press on the legislation of midwifery. Both were written in 1986.

6 The proposal for midwives to be salaried employees of the state was not considered satisfactory, due to the Ministry's concerns about liability in the case of a malpractice claim.

7 The name Lebel was taken in honour of the midwife who delivered the first three of the Dionne Quintuplets in 1934 near North Bay, Ontario.

8 This recommendation followed the stipulation of two midwives at a birth regardless of birth setting.

9 Primary care nurses in a CHC in 1993 made between $42,000 and $56.000, physicians between $80,000 and $118,000 (plus an additional $5000 on-call allowance). Factored into this equation was the fact that midwives would work 22 per cent longer per week than a primary care nurse in a CHC.

10 There are still many areas where midwifery services are not available – and those areas where midwives are available have extensive waiting lists and in some cases end up turning away upwards of 500 women per year.

CHAPTER NINE

1 The tenure of the CDC was extended by two months to deal with the volume of work.

2 For an excellent retrospective on the creation of the Ontario Midwifery Education program, see Kaufman and Soderstrom (2004).

3 Ryerson later achieved university status.

CHAPTER TEN

1 The reason for the discrepancy for the ten midwives was not revealed in the source document.

2 The Task Force also made provisions for francophone applicants with the following recommendation: "The Midwifery Integration Program should

be conducted in both French and English if a sufficient number of francophone applicants apply for admission."

3 Many candidates would have to make arrangements to move, often with their families, and would also have to make arrangements for the coverage of their midwifery practice.

4 In its second cycle in 1997, this name of this program was changed to the Prior Learning and Experience Assessment (PLEA) program.

5 It should be noted that under the Midwifery Act, an exemption was made for Aboriginal midwives. That is, Aboriginal midwives not licensed under the Act could still legally continue practising.

6 Indeed, for a dramatically different account of a midwifery integration process see Kaufert and Robinson (2004).

7 For a description of the similar situation in nursing, see Williams (2001).

CONCLUSION

1 This is not to negate the importance of the issue of safety in determining who is qualified to practice midwifery but rather to point out the broader social factors involved in this process.

2 For an expanded discussion of the changes to midwifery through integration see Bourgeault, I.L. (2000). Delivering the "new" Canadian midwifery: the impact on midwifery of integration into the Ontario health care system. *Sociology of Health and Illness* 22(2), 172–96.

3 To be fair, the instructors and preceptors are still practising midwives.

4 Midwifery students, however, are now eligible for government student loans which they were not prior to having a formal education program.

5 According to the reporting in the *Guelph Mercury,* Midwife Kelly Dobbin testified that Namis yelled and swore at her over the phone, "I don't need your shit." Namis denied on the stand that he had been verbally abusive towards Dobbin.

6 This list is not meant to be exhaustive but rather representative.

APPENDIX

1 Navarro (1976, 1986) also describes a similar "congruence thesis."

2 This informant expressed some discomfort with being taped and potentially having quotes attributed to her/himself.

References

Abbott, Andrew (1988). *The System of Professions*. Chicago: University of Chicago Press.

Abercrombie, H. and J. Urry (1983). *Capital, Labour and the New Middle Classes*. London: Allen and Unwin.

Adams, Tracey (2000). *A Dentist and a Gentleman: Gender and the Rise of Dentistry in Ontario*. Toronto: University of Toronto Press.

Adams, Tracey and Ivy Lynn Bourgeault (2003). "Feminism and Female Health Professions." *Women's Health* 38(4), 73–90.

Alford, Robert (1975). *Health Care Politics*. Chicago: University of Chicago Press.

Allsop, Judith and Mike Saks (Eds.) (2002). *Regulating the Health Professions*. London: Sage Publications.

Anderson, D. (1986). "Midwifery Will Be a Practical Alternative." *The Toronto Star*, (December 27), Section E, Toronto. 1.

Annandale, Ellen C. (1988). "How Midwives Accomplish Natural Birth: Managing Risk and Balancing Expectations." *Social Problems* 35(2), 95–110.

– (1989). "Proletarianization or Restratification of the Medical Profession? The Case of Obstetrics." *International Journal of Health Services* 19(4), 611–34.

Arms, Suzanne (1975). *Immaculate Deception: A New Look at Women and Childbirth in America*. San Francisco: San Francisco Book Company.

Armstrong, Pat and Hugh Armstrong (1992a). "Lessons from Pay Equity." In M. Connelly and P. Armstrong (Eds.), *Feminism in Action*. Toronto: Canadian Scholars Press.

– (1992b). "Sex and the Professions in Canada." *Journal of Canadian Studies* 27(1), 118–35.

Arscott, Jane and Linda Trimble (Eds.) (1996). *In the Presence of Women: Representation in Canadian Governments*. Toronto: Harcourt Brace.

Atwood, Margaret (1985). *The Handmaid's Tale*. Toronto: McClelland and Stewart.

Baker, Margaret (1989). *Midwifery: A New Status* No. Library of Parliament.

Barickman, C., M. Bidgood-Wilson, and S. Ackley (1992). "Nurse-Midwifery Today: A Legislative Update Part 2." *Journal of Nurse-Midwifery* 37(3), 175–209.

Barnett, Z. (1979). "The Changing Pattern of Maternity Care and the Future Role of the Midwife." *Midwives' Chronicle and Nursing Notes* 92, 381–4.

Barrington, Eleanor (1984). *The Legalization of Midwifery in Canada*. National Action Committee on the Status of Women.

– (1985). *Midwifery is Catching*. Toronto: NC Press Limited.

Benoit, Cecilia (1987). "Uneasy Partners: Midwives and their Clients." *Canadian Journal of Sociology* 12(3), 275–84.

– (1990). "Mothering in a Newfoundland Community: 1900–1940." In K. Arnup, A. Levesque, and R. Roach Pierson (Eds.), *Delivering Motherhood: Maternal Ideologies in the 19th and 20th Centuries* (173–98). New York: Routledge.

– (1991). *Midwives in Passage*. St. John's, Newfoundland: Institute of Social and Economic Research.

– (1997). "Professionalizing Canadian Midwifery: Sociological Perspectives." In Farah Shroff (Ed.) *The New Midwifery: Reflections on Renaissance and Regulation* (41–9). Toronto: The Women's Press.

– (2000). *Women, Work and Social Rights: Canada in Historical and Comparative Perspective*. Scarborough, ON: Prentice Hall Allyn and Bacon Canada.

Benoit, Cecilia and Dena Carroll (1995). "Aboriginal Midwifery in British Columbia: A Narrative Untold." In P.H. Stephenson, S.J. Elliott, L.T. Foster, J.Harris (Eds.), *A Persistent Spirit: Towards Understanding Aboriginal Health in British Columbia* 31 (223–48). Victoria, BC: University of Victoria.

Benoit, Cecilia and Robbie Davis-Floyd (2004). "Becoming a Midwife in Canada: Models of Midwifery Education." In I. Bourgeault, C. Benoit, and R. Davis-Floyd (Eds.), *Reconceiving Midwifery* (169–86). McGill Queen's University Press: Kingston/Montreal.

Benoit Cecilia, Robbie Davis-Floyd, Jane Sandall, Edwin van Teijlingen, and Janielli Miller (2000). "Designing Midwives: A Comparison of Educational Models." In R. DeVries, C. Benoit, E. Van Teijlingen and S. Wrede (Eds.), *Birth by Design: Pregnancy, Maternity Care, and Midwifery in North America and Europe* (139–65). London: Routledge.

Bergqvist, Christina and Sue Findlay (1999). "Representing Women's Interests in the Policy Process: Women's Organizing and State Initiatives in Sweden and Canada, 1960s–1990s." In Linda Briskin and Mona Eliasson (Eds.), *Women's Organizing and Public Policy in Canada and Sweden*. Montreal: McGill-Queen's University Press.

Berlant, J.L. (1975). *Profession and Monopoly: A Study of Medicine in the United States and Great Britain*. Berkeley: University of California Press.

Bidgood-Wilson, M., D. Barickman, and S. Ackley (1992). "Nurse-Midwifery Today: A Legislative Update, Part i." *Journal of Nurse-Midwifery* 37(2), 96–140.

Biggs, C. Lesley (1983). "The Case of the Missing Midwives: A History of Midwifery in Ontario from 1795–1900." *Ontario History* 65(1), 21–35.

– (1989). *No Bones about Chiropractic? The Quest for Legitimacy by the Ontario Chiropractic Profession, 1895–1985.* PhD Dissertation, University of Toronto, Department of Behavioural Science.

– (2004). "Fragments of the History of Midwifery." In I. Bourgeault, C. Benoit, R. Davis-Floyd (Eds.), *Reconceiving Midwifery* (17–45). Montreal: McGill-Queen's University Press.

Biggs, C. Lesley, Brian Burtch, and Farah Shroff (Eds.) (1996/97) Special Issue on Midwifery in Canada. *Health and Canadian Society* 4(2).

Blais, Regis (2000). "Evaluation of the Midwifery Pilot-Projects in Quebec: An Overview." *Canadian Journal of Public Health* 91(1), 1–1 to 1–4.

Blais, Regis, Jean Lambert, and Brigitte Maheux. (1999). "What Accounts for Physician Options about Midwifery in Canada?" *Journal of Nurse-Midwifery* 44(4) (July/August): 399–407.

Bohme, G. (1984). "Midwifery as Science: An Essay on the Relation Between Scientific and Everyday Knowledge." In N. Stehr and V. Meja (Eds.), *Society and Knowledge* (365–85). London: Transaction.

Boon, Heather (1998). "Canadian Naturopathic Practitioners: Holistic and Scientific World Views." *Social Science and Medicine* 46(9), 1213–25.

Boreham, P. (1983). "Indetermination: Professional Knowledge, Organization and Control." *The Sociological Review* 31, 693–718.

Bourgeault, Ivy Lynn (1999). "Accessibility to Newly Integrated Professions: The Case of the 'New' Midwifery in Ontario." *Research in the Sociology of Health Care* 16, 205–21.

– (2000). "Delivering the 'New' Canadian Midwifery: The Impact on Midwifery of Integration into the Ontario Health Care System." *Sociology of Health and Illness* 22(2), 172–96.

– (2002). "The Evolution of the Social Science of Midwifery and its Canadian Contributions (Commentary)." *Canadian Journal of Midwifery Research and Practice* 1(2) (Winter), 4–8.

– (2005). Gendered Professionalization Strategies & the Rationalization of Health Care: Midwifery, Nurse Practitioners, and Hospital Nurse Staffing in Ontario, Canada. *Knowledge, Work and Society*, 3(1).

Bourgeault, Ivy Lynn, Cecilia Benoit, and Robbie Davis-Floyd (2004). *Reconceiving Midwifery*. McGill-Queen's University Press.

Bourgeault, Ivy Lynn, Eugene Declercq, and Jane Sandall (2001). "Changing Birth: Consumers, Politics and Policy." In R. DeVries et al., *Birth by Design: The Social and Cultural Aspects of Maternity Care in Europe and North America.* Routledge: New York.

Bourgeault, Ivy Lynn and Mary T. Fynes (1996/97). "Delivering Midwifery in Ontario: How and Why Midwifery was Integrated into the Provincial Health Care System." *Health and Canadian Society* 4(2), 227–62.

- (1997). "The Integration of Nurse- and Lay Midwives in the US and Canada." *Social Science and Medicine* 44(7), 1051–63.

Bourgeault, Ivy Lynn, Jacquelyne Luce, and Maggie MacDonald (1998). "The Integration of the 'New' Midwifery into Ontario Hospitals: The Views of Midwives, Nurses and Physicians." *Sociological Abstracts*, July, Supplement, 14th World Congress of Sociology, 46–7.

- (forthcoming). The Caring Dilemma in Midwifery: Balancing the Needs of Midwives and Clients in a Continuity of Care Model of Practice. *Community, Work and Family.*

Brante, R. (1988). "Sociological Approaches to the Professions." *Sociologica* 31(2), 119–42.

Briskin, Linda (1999). "Mapping Women's Organizing in Sweden and Canada: Some Thematic Considerations." In Linda Briskin and Mona Eliasson (Eds.), *Women's Organizing and Public Policy in Canada and Sweden* (3–47). Montreal: McGill-Queen's University Press.

Brownley, Martine W. (2000). *Deferrals of Domain: Contemporary Women Novelists and the State.* New York: St. Martin's Press.

Bucher, Rue (1988). "On the Natural History of Health Care Occupations." *Work and Occupations* 15(2), 131–7.

Buckley, Susan (1979). "Ladies or Midwives: Efforts to Reduce Infant and Maternal Mortality." In L. Kealey (Eds.), *A Not Unreasonable Claim: Women and Reform in Canada, 1880s–1920s,* Toronto: The Women's Press.

Buhler, L., N. Glick, and S.B. Sheps (1988). "Prenatal Care: A Comparative Evaluation of Nurse-Midwives and Family Physicians." *Canadian Medical Association Journal* 139, 397–403.

Burst, Helen V. (1977). "Harmonious Unity." *Journal of Nurse-Midwifery* 12(3), 10–11.

- (1981). "Two Roads – Which One?" *Journal of Nurse-Midwifery* 26(5), 7–12.

Burtch, Brian E. (1986). "Community Midwifery and State Measures: The New Midwifery in British Columbia." *Contemporary Crises* 10, 399–420.

- (1988a). "Midwifery and the State: The New Midwifery in Canada." In A.T. McLaren (Eds.), *Gender and Society: Creating a Canadian Women's Sociology* (349–71). Toronto: Copp Clark Pitman Ltd.

- (1988b). "Promoting Midwifery, Prosecuting Midwives: The State and the Midwifery Movement in Canada." In B.S. Bolaria and H.D. Dickinson (Eds.), *Sociology of Health Care in Canada* (313–27). Toronto: Harcourt Brace Jovanovich.

- (1994). *Trials of Labour: The Re-emergence of Midwifery.* Montreal and Kingston: McGill-Queen's University Press.

Butter, I.H., E.S., Carpenter, B.J. Kay, and R.S. Simmons (1985). *Sex and Status: Hierarchies in the Health Workforce.* Ann Arbor, Michigan: Department of Health Planning and Administration, School of Public Health, The University of Michigan.

- (1987). "Gender Hierarchies in the Health Labor Force." *International Journal of Health Services* 17(1), 133–49.
Butter, I.H. and B.J. Kay (1988). "State Laws and the Practice of Lay Midwifery." *American Journal of Public Health* 78(9), 1161–9.
- (1990). "Self-Certification in Lay Midwives' Organizations: A Vehicle for Professional Autonomy. *Social Science and Medicine* 30(12), 1329–39.
Cant, Sarah and Ursula Sharma (1996). "Demarcation and Transformation with Homeopathic Knowledge: Strategy of Professionalization." *Social Science and Medicine* 42(4), 579–88.
Carr, C. (1993). "The Effect of Third-party Payers on Provider Practice in a Hospital Based Maternity Service." *23rd International Congress of the International Confederation of Midwives* 1, Vancouver, British Columbia, 316–32.
Carroll, Dena and Cecilia Benoit (2004). "Aboriginal Midwifery in Canada: Ancient Traditions and Emerging Forms." In I. Bourgeault, C. Benoit, and R. tDavis-Floyd (Eds.), *Reconceiving Midwifery* (263–86). McGill Queen's University Press: Kingston/Montreal.
Charles, Nickie (2000). *Feminism, the State and Social Policy.* New York: St. Martin's Press.
Cherry, J. and J.C. Foster (1982). "Comparison of Hospital Charges Generated by Certified Nurse-midwives and Physicians' Clients." *Journal of Nurse-Midwifery* 27, 7–11.
Coburn, David (1988). "The Development of Nursing in Canada: Professionalization and Proletarianization." *International Journal of Health Services* 18, 437–56.
- (1993). "State Authority, Medical Dominance, and Trends in the Regulation of the Health Professions." *Social Science and Medicine* 37, 129–38.
- (1994). "Professionalization and Proleterianization: Medicine, Nursing, and Chropractic in Historical Perspective." *Labour/Le Travail* 34, 139–62.
Coburn, David and C. Lesley Biggs (1986). "Limits to Medical Dominance: The Case of Chiropractic." *Social Science and Medicine* 22, 1035–46.
Coburn David, Susan Rappolt, and Ivy Lynn Bourgeault (1997). "Decline Versus Retention of Power through Restratification: The Case of Medicine in Ontario." *Sociology of Health and Illness* 19(1), 1–22.
Coburn, David, Susan Rappolt, Ivy Lynn Bourgeault, and J. Angus. (1999). *Medicine, Nursing and the State.* Garamond Press: Toronto.
Coburn, David, George Torrance, and Joe Kaufert (1983). "Medical Dominance in Canada in Historical Perspective: The Rise and Fall of Medicine?" *International Journal of Health Services* 13, 407–32.
Cohen L. (1991). "Looming Manpower Shortage Has Canada's Obstetricians Worried." *Canadian Medical Association Journal* 144(4), 478–9, 482.
Collin, J., Regis Blais, D. White, et al. (2000). "Integration of Midwives into the Quebec Health Care System." *Canadian Journal of Public Health* 91(1), 1–16 to 1–20.

Connell, R. W. (1990). "The state, gender, and sexual politics: Theory and appraisal." *Theory and Society,* 19, 507–44.

Connor, Jim T.H. (1989). *Minority Medicine in Ontario, 1795–1903: A Study of Medical Pluralism and Its Decline.* PhD Dissertation, University of Waterloo.

– (1994). "Larger Fish to Catch Here than Midwives: Midwifery and the Medical Profession in Nineteenth-Century Ontario." In D. Dodd and D. Gorham (Eds.), *Caring and Curing: Historical Perspectives on Women and Healing in Canada* (103–34). Ottawa: University of Ottawa Press.

Conway, Margaret, David Ahern, and Gertrude Sterernagel (1999). *Women and Public Policy: A Revolution in Progress.* 2nd Edition. Washington: CQ Press.

Corea, Gena (1977). *Hidden Malpractice: How American Medicine Mistreats Women* (Updated ed.). New York: Harper Colophon Books.

Couchie, Carol and Herbert Nabigon (1997). "A Path Towards Reclaiming Nishnawbe Birth Culture: Can the Midwifery Exemption Clause for Aboriginal Midwives Make a Difference?" In Farah Shroff (Ed.), *The New Midwifery: Reflections on Renaissance and Regulation* (41–9). Toronto: The Women's Press.

Crawford, M. (1968). "Nurse-midwifery – Licensure or Certification." *Bulletin of the American College of Nurse-Midwives* 13(2), 18–23.

Crompton, Rosemary (1987). "Gender, Status and Professionalism." *Social Science and Medicine* 21, 413–28.

Crompton, Rosemary and K. Sanderson (1990). "Gendered Jobs and Social Change." *Work, Employment and Society* 4, 623–4.

Davies, Celia (1983). "Professionalizing Strategies as Time- and Culture-Bound: American and British Nursing Circa 1893." In E. Condliffe Lagemann (Ed.), *Nursing History: New Perspectives, New Possibilities* (47–63). New York: Teachers College Press.

Davies, Celia and J. Rosser (1986). "Gendered Jobs in the Health Service: A Problem for Labour Process Analysis." In D. Knights and H. Willmott (Eds.), *Gender and the Labour Process* (94–116). Hampshire: Gower Publishing Co.

Davies, R. (1996). "Practitioners in Their Own Right: An Ethnographic Study of the Perceptions of Student Midwives." In S. Robinson and A. Thompson (Eds.), *Midwives, Research and Childbirth* 4 (85–107). London: Chapman and Hall.

Davis-Floyd, Robbie (1999). "Southern Discomfort: American Midwifery as a Cautionary Tale." Paper presented at *Reconceiving Midwifery in Canada* conference, Toronto. July.

Declercq, Eugene R. (1992). "The Transformation of American Midwifery: 1975–1988." *American Journal of Public Health* 82(5) (May), 680–4.

– (2004). "Percentage of Live Births Attended by CNMs in the United States, 1989–2001." *Journal of Midwifery and Women's Health* 1.

Devitt, Neal (1977). "The Transition from Home to Hospital Birth in the United States, 1930–1960." *Birth and the Family Journal* 4(2), 47–58.

DeVries, Raymond G. (1982). "Midwifery and the Problem of Licensure." *Research in the Sociology of Health Care* 2, 77–120.

– (1985). *Regulating Birth: Midwives, Medicine, and the Law.* Philadelphia: Temple University Press.

– (1986). "The Contest for Control: Regulating New and Expanding Health Occupations." *American Journal of Public Health* 76(9), 1147–50.

– (1996). *Making Midwives Legal.* 2nd Ed. Columbus, Ohio: Ohio State University Press.

– (2004). *A Pleasing Birth: Midwives and Maternity Care in the Netherlands.* Temple University Press: Philadelphia.

DeVries, Raymond G., Cecilia Benoit, Edwin van Teijlingen, Sirpa Wrede (2001). *Birth by Design: The Social and Cultural Aspects of Maternity Care in Europe and North America.* Routledge: New York.

Dingwall, Robert, Rafferty, Anne, and C. Webster (1988). *An Introduction to the Social History of Nursing.* Routledge, London.

Dobkin E. (1994) "Cost of midwifery." *Canadian Medical Association Journal* 151(5), 516–17.

Donnison, Jean (1977). *Midwives and Medical Men.* London: Heinemann.

Eastman, K.S. and M.O. Loustaunau (1987). "Reacting to the Medical Bureaucracy: Lay Midwifery as a Birthing Alternative." *Marriage and the Family Review* 11(3–4), 23–37.

Eberts, Mary, Allen Schwartz, Rachel Edney, and Karen Kaufman (1987). *Report of the Task Force on the Implementation of Midwifery in Ontario.* Queen's Park Printers: Toronto.

Eduards, Maud (1991). "Toward a Third Way: Women's Politics and Welfare Policies in Sweden." *Social Research* 58(3) (fall), 677–705.

Edwards, Margot and Mary Waldorf (1984). *Reclaiming Birth: History and Heroines of American Childbirth Reform.* Trumansburg, New York: The Crossing Press.

Ehrenreich, Barbara and Deidre English (1973). *Witches, Midwives and Nurses.*

– (1978). *For Her Own Good.* New York: Anchor Books.

Eisenstein, Hester (1996). *Inside Agitators: Australian Femocrats and the State.* Philadelphia: Temple University Press.

Eisenstein, Zillah (1984). On the Relative Autonomy of the Capitalist Patriarchal State. In Z. Eisenstein. *Feminism and Sexual Equality.* New York: Monthly Review Press.

Esland, G. (1980). "Professions and Professionalism." In G. Esland and G. Salaman (Eds.), *The Politics of Work and Occupations* (213–50). Toronto: University of Toronto Press.

Etzioni, Amitai (Ed.) (1969). *The Semi–Professions and Their Organization: Teachers, Nurses, and Social Workers.* New York: Free Press.

Evans, Robert. G. (1981). "The Economic Implications of Midwifery: Money, Midwives and Medical Men." In M.T.F.O.B. Columbia and B.C.M. Association (Eds.), *Midwifery Is a Labour of Love* (68–74). Vancouver: Interdisciplinary Task Force.

Evenson, D. (1982). "Midwives: Survival of an Ancient Profession." *Women's Rights Law Reporter* 7(4), 313–30.

Feldberg, Georgina and Marianne Carlson (1999). "Organized for Health: Women's Activism in Canada and Sweden." In Linda Briskin and Mona Eliasson (Eds.), *Women's Organizing and Public Policy in Canada and Sweden* (347–74). Montreal: McGill-Queen's University Press.

Ferguson, D. (1985a). "Juror is Dismissed in Home-Birth Inquest Over Possible Bias." *Toronto Star,* July 3, A22.

– (1985b). "Ontario Should Grant Midwives Official Status, Inquest is Told." *Toronto Star,* July 10, 1985, A15.

Fielding, A.G. and D. Portwood (1980). "Professions and the State – Towards a Typology of Bureaucratic Professions." *Sociological Review* 28(1), 23–53.

Flanagan, J.A. (1986). "Childbirth in the Eighties: What Next?" *Journal of Nurse-Midwifery* 31(4), 194–9.

Flint, C. (1986). "A Radical Blueprint." *Nursing Times* (Jan. 1), 14.

Flint, C., P. Poulengeris, and A. Grant (1989). "The 'Know You Midwife' Scheme – A Randomised Trial of Continuity of Care by a Team of Midwives." *Midwifery* 5, 11–16.

Fooks, Cathy and Bob Gardiner (1986). *The Implementation of Midwifery in Ontario.* Current Issue Paper #50. Legislative Research Services of the Government of Ontario, Toronto.

Fox Piven, Frances (1990). "Ideology and the State: Women, Power, and the Welfare State." In L. Gordon (Ed.), *Women, the State and Welfare* (250–64). Madison: The University of Wisconsin Press.

Freidson, Eliot (1970a). *Profession of Medicine: A Study of the Sociology of Applied Knowledge* (Second Ed.). Chicago: University of Chicago Press.

– (1970b). *Professional Dominance: The Social Structure of Medical Care.* New York: Atherton.

Fudge, Judy (1996). "Fragmentation and Feminization: the Challenge of Equity for Labour-Relations Policy." In J. Brodie (Ed.), *Women and Canadian Public Policy* (57–88). Toronto: Harcourt Brace.

Fynes, Mary. T. (1994). *The Legitimation of Midwifery in Ontario.* Master's Thesis, University of Toronto.

Garland Spindel, Peggy (1995). Coordinator, Midwifery Communication and Accountability Project, Personal Communication, August.

Gaskin, Ina May (1988). "Midwifery Reinvented." In S. Kitzinger (Eds.), *The Midwife Challenge* (42–60). London: Pandora Press.

Giacomini, Mita and M. Peters (1996). *The Introduction of Public Funding for Midwifery in Ontario: Interpreting the Meaning of the Financial Incentives.* McMaster University Centre for Health Economics and Policy Analysis Working Paper 96–9, August.

Goldman B. (1988). "Home Birth: 'We Did It, All of Us.'" *Canadian Medical Association Journal* 139(8), 773–4.

Gort, Elaine and David Coburn (1988). "Naturopathy in Canada: Changing Relationship to Medicine, Chiropractic and the State." *Social Science and Medicine* 26, 1061–72.

Gotell, Lisa (1996). "Policing Desire: Obscenity Law, Pornography Politics, and Feminism in Canada." In J. Brodie (Ed.), *Women and Canadian Public Policy* (279–318). Toronto: Harcourt Brace.

Grandjean, B.D. and H.H. Bernal (1979). "Sex and Centralization in a Semiprofession." *Sociology of Work and Occupations* 6(1), 84–102.

Haas J.E. and Judith P. Rooks (1986). "National Survey of Factors Contributing to and Hindering the Successful Practice of Nurse-Midwifery: Summary of the American College of Nurse-Midwives Foundation Study." *Journal of Nurse-Midwifery* 31(5) (September/October), 212–15.

Haire, Doris (1972). *The Cultural Warping of Childbirth.* Washington, DC: International Childbirth Education Association.

Halpern, Sydney. A. (1992). "Dynamics of Professional Control: Internal Coalitions and Crossprofessional Boundaries." *American Journal of Sociology* 97(4), 994–1021.

Hartley, Heather and Christina Gasbarro (2002)."Forces Promoting Health Insurance Coverage of Homebirth: A Case Study in Washington State." *Women and Health* 36(3), 13–30.

Haug, Marie (1973). "Deprofessionalization: An Alternate Hypothesis for the Future." *Sociological Review Monographs* 20, 195–211.

Haug, Marie and Bebe Lavin (1983). *Consumerism in Medicine.* Beverly Hills, Sage.

Hawkins, Miranda and Sarah Knox (2003). *The Midwifery Option: A Canadian Guide to the Birth Experience.* Toronto: Harper Collins.

Hays, Patricia (1971). "Midwives? In Canada? Let's Hope So!"*Canadian Nurse* (July), 17–19.

Heagerty, Brooke V. (1990). *Class, Gender and Professionalization: The Struggle for British Midwifery, 1900–1936.* Doctoral Dissertation, Michigan State University.

Health Professions Legislation Review (1989). *Striking a Balance.* Toronto: Queen's Park Printers.

Heap, Ruby and M. Stuart (1995). "Nurses and Physiotherapists: Issues in the Professionalization of Health Care Occupations During and After World War I." *Health and Canadian Society* 3(1 and 2), 179–93.

Hearn, Jeffrey (1982). "Notes on Patriarchy, Professionalization and the Semi-professions." *Sociology* 16(2), 186–202.

Heitlinger, Alena (1993). "Women's Equality, Childbearing and the State: An Overview." In *Women's Equality, Demography, and Public Policies: A Comparative Perspective* (1–21). New York: St. Martin's Press.

Hernes, Helga Maria (1987). "Women and the Welfare State: The Transition from Private to Public Dependence." In Anne Showstack Sassoon (Ed.), *Women and the State: The Shifting Boundaries of Public and Private.* Hutchinson.

Hingstman, L. (1994). "Primary Care Obstetrics and Perinatal Health in the Netherlands." *Journal of Nurse Midwifery* 39, 379–86.

Hogan, A. (1975). "A Tribute to the Pioneers." *Journal of Nurse-Midwifery* 10(2) (Summer), 6–11.

Hosford, Elizabeth (1976). "The Home Birth Movement." *Journal of Nurse-Midwifery* 21(3), 27–30.

Hossie, L. (1985a). "Mother in Home Birth Death Feared Hospitals." *The Globe and Mail,* June 27.

– (1985b). "OMA Paper on Childbirth Criticized." *The Globe and Mail,* July 6, 16.

– (1985c). "Rushed Newborn to Hospital, Midwife Testifies At Inquest." *The Globe and Mail,* June 25, M3.

Hurlburt, Jane (1981). "Midwifery in Canada: A Capsule in History." *The Canadian Nurse* (February), 30–1.

James, Susan and Ivy Lynn Bourgeault (2004). "To Fund or Not To Fund: The Alberta Decision." In I. Bourgeault, C. Benoit, and R. Davis-Floyd (Eds.), *Reconceiving Midwifery* (131–49). McGill Queen's University Press: Kingston/Montreal.

Jasen, Patricia. (1997). "Race, Culture, and the Colonization of Childbirth in Northern Canada." *Social History of Medicine* 10, 383–400.

Jenkins, J. Craig and Bert Klandermans (1995). "The Politics of Social Protest." In J. Craig Jenkins and Bert Klandermans (Eds.), *The Politics of Social Protest: Comparative Perspectives on States And Social Movements* (3–13). Minneapolis, MN: University of Minnesota Press.

Jezioranski, L. (1987). "Towards A New Status for the Midwifery Profession in Ontario." *McGill Law Journal* 33, 90–136.

Johnson, Terrance J. (1972). *Professions and Power.* London: Macmillan.

– (1977). "The Professions in the Class Structure." In R. Scase (Eds.), *Industrial Society, Class Cleavage and Control* (93–110). London: George Allen and Unwin.

– (1980). "Work and Power." In G. Esland and G. Solamon (eds.), *The Politics of Work and Occupations* (335–71). Toronto: University of Toronto Press.

– (1982). "The State and the Professions: Peculiarities of the British." In A. Giddens and G. MacKenzie (Eds.), *Social Class and the Division of Labour* (186–208). New York: Cambridge University Press.

– (1995). "Governmentality and the Institutionalization of Expertise." In T. Johnson, G. Larkin, and M. Saks (Eds.), *Health Professions and the State in Europe* (7–24). London: Routledge.

Kaufert, Patricia and John O'Neil (1993). "Analysis of a Dialogue on Risks in Childbirth: Clinicians, Epidemioglogists, and Inuit Women." In S. Lindenbaum and M. Lock (Eds.), *Knowledge, Power and Practice* (32–54). Berkeley: University of California Press.

Kaufert, Patricia and Kris Robinson (2004). "Midwifery on the Prairies: Visionaries and Realists in Manitoba." In I. Bourgeault, C. Benoit, and R. Davis-Floyd (Eds.), *Reconceiving Midwifery* (204–19). McGill Queen's University Press: Kingston/Montreal.

Kaufman, Karyn J. and Helen McDonald (1988). "A Retrospective Evaluation of a Model of Midwifery Care." *Birth* 15(2), 95–9.

Kaufman, Karyn J. and Bobbi Soderstrom (2004). "Midwifery Education in Ontario: Its Origins, Operation and Impact on the Profession." In I. Bourgeault, C. Benoit, and R. Davis-Floyd (Eds.), *Reconceiving Midwifery* (187–203). McGill Queen's University Press: Kingston/Montreal.

Kay, Bonnie J., Irene H. Butter, D. Chang, and K. Houlihan (1988). "Women's Health and Social Change: the Case of the Lay Midwives." *International Journal of Health Services* 18(2), 223–36.

Kazanjian, Arminée. (1993). "Health-Manpower Planning or Gender Relations? The Obvious and the Oblique." In E. Riska and K. Wegar (Eds.), *Gender, Work and Medicine: Women and the Medical Division of Labour* (147–71). Newbury Park: Sage.

Kilthei, Jane (1994). "The Cost of Midwifery Care." *Canadian Medical Association Journal* 151(5), 516.

Kinch RA. (1986). "Midwifery and Home Births." *Canadian Medical Association Journal* 135(4), 280–1.

Kirkham, Mavis (1989). "Midwives and Information-Giving During Labour." In S. Robinson and A.M. Thompson (Eds.), *Midwives, Research and Childbirth* (117–38). London: Chapman Hall.

Knuttila, Murray (1992). *State Theories: From Liberalism to the Challenge of Feminism.* Halifax: Fernwood Books.

Kornelsen, Jude and Elaine Carty (1999). *Midwives Experiences of Practice Post-Registration*, Part of the series Perspectives on Midwifery, Vancouver: British Columbia Centre of Excellence for Women's Health.

– (2004). "Challenges to Midwifery Integration: Interprofessional Relationships in British Columbia." In I. Bourgeault, C. Benoit, and R. Davis-Floyd (Eds.), *Reconceiving Midwifery* (111–30). McGill Queen's University Press: Kingston/Montreal.

Kraus, N. (1984). "Cost-effectiveness as Whose Cost?" *Journal of Nurse-Midwifery* 29, 1.

Laforce, Hélène (1990). "The Different Stages of the Elimination of Midwives in Quebec." In K. Arnup, S. Levesque, and R. Roach Pierson (Eds.), *Delivering Motherhood: Maternal Ideologies and Practices in the 19th and 20th Centuries* (36–50). New York: Routledge.

Lang, Raven (1972). *Birth Book.* Ben Lomond, CA: Genesis.

Langton, Phyllis A. (1991). "Competing Occupational Ideologies, Identities, and the Practice of Nurse-Midwifery." *Research on Occupations and Professions* 6, 149–77.

Larkin, Gerry (1983). *Occupational Monopoly and Modern Medicine.* London: Tavistock.

Larson, Margali S. (1977). *The Rise of Professionalism: A Sociological Analysis.* Berkeley: University of California Press.

– (1979). "Professionalism: Rise and Fall." *International Journal of Health Services* 9, 607–27.

Litoff, Judith B. (1978). *American Midwives: 1860 to the Present.* Westport, Connecticut: Greenwood Press.

Lofsky Stan. (1995). "Family Practice Obstetrics in Ontario Revisited." *Ontario Medical Review* May, 41–6.

Lorber, Judith (1993). "Why Women Physicians Will Never Be True Equals in the American Medical Profession." In E. Riska and K. Wegar (Eds.), *Gender, Work and Medicine* (62–76). Sage Studies in International Sociology.

Lubic, Ruth W. (1976). "The Childbearing Center: A Demonstration Project in Out-of-Hospital Care." *Journal of Nurse-Midwifery* 21(3), 24–5.

Lyons, Luba (1981). "Today – I'm Coming Out of the Closet." In Midwifery Task Force of British Columbia, British Columbia Association of Midwives (Eds.), *Midwifery Is a Labour of Love* (30–4). Vancouver: Interdisciplinary Midwifery Task Force.

Lyons, Luba and Elaine Carty. (1999). *Reality, Opinion and Uncertainty: Views on Midwifery in BC's Health Care System,* Part of the series Perspectives on Midwifery, Vancouver: British Columbia Centre of Excellence for Women's Health.

MacDonald, Keith (1985). *Social Closure and Occupational Registration.*

MacDonald, Keith and George Ritzer (1988). "The Sociology of the Professions: Dead or Alive?" *Work and Occupations* 15(3), 251–72.

MacDonald, Margaret (1999). *Expectations: The Cultural Construction of Nature in Midwifery Discourse in Ontario.* PhD Dissertation, Department of Anthropology, York University.

MacDonald, Margaret and Ivy L. Bourgeault (2000). "The Politics of Representation: Doing and Writing 'Interested' Research on Midwifery." *Resources for Feminist Research* 28 (1.2), 151–68.

Maillé, Chantal and Lena Wängnerud (1999). "Looking for New Opportunities in Politics: Women's Organizations and the Political Parties in Canada and Sweden." In Linda Briskin and Mona Eliasson (Eds.), *Women's Organizing and Public Policy in Canada and Sweden* (184–209). Montreal: McGill-Queen's University Press.

Martin, D. (1992). "The Midwife's Tale: Old Wisdom and a New Challenge to the Control of Reproduction." *Columbia Journal of Gender and Law* 3(1), 417–48.

Martin, Joyce A., Brady E. Hamilton, Stephanie J. Ventura, Fay Manacker, Melissa M. Park, and Paul D. Sutton (2002). *Births: Final Data for 2001*, National Vital Statistics Report, National Center for Health Statistics. http://www.cdc.gov/nchs/releases/02news/precare.htm.

Mason, Jutta (1987). "A History of Midwifery in Canada." In M. Eberts, A. Schwartz, R. Edney, and K. Kaufman (Eds.), *Report of the Task Force on the Implementation of Midwifery in Ontario*. Toronto: Queen's Park Printer.

– (1988) "Midwifery in Canada." In S. Kitzinger (Eds.), *The Midwife Challenge* (99–133). London: Pandora.

– (1989). *Reflections on the Alternative Birth Culture: Does Midwifery Pose a Problem?* Paper presented at Association of Ontario Midwives Meeting.

– (1990). *The Trouble with Licensing Midwives*. Ottawa: CRIAW/ICREF.

Mathews, Joan J. and Kathleen Zadak (1991). "The Alternative Birth Movement in the United States: History and Current Status." *Women and Health* 17(1), 39–56.

McCool, William F. and Sandi J. McCool (1989). "Feminism and Nurse-Midwifery: Historical Overview and Current Issues." *Journal of Nurse-Midwifery* 34(6), 323–34.

McCormick, (1983). "Childbearing and Nurse-Midwives: A Woman's Right to Choose." *New York University Law Review* 58, 661–713.

McCrea, H. and V. Crute (1991). "Midwife/Client Relationship: Midwives" Perspectives." *Midwifery* 7, 183–92.

McDermott, Patricia (1996). "Pay and Employment Equity: Why Separate Policies?" In J. Brodie (Ed.), *Women and Canadian Public Policy* (89–104). Toronto: Harcourt Brace.

McIntosh, Mary (1978). "The State and the Oppression of Women." In Annette Kuhn and Anne Marie Wolpe (Eds.), *Feminism and Materialism: Women and Modes of Production*. London: Routledge.

McKendry, Rachel and Tom Langford (2000). "Legalized, Regulated, but Unfunded: Midwifery's Laborious Professionalization in Alberta, Canada, 1975–99." *Social Science and Medicine* 53, 531–42.

McNaughton, J.E. (1989). *The Role of the Newfoundland Midwife in Traditional Care*, PhD Dissertation, Department of Folklore, Memorial University of Newfoundland.

Mehl, Lewis E., G.H. Peterson, M. Whitt, and W.E. Hawes (1977). "Outcomes of Elective Home Births: A Series of 1,146 Cases." *Journal of Reproductive Medicine* 19(5), 281–92.

Mickleburgh, R. (1994). "Ontario Delivers after Hard Push for Midwifery." *Globe and Mail*. Jan 1: A3.

Midwifery Alliance of North America <www.mana.org/statechart.html>.

Mitchinson, Wendy (1991). *The Nature of Their Bodies: Women and Their Doctors in Victorian Canada*. Toronto: University of Toronto Press.

– (2002). *Giving Birth in Canada: 1900–1950*. Toronto: University of Toronto Press.

Muzio, L.G. (1990). "Midwifery Education and Nursing: Curricular Revolution or Civil War?" *Nursing and Health Care* 12(7) (September), 376–9.

Navarro, Vicente (1976). *Medicine under Capitalism*. New York: Free Press.

– (1986). *Crisis, Health and Medicine: A Social Critique*. London: Tavistock.

Naylor, C.D. (1986). *Private Practice, Public Payment: Canadian Medicine and the Politics of Health Insurance, 1911-1966*. Montréal: McGill-Queen's University Press.

Nelson, M.K. (1983). "Working-class Women, Middle-Class Women, and Models of Childbirth." *Social Problems* 30(3), 284–97.

Nestel, Sheryl (1996/97). "A New Profession to the White Population in Canada": Ontario Midwifery and the Politics of Race. *Health and Canadian Society* 4(2), 315–41.

– (2000). *Obstructed Labour: Race and Gender in the Re-emergence of Midwifery in Ontario* Doctoral dissertation, Department of Sociology and Equity Studies in Education, Ontario Institute for Studies in Education of the University of Toronto.

– (2004). "The Boundaries of Professional Belonging: How Race has Shaped the Re-emergence of Midwifery in Ontario." In I. Bourgeault, C. Benoit, and R. Davis-Floyd (Eds.), *Reconceiving Midwifery* (287–305). McGill Queen's University Press: Kingston/Montreal.

O'Brien, Mary (1981). *The Politics of Reproduction*, New York: Routledge.

O'Connor, Bonnie Blair (1993). "The Home Birth Movement in the United States." *The Journal of Medicine and Philosophy* 18, 147–74.

O'Neil, John and Patricia L. Kaufert (1995). "Irniktakpunga! Sex Determination and the Inuit Struggle for Birthing Rights in Northern Canada." In F.D. Ginsburg and R. Rapp (Eds.), *Conceiving the New World Order* (59–73). Berkley: University of California Press.

– (1996). "The Politics of Obstetric Care: The Inuit Experience." In W. Mitchinson, P. Bourne, A. Prentice, G. Cuthbert Brandt, B. Light, and N. Black (Eds.), *Canadian Women: A Reader* (416–29). Toronto: Harcourt Brace. First published in *Births and Power: Social Change and the Politics of Reproduction*, In W. Penn Handwerker et al (Eds.), Boulder: Westview Press (1990).

Oakley, Anne (1984). *The Captured Womb: A History of the Medical Care of Pregnant Women*. Oxford: Basil Blackwell.

Ontario Committee on the Healing Arts (1970). *Report of the Committee on the Healing Arts*. Queen's Park Printers, Toronto.

Oppenheimer, Jo (1983). "Childbirth in Ontario: The Transition from Home to Hospital in the Early Twentieth Century." *Ontario History* 65(1), 36–60.

Parkin, Frank (1979). *Marxism and Class Theory: A Bourgeois Critique*. London: Tavistock.

Parry, N. and J. Parry (1976). *The Rise of the Medical Profession*. London: Croom Helm.

Portwood, D. and A. Fielding (1981). "Privilege and the Professions." *Sociological Review* 29, 749–73.

Randall, Vicki (1998). "Gender and Power: Women Engage the State." In Vicky Randall and Georgina Waylen (Eds.), *Gender, Politics and the State* (185–205). New York: Routledge.

Reid, A.J. and J.G. Galbraith (1988). "Midwifery in a Family Practice: A Pilot Study." *Canadian Family Physician* 34, 1887–90.

Reid, M.L. and J.B. Morris (1979). "Perinatal Care and Cost Effectiveness: Changes in Health Expenditures and Birth Outcomes Following the Establishment of a Nurse-midwife Program." *Medical Care* 7, 491–500.

Reid, Margaret (1989). "Sisterhood and Professionalization: A Case Study of the American Lay Midwife." In C. Shepherd McClain (Eds.), *Women as Healers: Cross-Cultural Perspectives* (219–38). London: Rutgers University Press.

Reiger , Kereen (2001). *Our Bodies, Our Babies: The Forgotten Women's Movement*. Melbourne: Melbourne University Press.

Reinharz, D., R. Blais, W. Fraser, et al. (2000). "Cost-Effectiveness of Midwifery Services vs Medical Services in Canada." *Canadian Journal of Public Health* 91(1), 1–12 to 1–15.

Richards, M.P.M. (1982). "The Trouble with 'Choice' in Childbirth." *Birth* 9(4), 253–62.

Riska, Eliane and Katarina Wegar (Eds.) (1993). *Gender, Work and Medicine: Women and the Medical Division of Labour*. Sage Studies in International Sociology.

Robinson, Kris (1996/97). "Midwifery: An Australian Perspective." *Health and Canadian Society* 4(2), 343–65.

Robinson, S. (1990). "Maintaining the Independence of the Midwifery Profession: a Continuing Struggle." In J. Garcia, R. Kilpatrick, and R. Richards (Eds.), *The Politics of Maternity Care* (61–91). Oxford: Claredon Press.

Rooks, Judith P. (1983). "The Context of Nurse-Midwifery in the 1980s: Our Relationships with Medicine, Nursing, Lay-Midwives, Consumers and Health Care Economist." *Journal of Nurse-Midwifery* 28(5) (September/October), 3–8.

– (1986). "Cost-Effectiveness of Nurse-Midwifery Care." In J. Rooks and J.E. Hass (Eds.), *Nurse-Midwifery in America* (52–3). ACNM: Washington.

– (1990). "Nurse-Midwifery: The Window Is Wide Open." *American Journal of Nursing* (December), 30–6.

Rooks, Judith P. and S.H. Fischman (1980). "American Nurse-Midwifery Practice in 1976–77: Reflections of 50 Years of Growth and Development." *American Journal of Public Health* 70(9) (September), 990–6.

Rosser, Walter W. and Henry Muggah (1989). "Who Will Deliver Canada's Babies in the 1990s?" *Canadian Family Physician* 35, 2419–24.

Rothman, Barbara Katz (1981). "Awake and Aware, or False Consciousness: The Cooptation of Childbirth Reform in America." In S. Romalis (Eds.), *Childbirth: Alternatives to Medical Control* (150–80). Austin: University of Texas Press.

– (1982). *In Labor: Women and Power in the Birthplace*. New York: W.W. Norton and Company.

– (1989). *Recreating Motherhood*. New York: W.W. Norton and Company.

Rowley, M. (1993). "Team Midwifery – the Australian Experience." Paper presented at the *23rd Triennial Congress of the International Confederation of Midwives*, Vancouver, British Columbia.

Rushing, Beth (1991). "Market Explanations for Occupational Power: the Decline of Midwifery in Canada." *American Review of Canadian Studies* (Spring), 7–27.

– (1993). "Ideology and the Reemergence of North American Midwifery." *Work and Occupations* 20(1), 46–67.

Ruzek, Sheryl Burt (1978). *The Women's Health Movement: Feminist Alternatives to Medical Control*. New York: Praeger Publishers.

Saks, Mike (1983). "Removing the Blinkers? A Critique of Recent Contributions to the Sociology of Professions." *Sociology Review* 31, 1–21.

– (1994). "Nursing Education and the British Health Care Market: Educational Change and the Professionalisation of Nursing." Paper presented at *European Society of Medical Sociology on Health and Medicine in the New Europe*. Vienna, September 16–19th.

Sandall, Jane (1996). "Continuity of Midwifery Care in England: A New Professional Project?" *Gender, Work, and Organization* 3(4), 215–26.

Schlinger, Hiliary (1992). *Circle of Midwives*. LaFayette, N.Y: Hilary Schlinger.

Schneider, D. (1986). "Planned Out-of-Hospital Births, New Jersey, 1978–1980." *Social Science and Medicine* 23(10), 1011–15.

Schneider, G. and Bobbi Soderstrom (1987). "Analysis of 275 Planned and 10 Unplanned Home Births." *Canadian Family Physician* 33 (May), 1163–71.

Shah, M.A (1982). "The Unification of Midwives: A Time for Dialogue." *Journal of Nurse-Midwifery* 27(5) (September, October), 1–2.

Sharp, E.S. (1980). "Interdependence Reexamined." *Journal of Nurse-Midwifery* 25(5), 1–3.

Sharpe, Mary. (2001). "Exploring Legislated Ontario Midwifery: Texts, Ruling Relations and Ideological Practices." *Resources for Feminist Research* 28 (3/4), 39–63.

Shroff, Farah (Ed.) (1997). *The New Midwifery: Reflections on Renaissance and Regulation.* Toronto: The Women's Press.

Sides, B. (1981). "Problems and Trends of Home Confinements: A 15-year Survey (1966–1980) of Obstetrical Practice in an Urban Area." *The Practitioner* 225 (September), 1231–4.

Simmons, A.B. and K. Keohane (1992). "Canadian Immigration Policy: State Strategies and the Quest for Legitimacy." *Canadian Review of Sociology and Anthropology* 29(4), 421–52.

Simpson, R.L. and I.H. Simpson (1969). "Women and Bureaucracy in the Semi-professions." In A. Etzioni (Eds.), *The Semi-Professions and Their Organization* (196–265). New York: Free Press.

Smart, C. (1989). *Feminism and the Power of the Law.* London: Routledge.

Smulders, B. and A. Limburg (1988). "Obstetrics and midwifery in the Netherlands." In Sheila Kitzinger (Ed.), *The Midwife Challenge.* London: Pandora.

Stewart, Dianne and Raymond Pong (1999a). *Summary Report of the 1996 and 1997 Cohorts of Graduates of the Midwifery Education Programme.* Centre for Rural and Northern Health Research, Laurentian University (Unpublished report).

– (1999b). *Summary Report of the 1998 Cohort of Graduates of the Midwifery Education Programme.* Centre for Rural and Northern Health Research, Laurentian University (Unpublished report).

Sullivan, Deborah A. and Ruth Beeman (1983). "Four Years' Experience with Home Birth by Licensed Midwives in Arizona." *American Journal of Public Health* 73(6), 641–5.

Sullivan, Deborah A. and Rose Weitz (1984). "Obstacles to the Practice of Licensed Lay Midwifery." *Social Science and Medicine* 19(11), 1189–96.

– (1988). *Labor Pains: Modern Midwives and Home Birth.* New Haven: Yale University Press.

Sweet, Lois (1985). "Inquest Will Raise Key Questions about Midwives." *The Toronto Star*, June 21, F1.

– (1993). "Province to Pay for Midwives, Grier Says." *The Toronto Star*, October 3, A3.

Tate, Merryn (1988). "A Model of Continuity of Care." MIDIRS *Information Pack*, (April) 7.

Teasley, Regi (1983). *Birth and the Division of Labor: the Movement to Professionalize Nurse-midwifery, and its Relationship to the Movement for Home Birth and Lay Midwifery a Case Study of Vermont.* Doctoral Dissertation, Michigan State University.

322   References

Tedesco, Teresa (1985a). "Coroner Would Legalize Midwifery." *Globe and Mail*, July 16, 1985, 18.
– (1985b). "Crown Joins Defence in Urging Midwifery Be Legalized." *The Globe and Mail*, July 13, 1.
– (1985c). "Legalized Midwifery Is Urged to Reallocate Health Budget". *The Globe and Mail*, July 12.
– (1985d). "Make Midwifery Legal, Coroner's Panel Urges." *The Globe and Mail*, July 18, 1985, 1–2.
– (1985e). "Midwifery is Termed Essential by Us Pediatrician At Inquest." *The Globe and Mail*, July 9.
Tjaden, P.G. (1987). "Midwifery in Colorado: A Case Study in the Politics of Professionalization." *Qualitative Sociology* 10(1), 29–45.
Tom, S. (1982). "Nurse-midwifery: A Developing Profession." *Law, Medicine and Health Care* (December), 262–6.
Tuohy, Carolyn (1988). "Medicine and the State in Canada: The Extra-Billing Issue in Perspective." *Canadian Journal of Political Science* 21(2), 267–96.
Tyson, Holiday (1991). "Outcomes of 1001 Midwife–attended Home Births in Toronto, 1983–1988." Birth, 18(1), 14–19.
Vadeb--cœur, Hélène (2000). "Quebec and the legalisation of midwifery." MIDIRS *Midwifery Digest*, 10(1), 24–8.
– (2004). "Delaying Legislation: The Quebec Experiment." In I. Bourgeault, C. Benoit, and R. Davis-Floyd (Eds.), *Reconceiving Midwifery* (71–90). McGill Queen's University Press: Kingston/Montreal.
Vadeb--cœur, Hélène, Brigitte Maheux, and Régis Blais (1996/97). "Why Did Quebec Decide to Experiment with the Practice of Midwifery Rather Than Legalise the Profesion?" *Health and Canadian Society* 4(2), 447–80.
van Teijlinden, Edwin, Jane Sandall, Raymond DeVries, Cecilia Benoit, Sirpa Wrede, and Ivy Lynn Bourgeault (2003). "Comparative Methods in Midwifery Research." RCM *Midwives Journal* August, 18–21.
van Teijlinden, Edwin and Leonie van der Hulst (1995). "Midwifery in the Netherlands: More Than a Semi–Profession?" In G. Larkin, T. Johnson, and M. Saks (Eds.), *Health Professions and the State in Europe* (178–86). London: Routledge.
Van Wagner, Vicki (1988). "Women Organizing for Midwifery in Ontario." *Resources for Feminist Research* 17(3), 115–18.
– (1991). *With Woman: Community Midwifery.* Unpublished Master's Thesis, York University.
– (2004). "Why Legislation?: Using Regulation to Strengthen Midwifery." In I. Bourgeault, C. Benoit, and R. Davis-Floyd (Eds.), *Reconceiving Midwifery* (71–90). McGill Queen's University Press: Kingston/Montreal.

Ventre, Fran (1976). "The Making of a Legalized Lay Midwife." *Birth and the Family Review* 3(3), 109–17.

Ventre, Fran and Carol Leonard (1982). "The Future of Midwifery – An Alliance." *Journal of Nurse-Midwifery* 27(5) (September, October), 23–4.

Walsh, L.V. and A.L. Jaspan (1990). "Lay Midwifery to Nurse-Midwife: Perceived Learning Needs and Attitudes Toward to the Learning Experience." *Journal of Nurse-Midwifery* 35(4), 204–13.

Walzer, M. (1987). *Interpretation and Social Criticism*. Cambridge MA: Harvard University Press

Wardwell, Walter I. (1981). "Chiropractors: Challengers of Medical Dominance." *Research in the Sociology of Health Care* 2, 207–50.

Waylen, Georgina (1998). "Gender, Feminism and the State." In Vicky Randall and Georgina Waylen (Eds.), *Gender, Politics and the State* (1–77). New York: Routledge.

Weatherston, L. (1985). "Midwifery in the Hospital: Team Approach to Perinatal Care." *Dimensions* (April), 15–16, 22.

Weitz, Rose (1987). "English Midwives and the Association of Radical Midwives." *Women and Health* 12(1), 79–89.

Weitz, Rose, and Deborah A. Sullivan (1985). "Licensed Lay Midwifery and the Medical Model of Childbirth." *Sociology of Health and Illness* 7(1), 36–54.

– (1986). "The Politics of Childbirth: The Re-emergence of Midwifery in Arizona." *Social Problems* 33(3), 163–75.

Williams, C.L. (2001). "Black Women in White: Racial Conflict and Cooperation in the Nursing Profession, 1890–1950." *Contemporary Sociology* 19(5), 698–700.

Willis, Evan (1989). *Medical Dominance: The Division of Labour in the Australian Health Care System* (2nd Ed.). Sydney: George Allen and Unwin.

Witz, Anne (1990). "Patriarchy and Professions: The Gendered Politics of Occupational Closure." *Sociology* 24(4), 675–90.

– (1992) *Professions and Patriarchy.* London: Routledge.

Wysong, Pippa (1998). "Obstetrics Crisis Looms." *The Medical Post*, July 7. http://www.cofp.com/media/obstetrics.asp.

Index

AUTHORS